HE 630-2 (ENG N2)

Quality Improvement in Healthcare

Book N

D0417774

30121 0 03968862

Quality Improvement in Healthcare: Putting evidence into practice

Second edition

Karen Parsley
RGN, RSCN, BSc (Hons), MA
Director of Nursing, Brighton Health Care NHS Trust,
Royal Sussex County Hospital

and

Philomena Corrigan
RGN, BSc (Hons), MSc
Director of Nursing,
Calderdale Healthcare NHS Trust, Halifax

STAFFORDSHIRE
UNIVERSITY
LIBRARY

Stanley Thornes (Publishers) Ltd

© 1999 Stanley Thornes (Publishers) Ltd

All rights reserved. No part of this publication may be reproduced or transmitted in any form or by any means, electronic or mechanical, including photocopying, recording or any information storage and retrieval system, without permission in writing from the publisher or under licence from the Copyright Licensing Agency Limited. Further details of such licences (for reprographic reproduction) may be obtained from the Copyright Licensing Agency Limited of 90 Tottenham Court Road, London W1P 0LP.

First edition published by Chapman & Hall in 1994
(ISBN 0 412 48360 2)

Second edition published in 1999 by:
Stanley Thornes (Publishers) Ltd
Ellenborough House
Wellington Street
Cheltenham
Glos.
GL50 1YW
United Kingdom   **03968862**

99 00 01 02 03 / 10 9 8 7 6 5 4 3 2 1

A catalogue record for this book is available from the British Library

ISBN 0 7487 3355 8

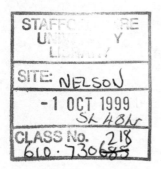
STAFF   RE
U   Y
L
SITE: NELSON
-1 OCT 1999
       SL48N
CLASS No. 218
610·730685

Typeset by The Florence Group, Stoodleigh, Devon
Printed and bound in Great Britain by T.J. International Ltd, Padstow, Cornwall

*For our mums, who taught us the importance of going the extra mile
Diny Norman-Ter Horst and Agnes Heffernan*

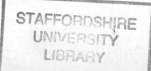
STAFFORDSHIRE
UNIVERSITY
LIBRARY

Contents

Acknowledgements

The authors would like to thank the following people for their important contributions to this book:

- Alison Ginsberg, for her sterling assistance with proofreading and preparation of the manuscript;
- Mark Renshaw for significant contributions to Chapters 2 (the case study of malignant pain) and 3 (the case study for clinical audit);
- Sister Kay Hyde and Staff Nurse Alison Lowe for allowing me to reproduce their patient care pathway and Strategy for Nursing and Midwifery work;
- Brian James for his case study on oesophageal cancer pathways;
- Shona Brown and Alan Stacey for their Quality Pointers Toolwork;
- Joanne Barnes and Kieran Walshe, who co-authored (with Karen Parsley) the first edition of the Brighton Health Care *Quality Matters* course, extracts from which are used in Chapter 3;
- Dr Keith Hurst for his constructive criticism of the first draft of the manuscript;
- John Towers and the IPC team for contributing to the case study in Chapter 7;
- Amanda Coleman for the excellent clinical care pathway, patient care plan, and nursing admission formats developed and used by St John of God Health Care, Subiaco, Western Australia;
- Colleagues past and present from Brighton Health Care NHS Trust, Doncaster Royal Infirmary and Montague Hospital NHS Trust; Crosby Associates and Newark General Hospital.

Every effort has been made to contact copyright holders and we apologise if any have been overlooked

PREFACE

This second edition of *Quality Improvement in Nursing and Healthcare: A Practical Approach* has been rewritten five years after the first edition. It is perhaps testimony to the enormous developments that have taken place in approaches to quality improvement and in healthcare itself that we had to undertake such a substantial rewrite of our original material. An encouraging development over the past five years has been the increasing shift towards a multidisciplinary approach to improving the quality of clinical practice. For this reason, we have also updated the title of our book to reflect this change, and have attempted to focus on a more generic approach to quality improvement. Perhaps inevitably (because of our professional backgrounds), many of the practical examples of transferring the theory of quality improvement into practice are based upon our own experiences as nurses within a multidisciplinary team within an acute setting. The subtitle reflects our continuing wish to integrate theory into practice and to provide readers with what we hope are very practical examples based on our own experiences of using quality improvement theories to change and improve clinical practice.

The first chapter provides an introduction to evidence-based practice (we use this term rather than 'evidence-based medicine' to reflect the importance of underpinning practice with research findings for all professions). This chapter defines the terms 'evidence-based practice' and 'clinical effectiveness'; describes the steps clinicians need to take to put evidence into practice; gives practical guidance on how to find and appraise the evidence and evaluate its impact on patient care. Chapter 1 also outlines some of the difficulties of this approach, and its limitations. One of these criticisms is that much of the research literature is not in a user-friendly format, and is generally inaccessible at the point where it is most needed – at the time of the consultation with the patient. The challenge for health professionals is therefore how to consolidate this vast range of evidence into a concise summary that is available at the point of healthcare delivery.

Chapter 2 describes different methods of documenting best practice in a user-friendly way to address the latter problems. Methods described for documenting practice include standards, procedures, guidelines, protocols and patient care pathways. Techniques on how to write these documents so that they are specific, measurable, achievable, relevant, timely, effective and research based are also outlined in this chapter.

We are all familiar with the numerous policies and procedures that are written and then gather dust on a shelf. The challenge is to implement these into practice and then to make measurements to ensure improvements have been made. Chapter 3 therefore introduces clinical audit as a mechanism for achieving this.

The first three chapters therefore deal predominantly with assisting individual or groups of clinicians to work together to improve their local practice. We recognized early in our careers that clinicians' efforts to improve their practice could be helped or hindered by policy and management practice at a local and a national level. Chapter 4 therefore looks at a broader context of quality improvement, describing both organizational approaches and national initiatives.

The danger in writing about our attempts to improve the quality of patient care is that some may misconstrue that we are setting ourselves up as experts in the field. On the contrary, much of our learning has come from well-meaning efforts which all too often did not go according to plan. Indeed, on reflection we recognize that this is probably because we didn't even have a plan. Fortunately, we were pursuing further academic study and had taken up more senior positions which gave us the opportunity of learning about strategic planning and project management. Chapter 5 sets out some of the underpinning theories we have found useful in helping us develop clinical practice and make improvements in patient care. We used the case study of developing and implementing a strategy for nursing, which we feel is relevant in the light of the new national strategy for nursing. Although this is a nursing example, we feel the theories presented and techniques used would be equally helpful in implementing other strategic initiatives by other professional groups.

Many of the techniques described in quality improvement texts and journals for the health professions have drawn heavily on the experience of industry. In particular, total quality management is one that is often specifically mentioned. Chapter 6 therefore describes this approach and offers a case study of implementing this in an NHS setting. Although this was presented in the first edition, we feel it is still very relevant today.

The final chapter describes a healthcare adaptation of the TQM approach, namely patient focused care. This was developed in the United States and has been adapted for use in some hospitals in the UK. This chapter describes the principles of patient focused care and offers a case study of implementing it within an NHS Trust.

As we completed the book, it was heartening to note just how much both the art and the science of improving the quality of healthcare have developed over the last five years. The final draft of the book proved an ever-moving feast, as each time we thought we had brought it up to date another national document emerged to move the agenda on still further. Hence we had *The New NHS: Modern, Dependable*, the Green Paper *Our Healthier Nation*, the consultation document *A First Class Service* and the Strategy for Nursing, Midwifery and Health Visiting imminent at the time of publication. Although causing us a headache in completing the text, it was enormously encouraging to see the importance of quality being noted and strengthened at all levels throughout the health service.

Of course, in the purist sense we have yet to see the evidence that this is making a genuine and lasting impact on patient care. However, we are optimistic that even without this concrete evidence there are significant opportunities for clinicians to get involved in improving the quality of patient care. As Henry VIII says in William Nicholson's play *Katherine Howard*,[1] 'What is faith but certainty without evidence?'

---

[1] Written for the Chichester Theatre, 1998.

1 DETERMINING 'BEST PRACTICE'

There is more that we'll never know, than we'll ever know.

(Marlin, 1995, p. 30)

This is the challenge for health professionals seeking to answer the question 'What is the best intervention for this patient?'

INTRODUCTION

It is difficult to consider the whole issue of quality improvement in healthcare without giving consideration to the unique relationship between the healthcare professional and the patient. The effectiveness of an intervention aimed at improving the patient's well-being will be influenced both by the skills and knowledge of the individual administering the care and by the individual physical and psychological response of the patient who receives the care. In the words of one author,

> *The quality of care can only be as high as the competence level of the person providing that care.*

(Harper, 1987, p.11)

The actions of a health professional can have an impact far greater than their influence on patient treatment. They have the ability to profoundly influence patterns of care and use of resources:

> *The practice patterns of individual clinicians are fundamental determinants of the quality, ethical standards, and cost effectiveness of health services.*

(Logan and Scott, 1996, p.595).

It is therefore logical that we start our journey on our quest for quality improvement in healthcare with the professionals themselves, since whatever other grand organizational schemes may be in place to promote 'quality', or control costs, they will ultimately be reliant on the skills and competence of the staff within the organization.

Defining 'the professions'

If we start with the healthcare professionals themselves, it is useful to understand the characteristics that distinguish professionals from other groups of workers. Essential elements of a profession are that it has recognizable ethics and a strong element of self-regulation. Many members of a profession will also have a vocation. The professional accepts several obligations (Royal College of Physicians, 1996):

- to maintain knowledge and proficiency in the professional fields;
- to comply with standards and ethics accepted by the profession;
- to acknowledge that the duties and obligations to public and clients transcend those contained in legal contracts of employment;
- to contribute to education and training of professional aspirants;
- to support the professionalism of others.

The first of these obligations refers to the maintenance of knowledge and proficiency in the professional field. This is a particular challenge to professionals where new knowledge is growing at a rapid rate. Doctors can face difficulties in keeping abreast of all the medical advances reported in primary journals. If one compares the time required for reading (for general medicine, sufficient to examine 19 articles per day, 365 days per year) with the time available (well under an hour a week by British medical consultants, even on self-reports), the difficulties of keeping abreast of contemporary practice are self-evident (Davidoff *et al.*, 1995; Sackett *et al.* 1996). This problem is compounded for other clinical professionals, nurses and professions allied to medicine, who need to keep abreast not only of advances in diagnosis and treatment but also of the associated changes in their professional knowledge. For example, the rapid growth of endoscopy as a diagnostic procedure required nurses to develop skills in caring for patients undertaking the procedure and also to learn how to prepare and clean the equipment. More recently, a number of nurses have expanded their scope of professional practice still further by training as nurse endoscopists, resulting in the development of courses such as ENB9N81 (Flexible Sigmoidoscopy) and ENB A87 (Upper GI).

The quest for knowledge about the efficacy of treatment is not solely confined to the professions themselves. As more treatments for historically untreatable diseases become available, the demand from the public for healthcare continues to rise. Governments are coming under increasing pressure to contain expenditure on healthcare. Within this context it is perhaps not surprising that assurances are being sought that treatments offered are beneficial to the health of the nation. In the literature on these related issues, two phrases have come to dominate both the professional and the health economist literature of the past five years:

- evidence-based medicine
- clinical effectiveness

This chapter sets out to define what is meant by these terms and to review how they can be applied in practice. Evidence-based medicine is not without its critics, and there are some alleged inherent weaknesses in its wholesale application. The final section of this chapter therefore outlines what some of these weaknesses are and some of the difficulties of attempting to apply the principles of evidence-based practice and clinical effectiveness to clinical practice.

Throughout this book we have chosen to use the term 'evidence-based practice' rather than 'evidence-based medicine', since the latter term is skewed towards the medical profession and excludes, by definition, other healthcare professionals. For a true quality service, all those delivering care need to ensure that their care is grounded in the knowledge that they are doing something that will benefit the patient.

Is treatment based on evidence?

There is often a misplaced assumption by the public that the treatment they are offered by professionals is based on sound scientific knowledge. Estimates of how much healthcare is based on research evidence vary from 15% to 82% (Ellis *et al.*, 1995). The challenge for basing practice on scientific evidence is twofold: first, generating the 'proof' that validates the treatment; and second, even when efficacy is proven, ensuring that clinicians use this knowledge to influence their practice. There is evidence to suggest that even if best practice is identified through research findings, application of the evidence does not always occur. Examples include:

- Dilatation and curettage (D&C) has been shown to be 'therapeutically useless and diagnostically inaccurate' (Lewis, 1993). In 1992–93 it was still the fourth most commonly performed procedure in the NHS.
- Thrombolytic treatment for myocardial infarction was shown to be clinically effective more than a decade before it became widely advocated (Haines and Jones, 1994).
- In spite of clear evidence on the most efficacious methods for treatment of leg ulcers, these have been poorly implemented in clinical practice (Naish, 1997, pp.64–66).
- Despite being a condition with a strong evidence base identifying best practice for prevention and treatment (Hibbs, 1988; Dealey, 1994; Collier, 1995), pressure sores continue to cost the NHS significant sums of money because these findings are not put into practice.

Defining 'evidence-based practice' and 'clinical effectiveness'

In reviewing the literature to seek to understand evidence-based practice, a useful summary is offered by Walshe (1996):

> *The evidence-based healthcare movement is an attempt to shed the clinical mindset of the past, dominated by expert opinion, precedent, uncontrolled case series and personal clinical experience, and to replace it with one based on science, epidemiology, the evidence of randomised controlled trials, meta-analysis of the findings from multiple research studies, and systematic reviews of the research literature.*

Walshe notes in this article that as the quality and accessibility of such evidence improve it will be increasingly difficult to defend practice that is not in line with the evidence. He identifies that in future the focus may shift from whether or not a procedure was carried out competently to whether or not a competent clinician would have performed the procedure at all.

This an important distinction when considering a definition for the term 'clinical effectiveness'. The literature can be confusing, since clinicians use the terms 'evidence-based medicine' and 'clinical effectiveness' interchangeably.

We make the distinction between efficiency – 'doing things right' – and effectiveness – 'doing the right things'. It is essential when embarking on any quality improvement programme that this distinction is appreciated. It has been our experience that quality assurance and accreditation tools often seek to measure whether things are done right, rather than challenging whether they should be done at all. For example, a ward scored 100% on compliance with a standard that patients on four-hourly measurement of temperature, pulse, respiration and blood pressure had these completed correctly and documented. The ward in question was a rehabilitation ward and, with the exception of one patient, there were no clinical reasons why the others needed these measurements taken. Hence it was efficient (the nurses carried out the observations competently, i.e. did things right), but not effective (there was no clinical reason for undertaking observations, i.e. they were not doing the right things).

Using Walshe's vision of development of evidence-based practice, there will be an increasing emphasis on challenging whether competent professionals should have carried out treatments and procedures at all; proof of competence in carrying out an intervention will not be sufficient under this model of practice.

The application of evidence-based practice can be conceptualized as a continuum: at one extreme the practitioner practising in a highly individualized way, and at the other extreme the clinician merely applying the evidence. As the section at the end of this chapter outlines, this perception has led to a number of critics regarding evidence-based practice as 'cookbook' medicine, suggesting that for each condition or set of symptoms there is a predetermined recipe of care. Critics are cynical about the rationale for the whole evidence-based practice agenda, viewing it as an attempt by managers and politicians to undermine the autonomy of the professional and to control the use of resources.

Others refute this assumption, claiming that it is the expertise of the clinician which drives the application of evidence-based practice, rather than the other way round. Sackett and colleagues note that evidence-based medicine is not 'cookbook' medicine because it requires a 'bottom-up' approach that integrates the external evidence with individual clinical expertise and patient choice. It therefore cannot result in slavish 'cookbook' approaches to patient care. His view is that external clinical evidence can inform, but can never replace, individual clinical expertise; and it is this expertise that decides whether the external evidence applies to the individual patient at all and, if so, how it should be integrated into a clinical decision (Sackett *et al.*, 1996). Guidelines therefore are just that; the Institute of Medicine definition states that they are 'systematically developed statements to *assist* the practitioner and patient decisions about appropriate healthcare for specific clinical circumstances' (author's emphasis).

As for the fear that evidence-based medicine will be hijacked by purchasers and managers to cut the costs of healthcare, Sackett and colleagues argue not only that this would be a misuse of evidence-based medicine, but also that it represents a fundamental misunderstanding of its financial consequences.

The latter point is an important one, and can also be helpful in seeking to explore the differences between what is meant by evidence-based medicine and by clinical effectiveness. In the literature reviewed, the term 'evidence-based practice' refers to 'the process of systematically finding, appraising and using contemporaneous research findings as the basis for clinical decisions' (Rosenberg and Donald, 1995).

The term 'clinical effectiveness' not only embraces the clinical impact of the treatment, but incorporates the view of health economists that there is a financial imperative to evaluate the economic implications (costs) of achieving changes in health status (benefits or effects) through clinical interventions. Hence evidence-based practice is what the clinician practises when faced with an individual patient. Clinical effectiveness is about treatment decisions for populations, i.e. what is best for the most. As noted above, excessive demands are being placed on health services. The health economists argue that a primary goal of any health service has to be to maximize its outcome (measured in 'healthiness' or quality-adjusted life years), and it is essential to choose the treatments that minimize costs and maximize benefits. Or, as the Americans so dramatically put it, 'getting the biggest bang for your buck'.

Hence implicit in much of the literature on clinical effectiveness is the assumption that, following a review of the evidence, some courses of treatment are judged not to have any therapeutic benefit. Other treatments may have dubious or unclear benefits. The argument of the health economist is that in a world of rising healthcare costs, diagnostic and treatment regimes that fall into the former category should not be publicly funded.

In practice, the evidence may be less clear-cut, and clinical guidelines for patients with the same condition may vary significantly depending on the view of either individual clinicians or professional colleges in different countries. For example, US guidelines for HIV recommend treatment far earlier than the UK equivalent. The US guidelines would significantly increase the UK drugs bill if adopted in the UK (Naish, 1997).

The health economists also differentiate between 'doing things right', which they refer to as 'improving technical efficiency', and 'doing the right things', defined as 'improving allocative efficiency'.

Doing things right: improving technical efficiency

Those who have worked in the National Health Service in recent years will be well aware of the annual targets of efficiency savings. The Department of Health can demonstrate that over the last 10–15 years it has been able to achieve a 1–2% reduction in unit costs year on year across the acute sector and some sectors outside it (Riley *et al.*, 1995). There has been progress in reducing lengths of stay and increasing day case surgery rates, both of which are important components of increasing technical efficiency.

Addressing technical efficiency appears seductive, as it is often easier to identify. The question has to be posed whether this can continue or if the obvious opportunities have now all been exploited. It can be argued that there must come a point of diminishing returns. However, other authors note that there are no special reasons why there should be a greater tailing off in productivity gains than in any other service industry that is subject to significant technical advances and rising overall resources (Riley *et al.*, 1995). It could be argued that technology used in other service industries (e.g. British Telecom) can replace or reduce human labour costs. However, technological advances in medicine have a tendency to create increased demand from the public and require additional staff, both to care for the patients undergoing the new treatment and to look after the new machine.

Doing the right things: improving allocative efficiency

Interest in allocative efficiency has been stimulated by the growing concern with appropriateness of treatment and care. Some examples were cited earlier; another includes the finding that, in the view of a UK panel, around a fifth of interventions for angiographies and coronary bypass grafts were inappropriate (Riley *et al.*, 1995). The difficulty in using this approach is in defining what is meant by 'appropriate'.

Weinberg (1993) defined the appropriate rate of intervention as 'a rate of service that would occur if patients were fully and neutrally informed about the state of medical progress, what works and what are the uncertainties; and if they were free to choose the treatments they wanted'. It can be appreciated that being able to reach such a judgement will be impossible without sound evidence on which to base a decision on appropriateness. Thus one clearly cannot make judgements on *clinical effectiveness* without a simultaneous move towards *evidence-based practice*.

The application of general incentives (tight budgets, broad performance and efficiency targets, and competition) can focus on driving out technical inefficiency. The weakness of these approaches is that they do not tackle the uncertainty of medical or other professional groups. There is a growing recognition that as well as looking at general efficiency incentives, one should simultaneously encourage specific or micro incentive mechanisms to encourage more appropriate care (Riley *et al.*, 1995). Such micro measures include:

- an upsurge of interest in service and clinical guidelines and protocols that can be linked to purchasing plans and contracts;
- the development and use of clinical outcomes;
- expansion of clinical audit, including the incorporation of cost and cost-effectiveness implications;
- health technology assessments.

It is important to appreciate that the development of guidelines and protocols, clinical outcomes, audit and the numerous other approaches to improving individual and organizational quality are all legitimate in their own right. They all serve different purposes. It is important that when seeking to improve quality an informed decision is made which selects the right one of the many quality improvement tools covered in this book. In practice, a combination of these approaches is likely to have the most impact, preferably occurring within a strategic framework for quality improvement.

It has been our experience that when implementing any of these mutually interdependent approaches to improving the quality of healthcare, there are a number of steps that need to be followed, regardless of which approach is being adopted. Examining the available evidence is as important when considering changes in health policy as in clinical practice. Politicians and health service managers have come under much criticism from clinicians for introducing wide-ranging health reforms with limited evidence to support the potential benefits to the health of the nation (Hayward, 1996).

Phases of evidence-based practice

The literature commonly cites four distinct phases in the performance of an evidence-based review:

- Formulate a clear clinical question.
- Search the literature for relevant clinical articles.
- Critically appraise the evidence.
- Implement useful findings.

Now that we have explored what evidence-based practice and clinical effectiveness are, the next section will identify how to put the evidence into practice, based on the phases identified above. In compiling this section we have drawn on the literature and our own practical application of the theory. What follows, therefore, is a pragmatic approach which is intended to assist individual clinicians and multidisciplinary teams seeking to improve the quality of care they give their patient.

Putting the evidence into practice

Although a variety of approaches are offered in the literature (Rosenberg and Donald, 1995; Sackett and Rosenberg, 1995), we have built our framework for implementing evidence-based practice on that of Summerton and colleagues (1995).

Table 1.1 summarizes the key questions to be answered when seeking the best solution to a clinical problem. Hence, inherent in this approach is the ability of the health professional to use his or her clinical judgement in seeking a diagnosis on the nature of the patient's problem. The expertise of the individual in making this diagnosis is therefore fundamental to the application of evidence-based practice. If the incorrect diagnosis is made, the application of the framework below is ineffective. The model can be applied by nurses, physiotherapists, dietitians and other healthcare professionals as well as doctors. However, it is our experience that the greatest impact can be made when a multidisciplinary team works together with the patient to determine the most appropriate interventions.

Table 1.1	Question to ask	Action required to answer question
Steps to evaluate evidence-based practice	What is the diagnosis or problem?	Examination and assessment
	How do we find information?	Literature searching
	Is the information of good quality?	Validation
	Is it right for the population we treat?	Applicability
	How do we tell people about it?	Dissemination/education
	How do we make it happen?	Implementation/change management
	Have we got the new treatment working?	Audit of process
	Is it doing what we wanted it to?	Audit of outcome
	Is appropriate evidence lacking?	Research questions
	Is it value for effort?	
	Is it value for resources?	Economics and statistics
	Is it best use of resources?	

Adapted from Summerton (1995).

The next section will outline how to seek the answers to the above questions and identify some tools and techniques and sources of information that can be used to help.

HOW DO WE FIND THE INFORMATION?

As the quantity of well-validated research evidence increases, it is essential that health professionals develop the skills necessary to assimilate, evaluate and make best use of that evidence for the benefit of patients. It was identified earlier that it is one of the tenets of a profession that those who practise within it maintain knowledge and proficiency in their professional field. It was also identified that this is an enormous challenge to professionals faced with a plethora of literature. When we seek knowledge from traditional sources of information, such as textbooks and journals, these are often difficult to access or may be out of date. One study that looked at a group of general physicians identified that in a typical halfday of practice four clinical decisions would have been altered if clinically useful information about them had been available and employed. Only 30% of these information needs were met in clinics and offices where these clinicians worked, and, despite the claim by clinicians that they predominantly used textbooks and journals to gain knowledge, direct observation identified that most of it was obtained by asking colleagues. The clinicians in this study identified three barriers to obtaining clinically important information (Covell, Uman and Manning, 1995):

- They lack the time necessary for keeping up to date.
- Their textbooks were out of date.
- Their journals were too disorganized to be useful.

Similar difficulties are experienced by other professional groups, and a review of the nursing literature identifies that evidence-based practice in the nursing profession is still comparatively underdeveloped.

For the practitioner seeking information about best practice, the straightforward literature search can prove time consuming and frustrating given the constraints identified above. In response to this difficulty, a number of different organizations and publications have been established to help clinicians access current information about best practice. These are summarized in Table 1.2.

It can be seen in Table 1.2 that there is a diverse range of information on evidence-based practice. This spans a wide spectrum from highly specialist refereed clinical journals publishing the results of trials, evaluations, views and reviews of specific editions, to publications concerned solely with clinical and cost effectiveness information regarding a particular treatment or condition. Information on clinical effectiveness is not communicated only through published work. There is increasing use

Table 1.2

Sources of effectiveness information: selected publications and organizations

National/international technical publications	Academic/independent health service research publications
• *New England Journal of Medicine*	• *Effective Healthcare* bulletins
• *American College of Physicians Journal Club*	• *Evidence-Based Medicine Newsletter*
• *British Medical Journal*	• *Outcomes Briefing Newsletter*
• *The Lancet*	• R&D Briefing Papers
• *Drugs and Therapeutics Bulletin*	• Topic-Based Effectiveness Reviews
• *Health Trends*	• Office of Health Economics Monographs
• *Journal of Health Economics*	• Centre for Health Economics Monographs
• *Health Economics*	• Centre for Health Economics Discussion Papers
• *Quality in Healthcare*	• Health Economics Research Unit Discussion Papers
• *Journal of Clinical Effectiveness in Nursing*	• Observatory Report series

UK NHS publications	Organizations
• Health of the Nation Information Packs	• NHS Centre for Reviews and Dissemination
• *Register of Cost Effectiveness Studies*	• The Cochrane Collaboration Centre / The Cochrane Collaboration
• Executive letters (e.g. EL(93)115 and EL(94)74)	• Centre for Evidence-Based Medicine
• Clinical Standards Advisory Group Reports	• UK Clearing House for Information on the Assessment of Health Outcomes
• *Healthcare Needs Assessments* (vols 1 and 2)	• Medical Royal Colleges
• *National Confidential Enquiry into Perioperative Deaths Reports*	• Central Health Outcomes Unit
• Bandolier newsletter and other regional R&D newsletters	• Royal College of Nursing Clinical Effectiveness Initiative

Reproduced with the permission of K. Walshe, from *Acting on the Evidence*, Appleby *et al.* (1995).

of information technology and on-line databases as effective methods of dissemination, as well as conferences, workshops, videos and other forms of media. It has been our experience that, when attempting to disseminate this information locally, one needs to encourage the use of as broad a range of different media as possible.

The presentation and content of effectiveness information is also varied to take account of the target audience. Some clinical journals are aimed at specialists in their field, with information presented in a way that is incomprehensible to the non-specialist. Similar difficulties can be experienced with publications examining the economic perspective. Other publications seek to present in a more user-friendly format the key findings from technical journals about the clinical and cost effectiveness of particular healthcare services, treatments and procedures.

There are three key sources of information we have found useful. These are:

- organizations dedicated to the production and dissemination of information regarding the clinical and cost effectiveness of healthcare interventions;
- publications;
- reports, guidelines and briefings.

These are summarized below.

Organizations

There is a growing number of national organizations who produce, commission and disseminate information regarding the clinical and cost effectiveness of healthcare interventions. These include the following.

The NHS Centre for Reviews and Dissemination

The NHS Centre for Reviews and Dissemination was funded by the Department of Health and set up in January 1995 to disseminate the results of healthcare research to the NHS and the consumers of its services. It is also responsible for increasing the knowledge base of the NHS on the clinical and cost effectiveness of healthcare interventions. Based at the University of York, it maintains two major databases for disseminating the results of its own studies and studies undertaken elsewhere.

The *Database of Abstracts of Reviews of Effectiveness* was created in 1994 and focuses primarily on the effectiveness of treatments for Health of the Nation topics. It is compiled by the Centre for Reviews and Dissemination, and includes records from two other sources, namely the international network of agencies for health technology assessment (INAHTA) and the UK Cochrane Centre.

The second database, the *NHS Economic Evaluations Database*, is based on studies of cost-effectiveness. Its initial focus was on primary care evaluations, but it has now expanded to encompass a broad range of topics. These databases serve as an on-line, continually updated resource for anyone within the NHS.

UK Cochrane Centre/Cochrane Collaboration

The Cochrane Centre was established as one of the first initiatives of the NHS Research and Development strategy, with the remit to prepare and disseminate systematic reviews of evidence-based practice. Based in Oxford, it was established in 1994. Under the umbrella of the Cochrane Collaboration, the Centre links with others around the world to construct, update and maintain a database of systematically reviewed, randomized controlled trials relevant to healthcare. Dissemination occurs primarily through the *Cochrane Database of Systematic Reviews*.

The UK Clearing House for Information on the Assessment of Health Outcomes

The Clearing House was set up jointly by the Department of Health in England and the Health Departments in Northern Ireland, Wales and Scotland in 1992. It has developed in association with the Research Unit of the Royal College of Physicians, and is based within the Nuffield Institute for Health at the University of Leeds. The remit of the UK Clearing House is to provide an information and advisory service on health outcomes, to act as a focal point for the exchange of information and to raise awareness of the key issues in health outcome measurement. Although the library of publications is maintained at the Nuffield Institute, development work has moved to the University of Salford.

The Centre for Evidence-Based Medicine

This Centre opened in 1995, funded by the NHS Research & Development programme. It is a joint initiative between Anglia & Oxford Regional Health Authority; the NHS R&D programme; the Nuffield Department of Medicine at the University of Oxford; the Oxford Radcliffe Hospitals Trust; and the Oxford Institute of Health Sciences. The main objectives are to promote evidence-based healthcare throughout the UK, to conduct research and generate new knowledge and to train researchers to undertake randomized controlled trials and systematic reviews.

The Central Health Outcomes Unit

The Central Health Outcomes Unit was established by the Department of Health in 1993. It aims to promote and coordinate the development and use of information on health outcomes, including methodological aspects of outcome assessment; data collection systems; expertise; analytical skills; and interpretation. The work of this Unit is coordinated through four groups: the Chief Medical Officers Advisory Group; the Clinical Outcomes Group; the Public Health Network; and the NHS Executives Working Group on Information Management and Technology.

Royal Colleges

The medical Royal Colleges and the Royal College of Nursing have become involved in producing and disseminating clinical guidelines and other tools aimed at promoting more clinical and cost effective practice.

Promoting Action on Clinical Effectiveness (PACE)

This network is an initiative of the King's Fund. The network aims to spread awareness and information about developments in evidence-based practice so that members can learn from and support each other's work and interests. In March 1996 a number of projects were identified that form the main element of the PACE programme. These include:

- Stroke prevention
- *Helicobacter pylori* eradication
- Pressure sores
- Low back pain
- Menorrhagia
- Incontinence
- Stroke
- Cardiac rehabilitation
- Cardiac failure
- Postoperative pain control
- Leg ulcers
- Cardiac/stable angina
- Family therapy in schizophrenia

Council of International Hospitals and the Advisory Board Company

The Council of International Hospitals is a membership-based research organization dedicated to sharing information and best practices across the healthcare industry. It is the international arm of the Washington-based Advisory Board, a private firm whose Healthcare Division membership includes over 1300 of the world's hospitals and healthcare systems. Gathering data across and beyond the membership, the Advisory Board publishes 30 major studies and over 17,000 customized research reports each year on behalf of its membership. In general, the research focuses on the best (and worst) demonstrated management practices, helping member organizations benefit from each other's experiences and preventing them from having to reinvent the wheel. The firm employs professionals who undertake the research and serve its worldwide membership. The healthcare division of the Advisory Board includes four distinct membership programmes, each publishing a separate line of research:

- Healthcare Advisory Board
- Governance Committee
- Cardiology Pre-eminence Roundtable
- Medical Leadership Council

Each member, and everyone within a member organization, has virtually unlimited access to the services and research provided by the Council. A membership year runs for 12 months from the date an organization decides to join. The subscription costs of £12,000 are not insignificant given the budget allocation for many NHS Trust Quality departments.

Publications

The publications on clinical effectiveness and evidence-based practice continue to grow. Some of those we have found useful include:

Outcomes Briefing

Outcomes Briefing is the newsletter from the UK Clearing House for Information on the Assessment of Health Outcomes. It deals with reviews of general and specific topics (for example, outcome measurement related to particular illnesses or interventions). It also offers information on activities by the Clearing House, including seminars and workshops (see above).

Effective Healthcare bulletins

The *Effective Healthcare* bulletins were commissioned by the Department of Health and aim to provide an overall summary of the clinical and cost effectiveness of particular healthcare or service intervention. Bulletins published to date include:

- Screening for osteoporosis to prevent fractures/Rehabilitation
- The management of subfertility
- The treatment of persistent 'glue ear'
- The treatment of depression in primary care
- Cholesterol screening and treatment
- Brief interventions and alcohol use
- Implementing clinical practice guidelines
- Menorrhagia
- Benign prostatic hypertrophy
- Pressure sores
- Cataract surgery
- Hip replacement
- Venous ulcers

Bandolier

This monthly newsletter has been produced by the Anglia & Oxford Regional Health Authority since February 1994. It aims to summarize reports and reviews on clinical effectiveness, and was originally intended to assist effective purchasing in the Anglia & Oxford region. It is now circulated nationally.

Journal of Clinical Effectiveness

This journal seeks to address the linked concepts of evidence-based practice, clinical effectiveness, guidelines and clinical audit. It is aimed at meeting the wide-ranging needs of clinical and non-clinical professionals in primary, secondary and community care, as well as those in purchasing and education who have an interest in clinical audit and clinical effectiveness. The journal states that its focus is essentially practical and clinically based, and the scope of original articles will include issues of practical importance in the areas of evidence-based practice, guidelines, care pathways, changing clinical practice and clinical audit.

There are two new publications aimed specifically at the nursing profession:

Evidence Based Nursing

Evidence-Based Nursing: Linking Research to Practice is published by the RCN Publishing Company and the BMJ Publishing Group. It is published quarterly with the support of the Health Information Research Unit, Department of Clinical Epidemiology and Biostatistics, McMaster University. The journal aims to help nurses by identifying and appraising high-quality, clinically relevant research and by publishing succinct, informative critical abstracts of each article together with commentaries from practising nurses who can place the new research in context.

Clinical Effectiveness in Nursing

Clinical Effectiveness in Nursing aims to address the effects of interventions on patient well-being by publishing work from nursing, midwifery, health visiting and allied disciplines that is directly relevant to the clinical work of nursing. Papers aim to be of high academic quality, but presented in a manner accessible and relevant to clinicians. The journal is peer reviewed and also offers peer commentary, to which authors then respond in the same issue. A correspondence section is used to widen the debate.

Reports, guidance and briefings

Aside from other regular publications, there are other documents we have found useful when seeking information on best practice. These include:

Acting on the Evidence: A Review of Clinical Effectiveness; Sources of Information, Dissemination and Implementation (*Appleby, Walshe and Ham, 1995*)

This document serves as an invaluable reference for those interested in promoting evidence-based practice. Providing useful background reading, it identifies the stages in the process of evidence-based medicine; economic assessment; the diffi-culties in putting research into practice; useful sources of information; different approaches to using effectiveness information, with a case study on the GRiP (Getting Research into Practice) project initiated by the Oxford RHA in 1993. It provides a critique of current approaches and identifies a series of recom-mendations for action and an action checklist for health authorities and Trusts.

Promoting Clinical Effectiveness – A Framework for Action in and through the NHS (*NHS Executive, 1996a*)

Drawing heavily on the NAHAT document summarized above, this document was repackaged and published by the NHS Executive in 1996. Although it was broadly welcomed by the professional press, one author noted that many health profes-sionals may think that the promotion of effective clinical policy would be even more welcome if it were matched by an evidence-based culture in other areas of government health policy. Examples include the 'care programme' approach to looking after severely mentally ill people in the community, and challenging the apparent inequities posed by the growth of general practitioner fundholding, in particular the uncertainty about its transaction costs and its lack of significant impact on patient care (Hayward, 1996). This reiterates the point made earlier that it is not only the clinicians who should base their practice on sound evidence; it is essential for managers and policy makers to do likewise. This pack is an excellent resource providing contact names and addresses of relevant academic centres; centres offering cost effectiveness advice; national audits using confidential enquiries; national advisory committees; professional contacts; and contacts at the NHS Executive. It also provides a document listing various sources of information on clinical effectiveness relating to specific clinical subject areas.

Acting on the Evidence: Progress in the NHS *(NHS Confederation, 1997)*
This research paper presents the findings of a research study aimed at assessing progress of evidence-based healthcare in the NHS and identifying innovations and approaches to serve as models of good practice.
The key findings covered the following key areas:

- **Meeting the corporate challenge.** The report highlighted that although some progress had been made by NHS boards, there was a need for greater board involvement, understanding and rapport.
- **Making it happen.** There was some evidence of innovative approaches in some of the health authorities and Trusts, but it seems many still have a long way to go. Areas highlighted for further improvement include: good information resources; skill development in finding, appraising and using information on effectiveness; and systems for monitoring the progress of work on clinical effectiveness.
- **Measuring progress.** The impact of three *Effective Healthcare* bulletins was examined. Most organizations surveyed could not tell easily what they had done with them, nor what action had been taken, although they recognized their importance.

The report concludes that greater attention should be given to making sure that policy on clinical effectiveness is carried through and implemented by health authorities and Trusts, by making it a much higher priority in arrangements for monitoring and managing performance. It will be interesting to see if the new Commission for Health Improvement, outlined in the White Paper *The New NHS: Modern, Dependable* (NHS Executive, 1997), addresses this issue.

Achieving Effective Practice: The Clinical Effectiveness and Research Information Pack for Nurses, Midwives and Health Visitors *(NHS Executive, 1998a)*
This excellent resource pack is divided into ten extremely user-friendly subsections, which can be used independently or as a complete package. The sections are on the following themes:

1   Clinical effectiveness – what it is all about.
2   Clinical effectiveness – finding out more.
3   Searching the literature.
4   Critically appraising the literature.
5   Designing and carrying out a clinical audit.
6   Preparing a proposal for clinical audit.
7   Changing clinical practice.
8   Designing a research study.
9   Preparing a proposal for research.
10   Writing and publishing on clinically effective practice.

Although aimed at nurses, midwives and health visitors, it is a useful pack, which should prove helpful to all professional groups.

Confidential enquiries

A number of confidential enquiries that identified recommendations for best practice have drawn from anonymous information supplied by clinical staff. In the medical profession, examples include the National Confidential Enquiry into Peri-Operative Deaths (NCEPOD), 1993; the Confidential Enquiry into Stillbirths and Deaths in Infancy; and the Confidential Enquiry into Maternal Deaths in the UK. These have provided recommendations endorsed by the Royal Colleges for areas for improvement in medical intervention. For example, NCEPOD has shown that it is unacceptable for junior doctors to carry out operations without supervision from and in consultation with their seniors; vital information on perioperative deaths should not be absent from case records; surgeons should not undertake low volumes of specialist procedures; and emergency surgery should not be performed after midnight.

Executive letters

EL(93)115

This document, produced in 1993, made explicit the NHS Executive's commitment to improving clinical effectiveness and moving towards evidence-based practice. It identified sources of information which all chief executives and directors of public health could use to improve the effectiveness of services they had purchased or provided, and identified guidelines of value in seven specific clinical areas, namely:

- making best use of the radiology department;
- guidelines on the management of asthma;
- recommendations for the management of diabetes in primary care;
- investigation and management of stable angina;
- management of leg ulcers in the community;
- management of neonates with respiratory distress syndrome;
- management of head injuries.

Purchasers were asked to provide a summary of the action they were taking to use these guidelines in the 1994–95 contracting round.

EL(94)94
This was issued by the NHS Executive in September 1994, and provided updated details of development work on clinical effectiveness. It is a source of this effectiveness information and information on clinical guidelines and other associated initiatives, including the health technology assessment programme.

EL(96)110
This executive letter enclosed the *Clinical Effectiveness* pack summarized above. It reiterates that improving the clinical effectiveness of NHS services is one of the most important ways of securing significant improvements to the health of the people of the UK, underpinned by both the NHS Priorities and Planning Guidance (EL(96)45), where it features as a medium-term priority, and the White Paper 'A Service with Ambitions' (*NHS Executive, 1996b*). Health Authorities were asked to use the resource pack to inform and support local effectiveness initiatives, working with Trusts and clinical teams in primary and secondary care.

EL(97)81 – The New NHS White Paper (NHS Executive, 1997)
This circular sets out the government's plans for replacing the internal market and modernizing the NHS.

The White Paper reflects the government's commitment to abolish the internal market and replace it with a system of integrated care, based on partnership between NHS bodies and other local agencies. The changes it sets out are designed to deliver a better service to patients through improved quality and efficiency, offering prompt quality treatment and care built around the needs of the individual. *The New NHS* forms the basis for a ten-year programme to renew and improve the NHS through evolutionary change rather than organizational upheaval.

Six key principles underlie the changes:

- renewing the NHS as a genuinely national service;
- making the delivery of healthcare against national standards a matter of local responsibility;
- getting the NHS to work in partnership, breaking down organizational barriers and forging stronger links with local authorities;
- driving efficiency by a more rigorous approach to performance and by cutting bureaucracy;
- focusing on quality of care so that excellence becomes the norm;
- rebuilding public confidence in the NHS as a public service.

The White Paper makes numerous references to clinical effectiveness and quality. It promises to set up a National Institute for Clinical Excellence to produce and disseminate clinical guidelines and audit methodologies, and to bring together current work and organizations. The government also places great emphasis on the role of clinicians in this process, through what they refer to as 'clinical governance', outlined in Chapter 4.

At the time of writing, there is little more detail on this new Institute. However, the benefits of increasing coordination across the expanding range of sources for information for busy clinicians would seem to be a useful initiative.

A First Class Service: Quality in the New NHS

This document (NHS Executive, 1998b) provides further details on taking forward the policy proposals in *The New NHS*. It is divided into four sections:

- **Quality standards.** This section reinforces the importance of evidence-based practice and clinical effectiveness. It sets out proposals to ensure that clear national standards for services, supported by consistent evidence-based guidance, are put in place to raise quality standards. The emphasis is on ensuring consistency of quality throughout the NHS with sensitivity to the needs of individual patients and local communities. It details the establishment of the new National Institute for Clinical Excellence (NICE) and the National Service Frameworks. Details of these are outlined further in Chapter 4.
- **Delivering quality standards.** This section describes mechanisms to ensure the new national quality standards are applied consistently at a local level through a system of clinical governance; through extended life-long learning to ensure NHS staff are equipped to deliver change and are given the opportunity to maintain and develop their skills and expertise; and through modernized professional self-regulation. More detailed explanations of clinical governance are given in Chapter 4. With respect to professional self-regulation, it is emphasized that the government is committed to working with the professional regulatory bodies to ensure that self-regulation keeps pace with public expectations and is more open and accountable. For example, a modernized regulatory system will play a fuller part in the early identification of possible lapses in clinical quality.
- **Monitoring quality standards.** This section describes three mechanisms for monitoring standards:
  - A Commission for Health Improvement (detailed in Chapter 4).
  - A national framework for setting performance (detailed in Chapter 4).
  - An annual survey of patient and user experience.
  It states, 'Best practice will be identified and spread. Poor performance will be rooted out' (p. 5).
- **Action for quality.** The final section seeks further consultation to develop the proposals, and asks for views on how best these objectives can be achieved with the active participation and partnership of those who work in the NHS and those who use NHS services.

Public Health Common Data Set/Population Health Outcome Indicators

The *Public Health Common Data Set* includes data on trends in mortality, morbidity and the Health of the Nation targets. This document is published annually.

Register of Cost-Effectiveness Studies

Published in 1994 by the Department of Health, the *Register of Cost-Effectiveness Studies* lists around 150 economic evaluations of healthcare services, treatments, procedures and other medical technologies. The studies were selected on the basis of their quality. Although a useful summary, a knowledge of health economics is required to interpret these studies.

Epidemiologically Based Healthcare Needs Assessments

These assessments were aimed at public health physicians in purchasing authorities. The two-volume *Healthcare Needs Assessments* was published in 1994 and covered twenty conditions and services which account for over one-third of the 'burden of disease' in the Western world. Each of the 20 services/conditions was reviewed from an epidemiological viewpoint, which included an examination of the range and effectiveness of services currently available in the NHS. In conclusion, an agenda for change was recommended for each area. This included diabetes mellitus, stroke, coronary heart disease, colorectal cancer, cancer of the lung, total hip replacement, dementia, prostatectomy for benign prostatic hyperplasia, and mental illness.

Health of the Nation Target Effectiveness Documents

These documents are aimed at managers and directors in purchasing organizations to develop local strategies for achieving the Health of the Nation goals. Five Key Area Handbooks were produced, covering coronary heart disease, stroke, cancers, mental illness, accidents, and HIV and sexual health. The 1998 Green Paper outlines a number of new targets which are described in Chapter 4.

Clinical guidelines

There is a growing body of literature on the development and application of clinical guidelines. Further details of this topic are included in the next chapter. However, such guidelines are an important source of information when considering where to find information on best practice. Many of the Royal Medical Colleges along with the Royal College of Nursing have developed guidelines within their specialities. The Clinical Outcomes Group (COG) chaired jointly by the chief nursing and medical officers carries out a review to select robust clinical guidelines which are based on clear evidence.

Summary

In summary, it can be appreciated that there is a vast range of sources of information to help professionals maintain their knowledge and proficiency in their professional fields. Once the information has been collected, the challenge is how to analyse and interpret it. This will now be explored using the second criterion outlined in our model in Table 1.1, critiquing the evidence we have collected from our literature review and forming a judgement on its content.

IS INFORMATION OF GOOD QUALITY?

Appraising the evidence

Having collected the information available, the next step is to evaluate the evidence for its validity and clinical usefulness. This step is essential, as it enables the practitioner to make an informed decision on whether or not the article or data can be relied upon to give useful guidance. It is important to remember that just because something is published does not mean it is automatically true. A large proportion of published clinical research lacks either relevance or sufficient methodological rigour to be reliable enough in answering clinical questions (Rosenberg and Donald, 1995).

We have developed and utilized the systematic approach of asking the following questions when appraising the evidence (James, 1997):

- Have you explored all possible sources for evidence? (See last section on 'Finding the evidence' for many sources.)
- When were the articles published? (The more dated the article, the more likely that new literature has been published since.)
- Who was involved in producing the evidence? Was it one professional group? Could this influence the conclusions?
- Did anyone sponsor the work (e.g. drug companies, governments)? Could this influence either the research focus or the conclusions?
- Has your evidence stated the source of their evidence/research? Are they credible?
- Have positive and negative studies been taken into account? (Journals may focus on reports with significant findings; there may be larger, unpublished studies that contradict these but do not get published.)
- What sort of evidence is the literature based on? Is it:
  - **Meta-analysis.** The combination of many randomized controlled trials and viewed by many as the strongest form of evidence.
  - **Randomized controlled trial (RCT).** An attempt to isolate the effects of a clinical intervention through allocating patients at random to either a control or a trial group. If the sample size is large enough, the groups will be statistically identical in terms of average age, gender mix and other characteristics that may affect the final outcome of treatment. Ideally, the only difference between the groups is that the trial group receives the treatment to be tested and the control group does not. Any differences in health outcomes between the two groups can therefore be attributed to the medical intervention. Some RCTs are designed so that clinicians and patients are not told who is in the control and who is in the trial group (known as double-blind RCT), hence minimizing any conscious or unconscious bias, for example in the way clinicians deliver treatment under trial and/or any placebo effects.
  - **Non-randomized controlled trial.** Including observational studies and uncontrolled trials.

- **Expert opinion.** Including qualitative data or opinions.
- If the results of several studies are combined, was it reasonable to do this? Were they similar in the first place; are they described before and after combination and are the results of different studies similar? Are there any explanations for similarities or differences that are unexpected?
- What was the intervention being investigated? Is it relevant for your purposes?
- How were the outcomes measured? Are there any weaknesses in the approaches to measurement which may influence the results?
- What was the population to which it applied? How closely does this compare with your client group?
- Which databases were searched? Was the literature review comprehensive?
- Do the source references listed in the publication agree with the findings of the main article?
- How precise are the results of any study? What sort of confidence intervals (the range within which the value of the measure or numerical value of a population is estimated to exist) are there?
- What are the limitations (i.e. the theoretical and methodological restrictions in a study which may decrease the generalizability of the findings)?

Rosenberg and Donald (1995) present a structured framework developed by teams working in North America and the United Kingdom which enables individuals without research expertise to evaluate clinical articles. This is shown in Table 1.3.

Table 1.3

Critical appraisal questions used to evaluate a therapy article

	Yes	Can't tell	No
Are the results valid?			
Was the assignment of patients to treatments randomized?			
Were all patients who entered the trial properly accounted for and attributed at its conclusion?			
• Was follow-up complete?			
• Were patients analysed in the groups to which they were randomized?			
Were patients, health workers, and study personnel blinded to treatment?			
Were the groups similar at the start of the trial?			
Aside from the experimental intervention, were the groups treated equally?			
What are the results?			
How large was the treatment effect?			
How precise was the treatment effect?			
Will the results help me care for my patients?			
Can the results be applied to my patient care?			
Were all clinically important outcomes considered?			
Are the likely benefits worth the potential harm and costs?			

This table was first published in the *British Medical Journal* (*BMJ*) (Rosenberg, W. and Donald, A. (1995) Evidence based medicine: an approach to clinical problem-solving, *BMJ*, **310**, 1122–6) and is reproduced by permission of the *BMJ*.

The authors recommend that the fundamentals of application of this model be taught by those experienced in its use. They estimate that, following such training, experienced practitioners can learn to appraise critically most articles (depending on length) in under ten minutes, transforming themselves from passive opinion-based spectators to active, evidence-based clinicians.

Other authors (Sackett and Rosenberg, 1995) advocate that criteria for methodological rigour should be kept pure and simple. Suggested criteria for studies of diagnosis, treatment and review articles are:

- **Diagnosis.** Has the diagnostic test been evaluated in a patient sample that included an appropriate spectrum of mild and severe, treated and untreated disease, plus individuals with different but commonly confused disorders? Was there an independent, blind comparison with a 'gold standard' of diagnosis?
- **Treatment.** Was the assignment of patients to treatments randomized? Were all patients who entered the study accounted for at its conclusion?
- **Review articles.** Were explicit methods used to determine which articles to include in the review?

The authors of the above criteria stress it is important that these criteria should not be presented in such a way that fosters nihilism (if the study is not randomized, it is useless and provides no valuable information) but should provide a way of helping to work out the strength of inference associated with a clinical decision. This should point out instances in which criteria can be violated without reducing the strength of the inference.

This observation is a timely reminder that, even if there is clear conclusive evidence supporting a particular course of treatment, application of the findings to specific groups of patients can be problematic. Some of the weaknesses in oversimplifying the implementation of evidence-based practice are outlined later in this chapter. However, a key consideration at this point is whether or not the trial findings (even if they are found to be robust) are applicable to our specific client groups. Some of the complexities in considering this factor are outlined under the third criterion in our framework in Table 1.1; namely that of applicability.

Are the findings relevant for the population we treat?

When reviewing the literature to inform the section 'Where do we find the information', we found that the majority of publications focused on the randomized controlled trial as the gold standard when seeking to determine best practice. Many of the organizations outlined in the above section use meta-analysis. Meta-analysis uses specific statistical techniques to give greater confidence from a number of studies than can be achieved from the single study. It is thus regarded as a method to show a more specific, statistically higher-powered endpoint covering a number of experimental studies on a particular topic. Variations between trial designs have been seen as limiting factors in meta-analysis, and decisions on criteria for which trials to include and which to exclude are critical in the analytical process. However, it has been observed that these variations in sample selection for clinical trials may actually assist clinicians when using research findings in their everyday practice (Batstone and Edwards, 1997).

For example, such a heterogeneous approach was used in systematic reviews of thrombolytic therapy. The meta-analysis of data from these trials exploited the variation in time between onset of pain and randomization to treatment or control to show if time to thrombolytic therapy was a variable in response to treatment (Fibrinolytic Therapy Trialists Collaborative Group, 1994). The analysis identified that effectiveness in reducing death from myocardial infarction was greater the earlier the treatment was given, as demonstrated by the NNT (number needed to treat to gain benefit) being reduced from 140 at 17 hours to 25 at two hours. Hence it is not just the administration of the drug which influences outcome, but timelines of intervention.

Number needed to treat (NNT)

The 'number needed to treat' is the number of patients who must be treated in order to prevent one adverse event. NNT tells clinicians and patients how much effort they must expend to prevent one event, thus allowing comparisons with the amount of effort that must be expended to prevent the same or other events in patients with other disorders. The general principle of 'number needed to treat' can be used to assess clinical approaches including long-term drug therapy. You can calculate the number of patients needed to be operated on to prevent one adverse event by carrying out a similar analysis of randomized trials and surgical procedures. For example, in the European Coronary Study Group trial, only six patients with stable angina and stenosis of the left main coronary artery had to undergo coronary artery bypass surgery for one life to be saved after five years of follow-up (European Coronary Study Group, 1982). You can also calculate the number of people needed to be immunized by combining the incidence of infection with the results from vaccine trials. For example, over 200 people need to be immunized with hepatitis B vaccine in order to prevent one case of hepatitis in the low-risk general population of the United States, as compared with only eight persons in a high-risk population of homosexual men (Szmuness et al., 1980; Health & Public Safety Committee, American College of Physicians, 1984; Mulley, Silverstein and Dienstag, 1982). This technique can also be adapted to diagnosis and screening by calculating the number of patients needed to be examined to prevent one death from breast cancer. A comparison of screened and unscreened women in the Swedish National Board of Health & Welfare study showed that approximately 1592 women between 50 and 74 years of age had to be screened with mammography in order to prevent one death from breast cancer seven years after the screening was instituted (Tabar et al., 1985; Laupacis, Sackett and Roberts, 1988).

Glasziou and Irwig (1993) asked the question 'To which groups of patients can the results of clinical trials be applied?' They summarized that this question is often inappropriately answered by reference to the trial entry criteria. They state that relying on the eligibility criteria for a clinical trial is both erroneous and limiting; they warn against restrictive generalization, and advise that we ask, 'Are the patients in this study so different from my patients that I could not apply the study results?' Accepting this advice, they then questioned how to decide when a patient is too different to benefit from treatment. They note that the search for differences should be based on features of the disease process or risk, rather than any differences in sociodemographic characteristics.

They ask the converse of the above question, 'Can the study results be generalized to all patients who would be eligible for the trial?' The answer would seem to be, obviously, 'Yes'; however, they refute this by application of Lubsen and Tijssens' model (the basic model: separating benefit and harm; 1989; in Glasziou and Irwig, 1993).

This model suggests that patient benefit increases with risk from the disease – those most at risk have most to gain – but that harm, or risk of adverse events, will remain comparatively fixed. Thus, at some low level of risk, the benefits will only just balance the harm, and we should refrain from treatment. They therefore advocate that clinicians deciding whether a trial's results apply to a particular patient should not focus on the inclusion and exclusion criteria of the trial – which are usually designed for improving the power of the study or maximizing safety – but should try to predict whether each patient would benefit.

Making this decision involves piecing together three types of information about the benefit and harm:

- the reduction in relative risk
- the risk
- the relative evaluation of the outcome

This method suggests that the application of trial results need not be confined by eligibility criteria or the trial setting.

Another important factor when considering applicability of findings for our patient group deals with the nature of the intervention. A study investigating the use of drug regimens for *H. pylori* eradication found that the most notable feature in a drug regimen comparison was the high compliance rate of the study participants (Schoenfeld and Butler, 1996). As Batstone and Edwards (1997) note, gaining a high compliance rate by selection of motivated subjects, patient information, nurses recruited to explain the study, and telephone access to deal with problems, etc. is legitimate to exclude undesirable variations when investigating whether drug A works better than drug B. This does not invalidate the applicability of the research findings, but does mean that the intervention should be seen not just as prescription of drugs, but as how to motivate patients to comply, together with provision of patient information and staff to reinforce this and deal with problems. Hence it becomes a multifaceted intervention with costs greater than the drugs themselves.

In response to the issues regarding applicability: at the 3rd Cochrane Colloquium (held in October 1996), a Cochrane Applicability Methods Working

Group proposed a five-step approach to the application of results of systematic reviews. These are:

1 Consider all the patient-relevant endpoints by tabulating all the possible benefits and drawbacks, whether data are available or not.
2 Consider from the data whether there are any factors that may be responsible for variations in the effect of the intervention being considered, and think of the implications for both the individual patient and the population as a whole. Variations in effectiveness may be the result of:
   • patient features (sex, race, age, biochemical markers, selection criteria);
   • characteristics of the intervention (timing, intensity, compliance, location);
   • disease features (receptor status, grading, associated disorders included or excluded);
   • how the effect was assessed (relative risk, risk ratio, NNT);
   • factors associated with the healthcare system (incentives, limitations to prescribing, funding arrangements);
   • the level of certainty of diagnosis in trials versus anticipated clinical practice etc.
3 Clinicians should assess whether the effects vary with risk because low-risk patients usually gain less absolute benefit than high-risk patients.
4 There is a need to predict the absolute benefit or harm for patients by calculating the NNT for each outcome based on the individual patient's expected event rate.
5 Weigh up the overall benefits and disadvantages and consider the trade-offs for both the patient and society in general.

It can be appreciated that the assessment of applicability of research findings is in itself a complex process, yet this is what competent practitioners routinely do; the art rather than the science of healthcare. Lack of data to answer all the points in decision making is common, and practitioners routinely have to fill in the gaps. This is an important consideration when reflecting on the application of evidence-based practice. The McGibbon definition of evidence-based practice considers patient-reported, clinician-observed as well as research-derived evidence as an integral part of clinically effective decision making (in Batstone and Edwards, 1997).

Qualitative research

It can be appreciated from the previous section that much of the medical literature is dominated by the scientific method, with the gold standard of a randomized controlled trial and quantitative research methods being heavily dominant. It is important to note that other research methods are equally valid and may be more appropriate within certain contexts. Qualitative research is a comparatively new approach to healthcare, although it has been used within the social and behavioural sciences (Baumrind, 1980; Glaser and Strauss, 1967; Kaplin, 1964; and Scheffler, 1967; in Burns and Grove, 1995, p. 393). The purpose of qualitative research methods is to assist the researcher to gain insight through discovering meanings. These insights are obtained not (as in quantitative methods) through establishing cause and effect, but through improving our understanding of the whole. Within a holistic framework, qualitative research provides a way of exploring the richness and complexity of the situation being observed.

Qualitative research is conducted to describe and promote understanding of human experiences such as (for example) pain, caring, powerlessness and comfort. The scientific method and quantitative research do not always lend themselves well to such studies, since human emotions are more difficult to quantify and assign a numerical value to. Qualitative research offers different techniques to exploring these emotional responses. It also focuses on the understanding of the whole, which is consistent with the holistic philosophy of nursing and other healthcare professions (Baer, 1979; Leininger, 1985; Ludemann, 1979; Munhall, 1982, 1989; and Munhall and Oiler, 1986; in Burns and Grove, 1995, p. 393).

Qualitative research is an artistic and philosophical approach that is often described as a 'soft' science. It evolved from the behavioural and social sciences, with proponents of this approach believing that the truth is dynamic and can only be found by studying people as they interact with and in their sociohistoric settings (Tinkle and Beaton, 1983 in Riley *et al*., 1995, p.394). Differing characteristics between quantitative and qualitative research characteristics are shown in Table 1.4. It can be appreciated that these are substantively different research techniques, but both can provide valid evidence on which to underpin clinical practice.

A major challenge for the evidence-based practice movement is how, having identified how to find the information and assessed it for applicability, to tell people about it. These 'people' are not just the practitioners but also patients and carers making an effort to enter into a genuine partnership which allows informed choices to be made by the patient about their treatment and care.

Table 1.4	Quantitative research	Qualitative research
Quantitative and qualitative research characteristics	Hard science	Soft science
	Focus: concise and narrow	Focus: complex and broad
	Reductionistic	Holistic
	Objective	Subjective
	Reasoning: logistic, deductive	Reasoning: dialectic, inductive
	Basis of knowing: cause-and-effect relationships	Basis of knowing: meaning, discovery
	Tests theory	Develops theory
	Control	Shared interpretation
	Instruments	Communication and observation
	Basic element of analysis: numbers	Basic element of analysis: words
	Statistical analysis	Individual interpretation
	Generalization	Uniqueness

Source: Burns and Grove (1995).

Table 1.5 *An agenda for action*	• Is the board really involved in and committed to improving clinical effectiveness? • Is there an executive director on the board who takes full responsibility for improving clinical effectiveness? • Does the organization have a formal strategy for clinical effectiveness? • Is there a coordinating group responsible for leading on clinical effectiveness? • Is there a senior individual working with the lead executive director to implement the strategy on clinical effectiveness? • Has the organization reviewed its structures in the light of its strategy for improving clinical effectiveness? • Does the organization have adequate access to information resources? • How does the organization disseminate and follow up information on effectiveness? • Is appropriate training relating to clinical effectiveness being provided? • Are health authorities incorporating evidence on effectiveness into their key roles in assessing healthcare needs and commissioning services to meet those needs? • Are trusts incorporating evidence on effectiveness into their key roles in healthcare provision? • Is the progress of efforts to improve clinical effectiveness and to foster evidence-based healthcare regularly monitored and reviewed? • Are efforts to improve clinical effectiveness having a measurable impact?

Reproduced by kind permission of the Editor of the *Health Service Journal* from Walshe and Ham (1997).

How do we tell people about it?

The 'Agenda for Action' checklist, aimed at identifying key actions required to promote an evidence-based culture within healthcare organizations, highlighted key points to consider when communicating clinical effectiveness information (Walshe and Ham, 1997).

This action checklist was developed in a subsequent piece of work, and is reproduced in Table 1.5.

Organizational structures

We found this a useful organizational checklist when exploring the whole area of access to information by professional staff. Ultimately, for this to be truly effective, it is an issue that needs to be addressed corporately so that the organization creates a culture in which access to contemporary clinical knowledge is encouraged. This requires a strategy for developing and disseminating information on current best practice to its healthcare professionals, and an organizational structure to support this.

How do we make it happen?

Once we have identified the information available, assessed it for applicability and ensured people know about it, the challenge then is to make it happen in practice. The management of change is fundamental to the implementation of evidence-based practice. For this reason a separate section is devoted to this topic later in this book.

Have we got the new treatment working?

Assessment of whether or not best practice is being practised can be achieved through an audit of clinical processes. The use of process measures can provide a sensitive and valid assessment of quality of care (Davies and Combie, 1995). Mant and Hicks (1995) have shown that such process measures may be more sensitive than outcomes in detecting differences in quality of care between hospitals. Audit of clinical processes is addressed elsewhere in this book in the sections on clinical audit, variance analysis and documentation of best practice.

Is it doing what we wanted it to?

When we have identified the information available, assessed it for applicability, ensured people know about it, made it happen in practice and audited the process to ensure compliance with best practice, the next step is to identify whether or not the intervention is doing what we wanted it to. This can be achieved through the assessment of clinical outcomes. Again, this is fundamental to the application of evidence-based practice and, along with audit of clinical processes, a valuable tool for assessing the impact of our interventions and determining whether they benefit the patient. Identification and assessment of outcome measures are dealt with in a separate section of this book.

Is appropriate evidence lacking?

It was identified earlier that in seeking information on best practice it may be there is no definitive research that provides answers to the questions we pose. This may stimulate practitioners to pose new research questions in order to advance clinical knowledge. Advancing clinical knowledge is key in addressing the whole evidence-based agenda.

Is it value for effort/resources? Is it best use of resources?

The introductory section of this chapter outlined the growing role that health economists have to play in assessment of best practice. They pose more radical questions that are less about the benefit to individuals and more about choosing treatments that minimize costs and maximize benefits. In considering responses to these questions, some of the techniques referred to earlier (cost benefit analysis, cost effectiveness analysis, cost utility analysis and cost minimization analysis) can be useful in assessing value for effort and resources.

EVIDENCE-BASED PRACTICE: THE DIFFICULTIES IN APPLICATION OF PRINCIPLES INTO PRACTICE

It can be appreciated that in working through the above framework to apply evidence-based practice, there are a number of limitations to the clinical and cost effectiveness movement. The literature review highlighted a number of criticisms and weaknesses in this approach, which we will now explore.

It has been argued that evidence-based medicine takes too little account of the uncertainties inherent in clinical practice; that it seeks to impose a 'spurious rationality' on processes that may be inherently irrational (or at least not capable of being made wholly rational) (McKee and Clarke, in Appleby, Walshe and Ham, 1995). Naylor (1995) suggests that, despite the efforts of researchers and clinicians, the 'grey zone' of clinical practice, in which evidence is incomplete or absent altogether, remains stubbornly large. Clinicians have to be prepared to blend 'the art of uncertainty with the science of probability'.

Criticisms of the application of evidence-based medicine fall into three categories: limitations at the primary research stage, dissemination of findings and putting findings into practice (Appleby, Walshe and Ham, 1995, p. 6).

Limitations at the primary research stage

At the primary research stage (involving clinical trials) there may, quite simply, be no available research. It is only in the case of pharmaceuticals that there is a requirement for evidence of efficacy before a new intervention is introduced. It may often be the case that a treatment or technology has become accepted practice over time, with practitioners relying on their own personal experience of its impact on the health of their patients.

Other authors challenge the assumption that evidence-based medicine is solely a drive to apply findings from randomized controlled trials, believing those who advocate such views have a fundamental misunderstanding of what evidence-based medicine is seeking to achieve.

Sackett and colleagues note that evidence-based medicine is not restricted to randomized trials and meta-analysis (Sackett *et al.*, 1996), and conclude that it involves tracking down the best external evidence with which to answer our clinical questions:

> *To find out about the accuracy of a diagnostic test, we need to find proper cross-sectional studies of patients clinically suspected of harbouring the relevant disorder, not a randomised trial. For questions about prognosis, we need proper follow-up studies of patients assembled at a uniform, early point in the clinical course of their disease. And sometimes, the evidence we need will come from the basic sciences such as genetics or immunology. It is when asking questions about therapy that we should try and avoid the non-experimental approaches, since these routinely lead to false positive conclusions about efficacy. Because the randomised trial, and especially the systematic review of several randomised trials, is so much more likely to inform us and so much less likely to mislead us, it has become the 'gold standard' for judging whether a treatment does more good than harm. However, some questions about therapy do not require randomised trials (successful interventions for otherwise fatal conditions) or cannot wait for the trials to be conducted. And if no randomised trial has been carried out for the patient's*

predicament, we must follow the trail to the next best external evidence and work from there.

The criticisms regarding the quality and nature of research evidence highlighted by the medical profession are also relevant to nursing. The evidence cited from research is usually based on a well-defined population that is incompatible with what you would encounter as a practitioner, because, for example, most trials exclude co-morbidity, and nurses don't tend to treat people who have only one thing wrong with them.

In a (comparatively rare) article in the nursing press exploring this issue, Naish (1997) notes;

> *People argue that health professionals use far more unquantifiable evidence when making patient care decisions – that they take account of holistic elements such as the social, psychological and environmental issues, as well as using intuition. This applies very much to nursing. And if you only take into account the evidence of randomised controlled trials, you will be eliminating a lot of things that nurses use.*

This stresses the importance of considering qualitative as well as quantitative research methods as valid sources of evidence.

It is also important to remember that clinical trials can quickly become out of date, or the trials themselves may have been poorly constructed and of dubious validity and reliability. There may be significant pressure to introduce a new technology which overrides the need or capacity to carry out an RCT. When the clinical evidence of effectiveness is eventually collected, it is often the case that the new technology or treatment has already become well established within healthcare services (for example the use of keyhole surgery).

Another difficulty with randomized controlled trials is posed by the ethical issues surrounding their construction. In using this type of trial, there is the potential to deny 'effective' treatment to some patients. Another problem with respect to RCTs is the huge cost of such clinical trials and the difficulty in attracting the funding.

The challenge is therefore balancing the need to assess medical technology and practice in a more robust way than relying solely on personal experience or prejudice.

Review and dissemination of findings

The second stage of the process of evidence-based medicine, the review and dissemination of research findings, is also problematic. Even where robust studies exist, they are not always accessible to practitioners who require them. This issue is covered in more detail earlier in this chapter, and later in this book where we explore the use of clinical guidelines, pathways, protocols and procedures as a mechanism for summarizing best practice, based on best evidence from the literature in a format that is easily accessible to practitioners. Even this seemingly logical solution to the problem of dissemination of evidence is not without its difficulties. As one clinician observes,

There is a fear that, in the absence of evidence clearly applicable to the case in hand, the clinician might be forced by guidelines to make use of evidence which is only doubtfully relevant, generated perhaps in a different grouping of patients in another country at some other time and using a similar but not identical treatment. This is evidence-biased medicine: it is to use evidence in the manner of the fabled drunkard who searched under the streetlamp for his doorkey because that is where the light was, even though he had dropped the key somewhere else.

(Evans, 1995)

Putting research findings into clinical practice

Even if well-validated trials do exist, application of the findings into practice can also be fraught with difficulty. For example, Evans (1995) notes that the question of whether evidence derived from patients enrolled in published trials is relevant to the patient one is agonizing over is particularly serious in geriatrics, since too many RCTs have excluded older, and particularly older and iller, patients. He identifies the problem that clinicians for older people need more complex evidence than mega-trialists are ever able to provide. Even where the 'proof' is available, it often involves confidence intervals which then require the clinicians to make a further judgement on the value to the patient sitting in front of them. Is it good enough to be '95% confident' that a particular treatment will benefit them? He identifies that healthcare managers and trialists may be happy for treatments to work on average, but patients expect their doctors to do better than that. He notes that as clinicians we must not arrogate to ourselves decisions that properly belong to the patients. Our task is to present the evidence that can enable individual patients to make up their minds about what treatment they want.

Other difficulties in implementing findings into practice are driven by the way in which healthcare services are organized and managed in the UK. Commissioners and purchasers are not always in a position to induce providers to change their practice based on current evidence. There is debate around the extent to which purchasers of healthcare should dictate how providers should deliver their services, for example the use of guidelines and protocols for managed care. Certainly, in the United States and in some of the private sector healthcare organizations in the UK, there is a strong shift to adopt such models. The extent to which managers and health economists (often with no clinical background) should influence medical practice in this way is the subject for further debate.

Getting research into practice also depends on ensuring that the right audience actually understands what the evidence means or what changes it advocates or implies. This requires those making decisions to have a good understanding of how to critique research findings. Many RCT results are not clear-cut. The issue of appropriateness for certain populations also needs consideration, as outlined earlier.

In conclusion, it can be appreciated that moving towards an evidence-based health service, although laudable in itself, is nonetheless an extremely complex and difficult exercise. First there is a requirement to produce the evidence through clinical and economic evaluations of healthcare interventions. These need to be done in a rigorous, robust way. Second, there is a requirement to review and pull together the evidence from multiple trials and evaluations, to develop conclusions and recommendations for practice to be produced. Third, these findings then need to be disseminated in a way that it is accessible and user friendly for clinicians. Finally, the evidence has to be used to change behaviour and impact on decision making by all of those involved in healthcare, not just clinicians. The next chapter therefore looks at methods for documenting best practice in an attempt to make it more accessible and user friendly for clinicians.

REFERENCES AND BIBLIOGRAPHY

Appleby, J., Walshe, K. and Ham, C. (1995) *Acting on the Evidence*. NAHAT Research Paper No. 17, London.

Baer, E.D. (1979) Philosophy provides the rationale for nursing's multiple research directions. *Image*, 11(3), 72–4.

Batstone, G. and Edwards, M. (1997) Issues of applicability. *Journal of Clinical Effectiveness*, 2(1), 1–2.

Baumrind, D. (1980) New directions in socialization research. *American Psychologist*, 35(7), 639–52.

Burns, N. and Grove, S. (1995) *Understanding Nursing Research*, W.B. Saunders, Philadelphia.

Collier, M. (1995) *Pressure Sore Development and Prevention*. Educational leaflet no. 3, volume 1 (revised), Wound Care Society, London.

Covell, D.G., Uman, G.C. and Manning, P.R. (1995) Information needs in practice: are they being met? *Annals of Internal Medicine*, 103, 596–9.

Davidoff, F., Haynes, B., Sackett, D. and Smith, R. (1995) Evidence-based medicine: a new journal to help doctors identify the information they need. *British Medical Journal*, 310, 1085–6.

Davies, H.T.O. and Combie, I.K. (1995) Assessing the quality of care. *British Medical Journal*, 311, 766.

Dealey, C. (1994) *The Care of Wounds*. Blackwell Scientific Publications, London.

Department of Health (1994) *Register of Cost Effectiveness Studies*, Department of Health (Economics and Operational Research Division), London.

Ellis, J., Mulligan, I., Rowe, J. and Sackett, D.L. (1995) Inpatient general medicine is evidence-based. *Lancet*, 346, 407–10.

European Coronary Study Group (1982) Long-term results of prospective randomised study of coronary artery bypass surgery in stable angina pectoris. *Lancet*, 2, 1173–80.

Evans, J.G. (1995) Evidence based and evidence biased medicine. *Age and Ageing*, November, 461–3.

Fibrinolytic Therapy Trialists Collaborative Group (1994) Indications for fibrinolytic therapy in suspected acute MI; collaborative overview of early mortality and major co-morbidity results from all randomised controlled trials of more than 1000 patients. *Lancet*, 343, 311–22.

Glasziou, P.P. and Irwig, L.M. (1993) An evidence-based approach to individualising treatment. *British Medical Journal*, 311, 1356–8.

Haines, A. and Jones, R. (1994) Implementing the findings of research. *British Medical Journal*, 308, 1488–92.

Harper, T. (1987) Skill mix: all mixed up. *Nursing Times*, 82(48), 27–31.

Hayward, J. (1996) Promoting clinical effectiveness. *British Medical Journal*, 15 June, 1491–2.

Health & Public Safety Committee, American College of Physicians (1984) Hepatitis B vaccine. *Annals of Internal Medicine*, 100, 149–50.

Healthcare Needs Assessment (1994) in *The Epidemiologically Based Needs Assessment Review* (eds A. Stevens and J. Rafter). Radcliffe Medical Press, Oxford.

Hibbs, P.J. (1988) *Pressure Area Care for the City and Hackney Health Authority*. City and Hackney Health Authority, London.

James, B. (1997) Critical appraisal of evidence, in *Developing Clinical Guidelines and Patient Care Pathways*, Brighton Health Care NHS Trust, Brighton.

Laupacis, A., Sackett, D.L. and Roberts, R.S. (1988) An assessment of clinically useful measures of the consequences of treatment. *New England Journal of Medicine*, 318(26), 1728–33.

Leininger, M.M. (1985) *Qualitative Research Methods in Nursing*, Grune & Stratton, Orlando, FL.

Lewis, B.V. (1993) Diagnostic dilatation and curettage in young women should be replaced by outpatient endometrial biopsy. *British Medical Journal*, 306, 225–6.

Logan, R. and Scott, P.J. (1996) Uncertainty in clinical practice: implications for quality and costs of healthcare. *Lancet*, 347(9001), 595–8.

Lubsen, J. and Tijssen, J.G.P. (1989) Large trials with simple protocols: indications and contraindications. *Controlled Clinical Trials*, 10, S151–60.

Mant, J. and Hicks, N. (1995) Detecting differences in quality of care; the sensitivity of measures in process and outcome in treating myocardial infarction. *British Medical Journal*, 311, 793–6.

Marlin, M. (1995) The contemplative navel, part 1: the silliest prophesies. *Imagine Nations United*, p.30.

Mulley, A.G., Silverstein, M.D. and Dienstag, J.L. (1982) Indications for use of hepatitis B vaccine, based on cost-effectiveness analysis. *New England Journal of Medicine*, 307, 644–52.

Munhall, P.L. (1982) Ethical juxtapositions in nursing research. *Topics in Clinical Nursing*, 4(1), 66–73.

Munhall, P.L. (1989) Philosophical ponderings on qualitative research methods in nursing. *Nursing Science Quarterly*, 2(1): 20–28.

Munhall, P.L. and Oiler, C.J. (1986) Nursing research: a qualitative perspective, Appleton-Century-Crofts, Norwalk, CT.

Naish, J. (1997) So where is the evidence? *Nursing Times*, 19 March, 64–6.

Naylor, C.D. (1995) Grey zones of clinical practice: some limits to evidence-based medicine. *Lancet*, 345, 840–2.

NHS Confederation (1997) *Acting on the Evidence: Progress in the NHS*. University of Birmingham Health Services Management Centre, Birmingham.

NHS Executive (1996a) *Promoting Clinical Effectiveness – A Framework for Action in and through the NHS*. Department of Health, London.

NHS Executive (1996b) *The National Health Service: A Service with Ambitions*. Department of Health, London.

NHS Executive (1997) *The New NHS: Modern, Dependable*, Department of Health, London.

NHS Executive (1998a) *Achieving Effective Practice: The Clinical Effectiveness and Research Information Pack for Nurses, Midwives and Health Visitors*, Department of Health, London.

NHS Executive (1998b) *A First Class Service: Quality in the New NHS*. Department of Health, London.

Register of Cost-Effectiveness Studies (1994) Department of Health (Economics & Operational Research Division), London.

Riley, C., Morton, W., Pulle, A. and Semple Piggott, C. (1995) *Releasing Resources to Achieve Health Gain*, Radcliffe Medical Press, Oxford, New York.

Rosenberg, W. and Donald, A. (1995) Evidence based medicine: an approach to clinical problem-solving. *British Medical Journal*, 310, 1122–6.

Royal College of Physicians (1996) *The Consultant Physician: Responding to Change*.

Sackett, D.L. and Rosenberg, W.M.C. (1995a) Evidence-based medicine and guidelines, in *Clinical Effectiveness and Guidelines to Cost Effective Practice* (eds M. Deighan *et al.*), Health Services Management Unit, *The University of Manchester*, pp. 137–44.

Sackett, D.L. and Rosenberg, W.M.C. (1995b) On the need for evidence-based medicine. *Journal of Public Health Medicine*, 17(3), 330–4.

Sackett, D.L., Rosenberg, W., Richardson, W.S., Gray, J.A.M. and Haynes, R.B. (1996) Evidence-based medicine: what it is and what it isn't. *British Medical Journal*, 312, 71–2.

Scheffler, I. (1967) *Science and Subjectivity*, Indianapolis: Bobbs-Merrill.

Schoenfeld, P.S. and Butler, J.A. (1996) Commentary on papers of *H. Pylori* eradication. *Evidence Based Medicine*, 1, 109–10.

Summerton, N. (1995) The burden of proof. *Health Service Journal*, 105(5481), 33.

Szmuness, W., Stevens, C.E., Harley, E.J. *et al.* (1980) Hepatitis B vaccine: demonstration of efficacy in a controlled clinical trial in a high-risk population in the United States. *New England Journal of Medicine*, 303, 833–41.

Tabar, L., Fagerberg, C.J.G., Gad, A. *et al.* (1985) Reduction in mortality from breast cancer after mass screening with mammography: randomised trail from the Breast Cancer Screening Workshop Group of the Swedish National Board of Health and Welfare. *Lancet*, 1, 829–32.

Walshe, K. (1996) Evidence-based healthcare: Brave New World? *Healthcare Risk Report*, March, 16–18.

Walshe, K. and Ham, C. (1997) Who's acting on the evidence? *Health Service Journal*, 3 April, 22–5.

Weinberg, J. (1993). Future directions for small area variations. *Medical Care*, 31(5), S7575–80.

USEFUL ADDRESSES

The NHS Centre for Reviews and Dissemination (CRD) Information Service

NHS Centre for Reviews & Dissemination
University of York
York Y01 5DD
Tel. (01904) 433634
Fax (01904) 533661

Cochrane Centre
BMJ Publishing Group
PO Box 295
London WC1H 9TE
Fax (0171) 383 6662

UK Clearing House on Health Outcomes
Nuffield Institute for Health
71–75 Clarendon Road
Leeds LS2 9PL

Central Health Outcomes Unit
Department of Health
Wellington House
133–155 Waterloo Road
London SW1 8UG
Tel. (0171) 972 2000

Royal College of Nursing – Clinical Effectiveness Initiative
20 Cavendish Square
London W1M 0AB

Royal College of Physicians of London Research Unit
Royal College of Physicians
1 St Andrews Place
Regent's Park
London NW1 4LE

The Centre for Evidence-Based Medicine
University of Oxford
Nuffield Department of Clinical Medicine
The Oxford Radcliffe Hospital NHS Trust
Headley Way
Oxford OX3 9DU
Tel. (01865) 221321

2 Documenting 'best practice'

The previous chapter explored how to identify best practice. From the literature reviewed in Chapter 1, a major criticism of evidence-based practice was that much of the evidence is not in a user-friendly format. It is also generally inaccessible at the point where it is most needed – at the time of consultation with the patient. The challenge for health professionals is therefore how to consolidate this vast range of evidence into a concise summary which is available at the point of healthcare delivery. It is perhaps not surprising that in an attempt to meet this challenge a number of different methods have evolved that seek to document best practice.

A 'method' is defined in the Collins dictionary as 'a way of doing something . . . conscious regularity'. The attraction of methods such as policies, protocols, guidelines, etc. is that they provide a systematic way of summarizing what needs to be done for the patient. Once the particular method of documenting best practice has been learned, these methods offer a mental map for the professional which it is comparatively easy to apply to a range of clinical conditions and organizational processes. They provide a rigorous way of ensuring that all the factors identified as part of the method used are explored and written down. For example, the Donabedian method (1969) focuses the user on structure, process and outcome; Maxwell (1984) focuses on six other dimensions outlined later in this chapter. Other authors may use the terms 'frameworks', 'tools' or 'techniques'.

This chapter will give an overview and definition of the differing terms used and an explanation of how best to choose the appropriate method, depending on the purpose for which it is intended. We then examine the general principles that apply to documenting best practice, regardless of which method is selected. This will be followed by a more detailed examination of some of the most frequently used methods for documenting best practice in health services today – namely, standards, protocols, guidelines, pathways, policies and procedures. The authors will present case studies from their experience of implementing these in their own practice and identify the strengths and weaknesses of each approach.

Why document best practice?

Documenting best practice is a way to get information from research into clinical practice. The key points from the relevant research literature can be summarized in an easy-to-follow plan of action which is accessible to healthcare staff at the point of consultation. Documenting best practice can eliminate unnecessary variation in treatment. It is often found that patients with similar clinical conditions have large variations in the types of test they have, the length of time it takes for treatment to be carried out, and the information they receive. By identifying and documenting what best practice is, it is possible to reduce these variations.

Documentation of best practice is a useful teaching aid for new employees. The document is a source of reference for them and their teacher to help them understand how things need to be done. Documenting best practice can also be an excellent resource for the patient. It provides clear information on the recommended course of treatment. It can assist patients in reaching a decision of informed consent and participating in their programme of care. Best practice documents can maximize health gains through ensuring patients are being treated in the most efficacious way. Resources used for healthcare are then used efficiently and effectively.

Methods for documenting best practice

In healthcare, many different terms are used to describe the different methods for documenting best practice. The problem is, they often have different meanings to different professional groups, which causes confusion among a multidisciplinary team in developing a clearly documented programme of treatment and care for patients based on best evidence . Examples of terms used include 'standards', 'protocols', 'guidelines', 'patient care pathways', 'policies' and 'procedures'.

We offer our own set of definitions and interpretations of these different terms below. This is purely for clarity when explaining the similarities and differences between various concepts, and to put into context the case studies for each outlined later in this chapter. Other writers may choose to use different terms which are either already well understood within their own organization or more culturally accessible for certain professional groups. In our experience, the most important thing when adopting these methods is that the multidisciplinary team has a shared understanding of the approach being used, and selects the right one for the purpose in hand.

Definitions

A 'policy' is a statement of organizational intent for a given issue and gives a clear position statement for the organization's customers and employees on its values and beliefs. A 'standard' states what level of performance is expected. A 'guideline', 'procedure' or 'protocol' is a framework that stipulates the practice required to reach that standard.

For example, an organization may develop an equal opportunities 'policy'. This policy will be a statement of strategic intent, which sets out a clear position statement; for example: 'This hospital is committed to employing a workforce which reflects the diversity of the local community.'

A 'procedure' may describe the actions undertaken to implement the policy, such as procedures for recruitment and selection which target a diverse range of applicants. Typically procedures are intended to be adhered to fairly rigidly by employees, and in many organizations breach of procedure is a disciplinary offence. Other examples include fire and safety procedures; procedures for the disposal of clinical waste; and procedures for the safe storage of patients' money and valuables.

A 'guideline' or 'protocol' is often less prescriptive, and generally requires a certain level of professional judgement and decision making. In a clinical example (such as a protocol for cardiac arrest), it requires a level of professional expertise that enables a diagnosis of the problem to be made which then triggers a prescribed series of actions. An organization may develop a set of good practice guidelines for equal opportunities, such as advice for managers citing good practice to ensure that disabled job applicants are treated fairly and equally and that disabled patients have the same access to services as non-disabled users.

Finally, a 'standard' is a statement of a measurable level of performance which should be achieved. For example, 'The number of disabled employees will increase in X hospital by 1% within 12 months.'

All of the above methods seek ways to define requirements by writing down how and why things should be done, with the aim of ensuring that everyone is aware of what they are expected to do and the level of performance required by the organization. They should all cite the evidence and rationale for the course of action defined. This is essential if we are to avoid merely documenting what we have always done, without challenging the evidence base as to why we are actually doing it. The distinction was made in the last chapter between 'efficiency: doing things right' and 'effectiveness: doing the right things'. Merely documenting what we do, rather than what we ought to be doing, will undermine the whole point of such quality improvement programmes. Developing whole audit programmes around protocols and standards that are not empirically based is a worrying phenomenon in health services. It merely creates the illusion of valuing quality and is also a waste of resources that could be more effectively deployed.

Similarities between the methods

Some of the important similarities between these different methods are:

- All involve the development of a clear and definitive written statement which sets out explicitly and unambiguously the requirements for a specific process.
- All are used to identify the best practice and to communicate them to people and to encourage or ensure their use.
- All provide a basis for measurements of the quality of care to be made and so they can all be used in audit or quality improvement projects.
- All are designed with a specific and clearly defined goal in mind.

Differences

However, there are also some important differences in these approaches. A policy is made at a strategic level for the organization as a whole and indicates a set of values or beliefs. Procedures, protocols and guidelines and standards set out a series of actions and defined parameters for the employee to follow. They allow for different levels of divergence by individuals or groups from the best practice that they define. For example, a protocol may give considerable leeway for differences in practice, while a procedure tends to be much more prescriptive.

They come into play at different points in the quality improvement process. A policy may be used to frame the process through a statement of strategic intent; for example, 'Putting patients' interests first'. All procedures and standards therefore need to be congruent with this policy. This then requires the organization to develop the standards and procedures to ensure the intent is translated into practice.

Writing standards, guidelines, procedures, protocols and pathways

An essential prerequisite of developing any of the above methods is to follow the key steps outlined in the previous chapter, namely:

- Formulate a clear clinical/professional question.
- Search the literature for relevant clinical articles.
- Critically appraise the evidence.
- Implement useful findings.

Documenting best practice using one of the above methods is invaluable in the implementation step, as it provides an *aide-mémoire* for staff at the point of delivery.

There are numerous guidelines, standards, protocols, procedures or pathways that have already been developed, so carrying out a literature search is essential. In many cases there are national guidelines developed by the medical and nursing Royal Colleges and other professional bodies. There may also be regional guidelines, standards or pathways in existence, developed by other groups. Others in your own organization may already have tackled the subject you are looking at and developed some standards, guidelines or pathways.

GETTING STARTED: SELECTING YOUR METHOD

It is important first to decide what kind of statement of requirements you are developing. If you want to write a statement of principles or intent, which apply to the organization as a whole, a *policy* is the method best suited to your needs. If you want to set specific tasks to be performed for a particular process, with little or no deviation, a *procedure* is the best method. If you are developing a systematic approach to managing a particular process, which will require an element of expertise to apply and which will produce a clearly defined outcome, a *guideline* or *protocol* is the best method. A *protocol* (also known as an *algorithm*) is a set of instructions that have a conditional logic for solving a problem or accomplishing a task. Guideline algorithms relate to recommendations for patient care. Criteria algorithms concern rules for evaluation of criteria conformance. Protocols can be documented in words or in the form of a flowchart, as shown later in this chapter. If you want to define clearly the levels of performance or results to be achieved in a process or as a consequence of a process, a *standard* is the most appropriate method.

A more recent development in documenting best practice is the development of a multidisciplinary plan of care in diary format for a specific clinical condition. These are often referred to as patient care pathways, anticipated recovery paths, care maps, critical pathways, integrated care pathways, multidisciplinary care pathways of care or clinical pathways. We use the first term – 'patient care pathways'.

Pathways focus on the process of care. They outline (generally on a day-by-day basis) the activities, tasks and outcomes for a patient with a given diagnosis (Kennedy, 1995). They also include variance analysis, an inbuilt audit tool that records deviations from the prescribed pathway of care. Variance triggers a quality review to ensure corrective action is taken if there is a problem or new evidence-based practice in the process of care delivery. Pathways are useful for patients with a discrete condition that requires a predictable programme of treatment and care which would generally occur within timeframes that are reasonably consistent across the range of patient group. They are a useful way of identifying the responsibilities of each member of the multidisciplinary team and for providing a unitary patient record (i.e. all professionals write in the same document, thus reducing the risk of duplication through multiple record keeping). They tend to focus on all elements of the patient's needs and care, whereas guidelines and protocols tend to focus on professional practice.

It is essential that the right method is selected for the purpose you have in mind. It has been our experience that too little thought is given to choosing the most appropriate method. Selection of the wrong one will make audit difficult and can be time consuming and frustrating. An example of this was the rise in popularity at the end of the 1980s of using the Donabedian approach for setting standards in the nursing profession (a method outlined later in this chapter). This is a useful method for setting and auditing practice when used appropriately. However, in the authors' experience, this did in some cases lead to the almost slavish application of this approach without adequate reflection on the task in hand. One such example was a problem in a unit where it had been identified that oxygen cylinders were not being checked and consequently some were empty when they were needed. Some simple instructions for checking and changing the cylinder were required. A short procedure was the best method for doing this.

Instead, the staff, fresh back from their standard-setting course, had written a lengthy standard, listing

- the oxygen cylinder
- the porter
- the nurse
- the checking book
- a pen

under the structure column, a complex series of instructions under the process column, and the outcome cited as '100% of oxygen cylinders will be checked every 24 hours and be in working order when required.' A good clear outcome statement, but one can question the unnecessary complexity of going to such lengths on the structure and process or, indeed, of needing several hour-long meetings of nursing and portering staff to develop such a standard.

In practice, many of these methods exist in a mutually supportive manner. At the centre you have the core of policies that state the values and beliefs of the organization. This will be underpinned by the standards, procedures, guidelines and pathways which will all be congruent with policy in an organization with a robust quality strategy. For example, organizations that purport to value staff will set standards for staff development and training, have procedures for supporting them when sick, and guidelines for managers on good employment practices such as appraisal and supervision.

Many of these methods will be cross-referenced with each other; and often, when examining a new area of practice or concern, several different methods will need to be used. For example, when developing a care pathway for patients with oesophageal cancer, we first had to develop a guideline for clinical treatment. Once we had clearly established guidelines based on best practice, we also identified the need to set a standard for pain control. Underpinning the pain control standards were a number of procedures, for example the hospital procedure for the safe and secure handling of medicines. It was only when all of these building blocks were in place that we were able to begin constructing the care pathway.

Once you have selected the most appropriate method to fit your purpose (and the case studies later in this chapter will give examples of their application), regardless of the method selected, there are a number of important principles to consider when documenting practice. These are outlined below.

Setting the criteria

All the methods outlined later in this chapter comprise a collection of criteria (from the Greek meaning 'means of judging'). Criteria are standards or principles by which something is judged or evaluated. The criteria themselves all need to be based on best available evidence. Writing them in clear unambiguous language and avoiding excessive verbiage is an art form in itself. There follow some points for consideration when developing any of these methods.

Select target group

You need to determine a clearly defined target group (or resource) at whom each criterion is aimed. This is important for two reasons. First, it identifies clearly, to individuals who are involved in meeting the criteria, who or what the criteria apply to; for example, 'all postoperative patients' or 'patients with oesophageal cancer'. In instances where the criteria are not aimed at patient or staff groups, but at resources, the target group should be similarly stated; for example, 'all the wheelchairs in the outpatient department' or 'all the hospital budget statements'. Second, it identifies the sample group that needs to be audited to see whether the criterion is being met. (The process of auditing standards is discussed in more detail in the next chapter.)

The document (whatever form it takes) should state which individual, or group of individuals, is *responsible* for meeting the criteria. This is important, as it places the onus of responsibility for meeting the standard upon specific individuals, or groups (for example, 'all registered nurses'). In the event of the criterion not being met, it is the responsibility of these individuals to take action to rectify the problem. If the action required falls outside their sphere of responsibility, then it is up to them to inform others of the deficiency who are able to help. Failure to define spheres of responsibility in this way can cause problems in ensuring the criteria are followed. In practice, we have found it can lead to situations where everyone assumes that it is someone else's responsibility to ensure the criteria are met. This is particularly relevant in multidisciplinary pathways, which should make explicit which disciplines are responsible for specific criteria.

Meeting the criteria documented should be within the sphere of influence of those writing the document, or cooperation should be sought from others who are required to deliver against the criteria agreed. For example, nurses may write a technically excellent standard for planning patient discharge. However, to implement all the criteria, they require at least 48 hours' notice that the patient can go home (so that they can book appropriate community support, transport home and complete relevant Health Education Programmes). Medical staff may be unaware of this, and normal practice may be to tell the patients, at the time of the ward round, that they can go home that same day. The standard therefore cannot be met. A solution to this problem is to include other professionals whose cooperation is required in developing the standard.

The criteria should be a clear statement of intent. There is no place for 'weasel words'. These are phrases that attempt to 'weasel out' of commitment to the criteria. For example, 'The Charge Nurse will endeavour to ensure that most new staff on Nightingale ward receive instruction on safe lifting and handling techniques by the physiotherapist; preferably within five days of commencing employment.' Weasel words make it difficult to audit the criteria (in the last example there is no mandatory requirement to attend a lifting lecture because of the use of 'preferably', 'endeavour' and 'most'). They also absolve individuals of their responsibility for maintaining the standard, because they are not definitive.

USING 'SMARTER' CRITERIA WHEN DOCUMENTING BEST PRACTICE

All criteria listed in the document should be 'SMARTER', that is Specific, Measurable, Achievable, Relevant, Timely, Effective and Research based. These will now be explored in more detail.

Specific

Use exact and precise language and spell everything out. Do not assume people will understand what you mean. It should be clear when you read your document which patient group it applies to, what equipment is involved and which staff are responsible for that particular aspect of care. The criteria statements should be clear, understandable and unambiguous. When documenting best practice and developing the criteria, it helps to consider the following questions.

Why do we need to document best practice for this particular group of patients, procedure or practice?

The most common reason is that staff or patients have identified a problem. There may be specific complications arising for a particular patient group, or a national incident such as the inadequate cervical screening services in Kent & Canterbury NHS Trust (NHS Executive, 1997). Focusing on the root cause of the problem can ensure that criteria are included to eliminate the problem. For example, guidelines for lifting and handling could be developed as a result of an excessive number of lifting injuries sustained by nurses. Investigation may reveal that none of those injured had received instruction on lifting techniques. A mandatory standard could be set that 100% of new staff receive instruction on lifting and handling as part of their induction week. Other reasons for documenting best practice include areas of interest, an area for improvement, new research evidence or developing a service that appears desirable.

What are the criteria referring to?

This should be stated in specific terms. For example, 'Patients will be nursed with appropriate available equipment' is non-specific. It does not tell the reader which patients the criteria refer to, or what equipment is deemed appropriate. Conversely, 'All patients with a hemiplegia will be given a plateguard and wide-handled cutlery at mealtimes' is much more specific.

Who is involved?

This should include the individual or group for whom the method is written, and the individual or group who need to take action to meet the criteria.

When should specific criteria be met?

This falls into two categories. First, specific timings for actions that are stated in the method; for example, 'All patients will receive x analgesia following the onset of chest pain.' Other examples include criteria that need to occur on a regular basis, such as 'daily' or 'twice weekly'. It is quite clear to readers when, or how often, they are expected to comply with the criteria. Second, the timing for implementation of the method needs to be discussed. Those documenting practice should set a target date for its being met and should plan an audit after this date to measure its impact.

How will the criteria be met?

This needs to consider the resource implications of any changes in clinical practice and any education or training staff will require to meet the criteria.

Where does the overall area of practice covered in the document apply?

This can range from one specific ward to a hospital or regional or national standard. Working through the above checklist should ensure that criteria are specific.

Measurable

One of the reasons for documenting best practice is to make explicit the standard of performance on which the staff and the process will be judged. This implies some kind of measure against the criteria set, so that compliance with the set criteria can be judged. Setting criteria that cannot be measured is of limited value. It is helpful when designing measurement tools to ensure that criteria are specific.

Whether developing policies, standards, procedures, protocols or pathways, all should have a performance measure. The performance measure should define how it will be audited in practice. An example in the case study on pain management later in the chapter sets the performance measure as:

For consecutive surgical patients seen over a 6-month period, calculate the number of patients whose pain was assessed and documented every two hours while awake.

The performance measure is:

$$\frac{\text{no. of cases with criterion met} \times 100\%}{\% \text{ of surgery cases}}$$

Measuring criteria statements

Unless criteria statements are measurable, there is no way of knowing whether they are being met. If the performance measure is clear, but the criteria statements are unmeasurable, it is impossible to establish the reasons for failure in the event of the performance measure not being met. For example, the performance standard may state, 'A performance rate of hospital-acquired pressure damage of 3% or more triggers a review to improve assessing and implementing the patient's Waterlow score on admission and assessment twice daily, and reviews the adherence to the pressure damage protocol for patients identified at risk.' Provided the assessment tool (Waterlow score (Waterlow, 1988)) and the pressure damage protocol are clearly defined criteria, it is easy to audit to identify possible root causes for an increase in hospital-acquired pressure damage. Without such criteria, we can only note the symptoms (a poor performance measure) but cannot make a diagnosis of the cause. Formulating specific criteria is the easiest way of ensuring they are measurable.

Achievable

Policies, protocols, procedures, standards, guidelines or pathways define performance criteria that are achievable in practice. The level of their application in practice – i.e. whether you are aiming for an 'ideal', 'minimum' or 'highest realistic' standard – must be negotiated. This will depend on resources such as time and expertise available. An 'ideal' level of quality is the care it should be possible to give under ideal conditions when there are no constraints on resources. A 'minimum' level of quality is the minimum level of proper care for the patient to be maintained; the least that can be done. The 'highest realistic' level of quality spells out the best possible standard of care within known constraints. The level set is a compromise between clinical importance, practicability, affordability and acceptability. It is also worth remembering, as Tingle points out, that there may be legal implications if a statement setting out a standard of care is not reasonable or realistic (Tingle, 1992).

Opinion differs as to where the benchmark for standards should lie. Some consider that 'minimum standards' should be written, i.e. establishing the lowest acceptable standards. Others believe that standards should reflect what happens in practice, such as the pain performance measure above. A third approach to determining the standard involves defining an optimum level which the practitioner strives to attain.

Professional input is needed to identify the technical aspects of care that the customer is unable to define. For example, a patient with abdominal pain will not be able to identify the technical requirements to ensure that they have a successful operation. However, the patient will have requirements relating to their environment and comfort, such as adequate postoperative analgesia and assistance with hygiene. This may mean challenging current practice and attempting to secure increased resources.

In a time of resource constraint, professionals often find themselves compromising the care they wish to deliver. There are no easy answers to this, but a useful starting point can be to reach a consensus on what *should* be done through clearly agreed criteria. Competing for additional resources with a robust case based on clear research evidence is a lot more powerful. Ultimately a judgement will need to be made to assess the relative risks for either providing or withholding recommended treatments. It is perhaps not therefore surprising that clinical risk management is moving up Trust Boards' agenda. From 1999, the NHS Executive will require all Trust Boards and Health Authorities to include a 'controls assurance statement' confirming they have robust systems in place, not just (as to date) for financial risk, but also for clinical risk (NHS Executive, 1998).

Relevant

It has been our experience that many staff choose areas of practice or services to focus on of which they are the customer, rather than the provider, for example, nurses wanting to set performance criteria for turnaround times for medication to take out (TTOs) from pharmacy, or doctors wanting a sister or charge nurse present on all their ward rounds. Unless the people involved in the process are committed to making it work, and agree the criteria set are relevant, the impact of documenting practice using any method is likely to be limited. Criteria set need to be relevant to the sphere of influence of the professional developing them and the process they are trying to address. Criteria included in the statement must be relevant to achieving the stated outcome.

Timely

Specific timescales should be included within the criteria where appropriate, for example, 'four hourly' rather than 'frequently'. This also makes measuring the criteria easier. The date that the document (procedure, guideline, etc.) is agreed

STAFFORDSHIRE UNIVERSITY LIBRARY

should also be written on it, along with the review date. This ensures those following the document know whether it still applies to their area of practice. A clear review date also helps to ensure that the document does get reviewed against any new research findings since it was first written and agreed, to ensure that it is still a statement of best practice. Some accreditation systems (discussed later), such as ISO 9000, attach great importance to review dates.

Effective

Statements should describe care that is effective and based on best available evidence. These can be achieved using the steps set out in Chapter 1.

Time spent on documenting best practice, where there is consensus about a need to change and where a high level of care is both aspired to and feasible, is more likely to deliver successful changes in practice. Effective care also encompasses the social, physical, psychological and other patient needs which may not always have a body of evidence behind them that meets the gold standard of RCTs outlined in the last chapter, but are nonetheless crucial for the patient's well-being. Effective care may therefore be based on consensus about what is best practice rather than on research.

Research based

The performance standard and criteria should be theoretically sound. This covers several areas:

- Clinical criteria should be based on current research findings, where available.
- They should reflect the professional code of conduct, as defined by the professional bodies.
- They should incorporate legal and statutory requirements.
- They should be ethical.

Having examined the broad principles that apply to the documentation of best practice for any documentation method selected, the next section will examine in more detail the theory and application of documenting best practice using standards, protocols, guidelines, procedures and patient care pathways.

STANDARDS

A number of different methods are documented in the literature to assist in the setting, documentation and audit of standards. Of these, the Donabedian 'structure, process, outcome' has been most widely adopted by the nursing profession (Donabedian, 1969). This framework is outlined below. Other standard-setting frameworks are also explored in this chapter: the Crosby Process model worksheet, Maxwell's six dimensions of quality, and criteria listing (Crosby, 1989; Maxwell, 1984). Each of these is used to formulate a multidisciplinary discharge standard to explore the practical application of each framework, and to examine the differences and similarities between them. This will be followed by other methods used to document practice, namely guidelines and pathways.

The Donabedian 'structure, process, outcome' framework

Donabedian first published his framework for setting standards in 1969. His approach has been adopted, over 20 years later, by the nursing profession, with further development of the framework and production of a comprehensive teaching package by the Royal College of Nursing Standards of Care Project Team (1990). Much of the pioneering work in this field was done by Kitson (1988a, b) Kendall (1988) and Howell and Marr (1988). The next section introduces the terminology used and guidelines for using this approach. Its practical application is then discussed by means of a case study of a multidisciplinary team's attempt to develop a standard for patient discharge planning.

Donabedian referred to three different types of criteria necessary to meet the standard:

- structural criteria
- process criteria
- outcome criteria

We have found that the easiest way to understand these is to use the analogy of baking a cake. The standard statement might be 'An edible 10 inch chocolate sponge cake will be delivered to C ward before 6 p.m. every Friday.'

Structure criteria
These describe the resources in the system that are required to meet the standard. They include:

- equipment (the oven, mixer, cooking utensils)
- buildings (the kitchen)
- staff (the cook)
- agreed policies and procedures (the recipe, health and safety procedures)
- ancillary services (the porter to deliver the cake)
- materials (eggs, flour, etc.)
- money to buy the ingredients and pay wages

Process criteria
These describe the actions required by individuals in order to meet the standard. They include:

- Actions in implementing and monitoring the standard (for example, the cook reads the recipe; the cook weighs the ingredients; the cook mixes the ingredients).
- Assessment technique and procedure (for example, the cook assesses the oven temperature; the cook follows health and safety guidelines).

- Education, training and knowledge needed to meet the standard (for example, the cook has a City & Guilds certificate; the cook shows subordinates how to bake the cake).
- Methods of giving information (for example, the ward sends a written request for the cake on Wednesday before 6 p.m.).
- Evaluation activities to be performed by those involved in meeting the standard (for example, the cook checks that the cake is cooked).

Outcome criteria

These describe the desired effect of the standard in terms of behaviour, responses, level of knowledge and satisfaction (for example, 'The chocolate cake arrived on C ward at 17:30').

Case study

This case study applies the 'structure, process, outcome' framework in setting a multidisciplinary standard for patient discharge from hospital. Discharge planning was selected for the case study because it was a broad enough topic to show how the use of different frameworks can generate a different focus and affect what finally goes into the standards. A more clinically focused standard will be examined in the final case study in this chapter based on an example of developing a standard for the management of pain using an evidence-based approach.

Writing the standard

A multidisciplinary team was convened to set a standard aimed at improving discharge planning within the hospital. The team consisted of those professionals who were involved in planning and coordinating discharge of patients from hospital. The first task was to compile a standard statement that took account of the guidelines listed above. This proved difficult for two reasons. First, the term 'discharge' proved ambiguous. We were unsure whether this included patients discharged to other hospitals and of where the 'discharge' started or finished. (For example, was it when the patient left the hospital gates, when they arrived home safely or when they returned for their first outpatient appointment?) Defining the *scope* of the standard is important for the sake of clarity.

Second, we found it hard to set a standard that we could guarantee we could achieve. Impressive statements such as 'All patients will have their socioeconomic and health needs met on discharge from hospital' had to be discarded when we realized that they were outside our sphere of influence. If the patients wanted to go home to unsuitable circumstances, and to disregard all our well-intended health education, this was their prerogative. Our role (it was decided) was to ensure patients were offered the components of a planned discharge to enable them to make an informed choice. Providing we did this, the choice then lay with the patient. A statement that met the SMARTER criteria as closely as possible is shown on the completed standard in Table 2.1.

The structural components were then determined. This process involved all the professionals who had a role to play in planning patient discharge. The team

Table 2.1

Standard for discharge of patients from hospital using Donabedian's standard-setting framework

Performance standard: *'All patients will have a written discharge plan fulfilling the criteria identified in the hospital discharge procedure. The plan will be implemented within the timeframes stated.'*

Structure	Process	Outcome
• A multidisciplinary team including: consultant, senior house officer, RGN, community liaison sister, occupational therapist, physiotherapist, speech therapist, dietitian, social worker. • Staff pharmacist • Medical secretary • Medical records clerk • Ambulance service • A multidisciplinary discharge procedure	• The multidisciplinary team will assess the patient's social, medical and physical needs before discharge. • Members of the multidisciplinary team will follow the discharge procedure and maintain the discharge standard. • Members of the multidisciplinary team will offer the patient information and advice outlined in the discharge procedure. • Members of the multidisciplinary team will check the patient's understanding of information and advice. • Members of the multidisciplinary team will document a written plan of discharge for the patient. • The multidisciplinary team will audit the standard every 6 months.	• All discharges are implemented as planned. • Communication within the multidisciplinary team meets the criteria set out within the discharge procedure. • The patient's social, medical and physical needs are assessed, planned and implemented in preparation for discharge. • Discharges are audited. • The score on the audit tool improves.

debated other structural components, such as buildings and equipment. It was decided not to include all the wards and departments, telephones, typewriters, etc., as these were too numerous to mention. Also, it was felt at the time that the problems had arisen because of the lack of an established system for planning patient discharges, rather than from shortage of materials or equipment. The decision was taken to include specific essential items in the multidisciplinary discharge procedure rather than in the standard.

During the discussions it became apparent that no clear procedure incorporated all the disciplines relating to patient discharge. This was causing problems, as some aspects of patient discharge had never been assigned to a specific discipline. For example, everyone agreed that it was necessary to liaise with local authority rehabilitation officers for provision of disability equipment, house adaptations and other support services, but it had never been established who should do this. The team also became aware that even where there was an established procedure (such as in nursing), many staff were unaware of it, and some parts of the procedure required updating. There was clearly a need for a multidisciplinary discharge procedure to resolve these issues. Initially we were uncertain as to what constituted a standard and what constituted a procedure; an understandable confusion when neither of these two documents existed.

A *procedure* describes actions that need to be performed by an individual to complete a given task. A *standard* is a professionally agreed level of performance (that meets the components of the SMARTER guidelines). Hence a discharge *procedure* was required to inform individuals within each discipline of the actions they were required to undertake when discharging a patient. For example, 'The nurse will ensure the patient's valuables are returned to him or her on discharge.' The discharge *standard* was required to define an agreed level of service that patients discharged from hospital could expect to receive.

In the absence of a procedure, it is common to find procedural statements being incorporated into the process column on the standard. This was our first big mistake, with the initial process column in our standard being 12 pages long. This was resolved by starting again, this time writing a separate multidisciplinary discharge *procedure*, which was then mentioned under the structure column as a document that was essential for meeting the standard, so it was not necessary to repeat these criteria in the standard itself.

The process criteria were then compiled. These defined the prerequisites of meeting the standard, and are shown in Table 2.1. They proved relatively straightforward. A key consideration here was the need for both documents to be 'active' and not left to sit on a shelf gathering dust. This was resolved by including a representative from all areas as a link person, to explain the new standard and procedure to all staff. It was realized that the impact of these could be effectively monitored only through the use of an audit method. This was also included under the process element of the standard.

The outcome criteria were then agreed, as shown in Table 2.1. These were more difficult to formulate using the SMARTER criteria, as many of the original criteria suggested were subjective, impossible to measure or outside the sphere of influence of the team. The final five criteria were agreed, with the agreement on the meaning of these as follows:

Outcome 1 'All discharges were implemented as planned' referred to all the criteria within the patient's individual discharge plan being met. Each discharge plan had to fulfil the discharge standard and follow the steps set out in the discharge procedure.

Outcome 2 'Communication within the multidisciplinary team met the criteria set out within the discharge procedure.' The procedure set requirements on whose responsibility it was to contact (for example) the district nurse; required social workers to see the patient within 48 hours of a referral; and required nurses to give 48 hours' notice for transport if needed. Discharge assessment was to be made within 24 hours of admission so that the planning could begin as soon as possible. All these criteria can be audited by checking whether they were documented in the care plan and whether they were carried out within the agreed timeframe. The audit tool included criteria such as the amount of notice nurses were given by medical staff that the patient was to be discharged, and whether social workers received referrals within the agreed timeframe.

Outcome 3 '*The patient's social, medical and physical needs were assessed, planned and implemented in preparation for their discharge.*' This was rejected as the standard statement, as it was felt to be outside the sphere of influence of the team in the event of a patient refusing these services. However, it was felt to be a reasonable expected outcome. The important factor was that all these areas had been assessed, with the patient being offered the appropriate treatment or service. It was these factors that were measured in the audit tool.

Outcome 4[1] '*Discharges were audited.*' It was agreed that a randomized sample of six patients in every ward will be audited by the sister or charge nurse using the discharge audit tool on a monthly basis. A target was set that 'the score on the audit tool will increase to 95% over an 18 month period', with individual targets and action plans developed for each ward.

General comments on the practical application of this model

The Donabedian framework has several advantages when setting a standard. The first involves the ownership of the standard by those setting it, and the improved communications that arise from this exercise. We found the method a useful way of considering the different criteria required to meet the standard. Formulating the standard statement first helped in establishing relevant criteria required to meet it.

There were some difficulties in setting this particular standard. First, its more abstract nature made identifying structural components difficult. There is a difference of opinion as to how such components are identified by those using the standard. Some advocate the use of the structure to identify factors such as staff knowledge and information (Royal College of Nursing Standards of Care Project Team, 1990). Others refer to Donabedian's initial intention that structural factors should be those that do not change (such as buildings and equipment), and argue that knowledge and staffing levels can be viewed as either structure or process depending on one's position within the organization (Goldstone, 1991). This raises the problem of deciding which criteria belong in which column. Our final conclusion was that, provided that relevant criteria were identified (in terms of practical application of the standard), it made no difference whether criteria were listed in the structure, process or outcome column.

The second difficulty lay in the implied relationship that the three columns have to each other. Initially we made the mistake of trying to use the standard form layout shown in Table 2.1 as a flow sheet, where structural, process and outcome components were all linked across the page. We then identified the

---

[1] NB – These are strictly process measures, but they are used by proxy to ascertain outcomes.

problem (as in the example of the non-compliant patient) that the structure and process criteria may all be met, but the outcome not. This proved particularly problematic in our initial attempts at auditing only outcome measures. It was resolved by incorporating measures of structure, process and outcome into the audit method, which proved a far more effective gauge of how the standard was working. The converse of this scenario can present similar problems. For example, patients may achieve remarkable outcomes that mask the fact that the structural and process components are inadequate. Studies attempting to demonstrate a relationship between these three components have identified a poor, or non-existent, relationship between outcome measures and structural and process inputs (Overton and Stinson, 1977).

From an organizational perspective, widespread generation of a large number of standards proved logistically difficult to administrate. In the absence of a clearly defined mechanism for approving and maintaining the standards, their effectiveness can be impeded. At one extreme is the danger of poor standards being formulated and accepted locally in the absence of organizational and professional guidance and control. At the other extreme, standards that reflect current research and good practice may be set, but fail to be implemented because of a lack of management commitment necessary to release funding and resources. However, in future Trusts' intranets are likely to be a great advantage for coordinating and distributing local policies, procedures and standards, etc.

Absence of central coordination also led to a significant amount of duplication, with common interest areas such as care planning, wound care and pressure sore prevention producing numerous variations on the same theme. This in turn creates the risk that conflicting standards may be developed within one unit.

The Crosby process model worksheet

The process model worksheet is one of the methods used in the Crosby approach to total quality management (TQM), which is explained in a later chapter by means of a case study. It is included in this chapter as another framework that can be used to set standards. The Crosby approach also advocates the use of 'flowcharting', which can be used to determine standards criteria. This is outlined briefly below, as it is our experience that it can be used with any of the standard-setting approaches mentioned in this chapter, and may prove useful to those attempting to develop an eclectic approach to standard setting. It is also commonly used in a modified format to develop protocols or algorithms, as outlined later in this chapter.

Crosby (1989) uses slightly different terminology, referring to 'requirements' instead of 'standards'. His process model worksheet is designed to establish the requirements (or standards) for a given 'process'. The underlying concept of this approach is that 'All work is a process: a series of actions that produce a result' (Crosby, 1989). This means that, for all work processes, there will be inputs and outcomes, and customers and suppliers; as shown in the process model worksheet in Figure 2.1. For example, in the process 'discharging a patient', the outcome will be the patient being discharged. The inputs will be all the materials,

1

> *PROCESS NAME:*
> **Discharge of patients from hospital**

2 — SCOPE

First activity:
Consultant gives notice of discharge

Last activity:
Patient established in planned location

5

Facilities & equipment	Who provides	Requirements
Ambulance	Ambulance service	48 hrs notice
Storage of drugs	Management	Arrives on time
Internal transport	Porters	Conforms to drug storage procedure
Secure place for money	General office	1 hrs notice
		Arrives on time
		48 hrs notice of withdrawal
		Returned on time

6

Training & knowledge	Who provides	Requirements
Discharge procedure	MDT/time management	All staff aware of procedure
Induction for new staff re: discharge procedure	Departmental head	All staff follow procedure
Discharge audit tool	MDT	Within 2 days of appointment
		Used every 6 months

4a

Inputs	Suppliers	Requirements
Materials		
Drugs	Pharmacy	Correct 2hrs notice
Valuables	General office	Returned complete, on time
Patient transfer form	Nursing	Accurate/complete/ on time

4b

Inputs	Suppliers	Requirements
Information		
Notice of discharge	Doctor	12 hrs notice
Pt's social status	Patient/social worker	Accurate
Pt's physical status	Patient/nurse	On time
Pt's medical status	Doctor	Documented

4c

Inputs	Suppliers	Requirements
Patient	Consultant	Informed of discharge
		Involved in plan

3

Outcomes	Customers	Requirements
Patient discharged from hospital	Patient	Planned by MDT
		• with all materials and equipment
		• on time
		• to correct location
3a	3b	3c

7

Procedures	Who defines	Requirements
MDT Discharge procedure	MDT (approved by management)	Includes crown guidelines
		• current
		• validated
		• agreed
		• available

8

Performance criteria	Who defines	Requirements
Quality	Professionals, management	Right first time
Cost	Professionals, management	Within budget
Timescales	Professionals, management	On time

Figure 2.1

Process model worksheet (adapted from Crosby (1989))

information, facilities, equipment, training, knowledge, procedures and performance standards that are needed to achieve the desired result.

Customers

The notion of the 'customer and supplier' is one that is used in many approaches to total quality management. Processes have four types of 'customer': (i) internal; (ii) external; (iii) intermediate; and (iv) ultimate (Crosby, 1989). A 'customer' is the recipient of a service or product at a given stage of the process.

- 'Internal' customers are all the individuals who are internal to the organization. In the process of discharging a patient, these would include the nurses and doctors.
- 'External' customers are those individuals external to the organization who receive goods or services as part of the process. In the process of discharging a patient, these would include the general practitioner, who receives the discharge summary of the care of their patient from the hospital doctor, and the patient.
- The 'intermediate' customer refers to the recipient of the product or service during an intermediate stage of the process. In the process of discharging a patient, the pharmacy would be a customer of the prescription chart stating the discharge medication of the patient.
- The 'ultimate' customer is the individual who is the ultimate recipient of the service or product produced by the process. In the process of discharging a patient, the ultimate customer is the patient.

Suppliers

All processes also have 'suppliers'. 'Supplier' refers to the individual or department that delivers essential goods or services necessary for the process. For example, the pharmacy department is a supplier of the drugs necessary for the patient on discharge. It can be appreciated that, within a given process, one can be both a customer and a supplier. Hence the pharmacist is a customer when receiving the completed drug chart specifying the discharge medication, and a supplier when dispensing the medication. When examining a process using this approach, it is necessary to identify all the customers and suppliers within the process, because all these individuals need to agree the requirements necessary for making the process work (or, to use previous terminology, for meeting the criteria). For example, the pharmacist requires a certain amount of notice to enable the pharmacy to prepare the drugs for the patient's discharge. However, when examining this process, it became apparent that, in a significant proportion of cases, the prescription was written at the last minute, with the nurse having to go to the pharmacy to collect the drugs. The amount of notice required by the pharmacy to enable them to prepare the drugs had never been defined and, during this process, they were able to negotiate an acceptable amount of notice with the medical staff. The important factor in establishing requirements in this way is that they should be agreed between the customer and supplier. In cases where one area 'imposed' a new set of requirements without agreeing them with the supplier, they were (understandably) often never met. The benefit of establishing requirements in the process of discharging patients was that it gave all the individuals involved in the process an insight into the needs of their colleagues, which ultimately improved the process. Establishing clear requirements is a useful precursor for auditing the process, as these are easily transferred into audit criteria. For example, if it is agreed that the pharmacy requires two hours' notice for discharge prescriptions, it can easily measure the number of times this requirement (or standard) is not met.

Flowcharting

Flowcharting can be useful to identify components that need to be included in the standard framework. Flowcharts are also useful when examining work processes, as they enable the most likely source of potential problems in the process to be identified. Figure 2.2 shows an example of a flowchart completed by the multidisciplinary team dealing with one part of the discharge process – sending discharge letters to the patient's general practitioner (GP) on discharge. The initial agreed requirement (agreed between the medical staff and medical records) was that these should reach the GP within 21 days of the patient being discharged. (A discharge summary was always sent on the day of discharge; the discharge letter was a more detailed account of the patient's progress in hospital.) An audit of the process had identified that this requirement was not being met.

The flowchart shows the normal chain of events in the process of writing patient discharge letters. It identifies those involved in the process, and the

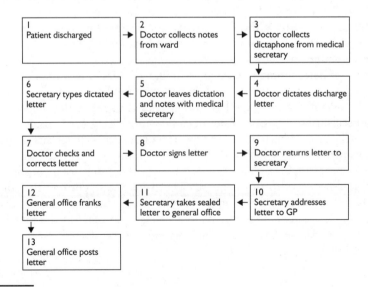

Figure 2.2

Flowchart showing process of compiling discharge letters to general practitioners

materials and equipment needed. Each stage offers potential clues as to where the errors in the system may be occurring. For example, in stage 2, if the notes are not available on the ward, the doctor will be unable to complete the process. Further understanding of the process can be gained by involving those identified by the flowchart as part of the process in completing a process model worksheet (explained below). The flowchart also offers a useful framework for different disciplines to examine a process that crosses both professional or departmental interfaces, where each area sees only a small part of the overall process. Many staff demonstrate little insight into the requirements of these other areas.

Completing the process model worksheet

For ease of explanation, the process model worksheet shown in Figure 2.1 is numbered in the order in which it is completed. Each of these steps is explained below:

Process name

This simply requires the name of the process under examination to be completed; in this case, 'Discharge of patients from hospital'.

Scope

This refers to the scope of the process being examined. The simplest way to determine the scope is to refer back to the flowchart for the process. For example, in the case of the discharge letter in Figure 2.2, it may be the whole process that needs exploring, in which case the contents from the first box 'Patient discharged' are entered under 'First activity', and from the last box 'General office post letter' under 'Last activity'. Conversely, one may wish to scrutinize a particular part of a complex process and narrow the scope. For example, in Figure 2.2 one could have the first activity as 'Doctor leaves dictation and notes with medical secretary', as shown in box 5, and the last activity as 'Doctor checks and corrects letter', as shown in box 7.

We think of determining the scope as similar to using a lens on a camera. One can either zoom in and examine a certain part in more detail, or take a wide-angled look at the overall process. We have often tended to make the scope too large, which unnecessarily complicated the documentation using the Crosby method.

It was helpful to determine the scope for the process of discharging patients because, as mentioned earlier, many of us were unsure where the process started and where it finished. Initially, this led to us attempting to incorporate every conceivable criterion into the standard. The team finally decided that the initial activity was 'the consultant giving notice that the patient was fit for discharge' and that the final activity was 'the patient being established in the planned location'. The latter phrase was used to include patients transferred to other hospitals or nursing homes.

Outcomes

It is necessary to consider the outcomes of the process before any inputs. Unless the outcomes of the process are clearly defined, it is difficult to establish what inputs are required. If you don't know what you want, you won't know what you need to get it!

In this example, the outcome of the process is the patient discharged, as shown in Figure 2.1 (3a).

Figure 2.1 (3b) asks who the customers of the outcome are. In this instance, this was limited to the patient, but there may be more than one customer for a given process. For example, another output that could be included from this process is the discharge letter; the customer in this instance would be the GP. Different customers will often have different requirements from the same process, as shown in Figure 2.1 (3c). The requirements of the patient are that:

- the discharge is planned by the multidisciplinary team with consideration of social, medical and physical needs;
- the patient is discharged to the correct location;
- the patient is given all necessary materials and equipment in preparation for discharge;
- the patient is discharged on time.

If the letter to the GP had been included in this section, then the requirements would be:

- The letter should arrive within 21 days.
- The letter should be accurate.
- The letter should be complete.

Inputs

This stage defines the material and information inputs required for the process. The model has been adapted for the health service to include a third box for the patient. This was because, for many of our processes, the patient is the 'input', and including them as a 'material' was regarded as inappropriate.

Material inputs (Figure 2.1 (4a)) are the inputs required by the process which are altered or consumed in some way by the process. Returning to the earlier cake-baking analogy, the material inputs would be the eggs, sugar, flour, etc. In this example, the material inputs are the drugs required on discharge, the money and valuables belonging to the patient that may be in safe keeping ('altered' by the process, as cash is returned as a cheque!) and the patient transfer form, which is altered by being written on. The suppliers of the material inputs are indicated. This proved a useful method of agreeing clear areas of responsibility for supplying certain inputs essential to the process which had not previously been established. For example, the general office agreed to return all money and valuables to the patient before discharge, but required 48 hours notice from nursing staff if a large cheque needed to be arranged. The requirements for each of the material inputs are then agreed, as shown in the final box in Figure 2.1 (4a).

Information input (Figure 2.1 (4b)) is the information required to operate the process. In this instance, this relies on the consultant informing the multidisciplinary team of the intention to discharge the patient; and information on the patient's social, physical and medical needs on discharge. The individuals responsible for supplying this information are shown in the following boxes (Figure 2.1). The requirements for each of these information inputs is shown in the final boxes.

The 'patient' input to the process (Figure 2.1 (4c)) identifies the supplier as the consultant, because once he or she gives notice of discharge the process begins. The patient's requirements of this information are shown in the final box.

Facilities and equipment
This box identifies all the facilities and equipment necessary for the discharge process. These are things that need to be present but, unlike the material inputs, are not altered or changed by the process. In the analogy of baking the cake, equipment would include the cake tin, the oven and the utensils, because these remain at the end of the process. The facilities would include the portering service, to deliver the cake, and the supplies department to deliver the ingredients. The facilities and equipment, as identified by the multidisciplinary team, for the discharge process are shown in box 5, along with the suppliers of these. Again, agreeing the requirements of these between different disciplines was an important part of improving the process.

Education and knowledge
It is at this stage that the staff required for the process are identified, along with any education or knowledge necessary. This was a useful step, as it forced the team to consider how all staff would be informed of the new multidisciplinary discharge procedure. This was important if it was not to be filed away to gather dust with all the other procedures.

Procedures
This box identifies any procedures necessary for the process. These may be already established or, as in the case of the multidisciplinary standard, require developing. It was an interesting observation that, in many of the processes we examined using this model, there were few defined procedures for many work processes. Many were carried out 'because they'd always been done like that', or were carried out differently (as with pressure area care), depending on who was involved in the process.

Performance criteria
This box determines the performance standard for quality, cost and timescales. Ideally, these should be defined by senior management and professionals. In terms of the performance standard for the quality of this process, the requirements identified should all be done right first time. The process should be carried out within the allocated budget, and the schedule for all the requirements identified is defined as all of them occurring 'on time'.

General comments on the practical application of this model

This framework also proved a useful method for identifying the different components necessary to meet the requirements in the process of discharging a patient. It concentrated the minds of the team on establishing requirements (or standards) for each of the components. This was useful both for improving the process and for ensuring that requirements were measurable. The use of the 'scope' was found to be advantageous, as it forced us to focus on the specific part of the process that was causing us difficulty.

The framework itself is more comprehensively laid out than that of the Donabedian model. Some staff preferred the more explicit headings, whereas others felt it was too complicated and difficult to understand. Educating staff to use the model was an important factor in its ease of use, and this is referred to in more detail in the general conclusions. Similar difficulties were identified to those highlighted with the Donabedian model with respect to the implied relationship between structure, process and outcome, although the process model does make the connections more explicit in each of the individual boxes where there is a chronological flow across each box.

Maxwell's 'dimensions of quality'

Maxwell first published his 'dimensions of quality' in 1984. He identified six components of quality standards:

- access to service
- relevance to need
- effectiveness
- equity
- social acceptability
- efficiency and economy

Discharge standard using Maxwell's dimensions

This framework can also be used in setting standards for patient discharge, as illustrated in Table 2.2.

General comments on the practical application of this model

Maxwell's dimensions offer an interesting alternative to the other two approaches outlined above. In the example of discharging a patient, it raised two areas not previously addressed by the team: 'equity' and 'relevance to need'. One of the overriding problems identified by team members based in the community was their inability to meet the increasing demands placed upon them by patients with greater needs being discharged earlier from hospital. This led ultimately to the prioritization of patients' needs.

'Relevance to need' was another new dimension. There was a danger that our well-intentioned attempts to offer everyone all the elements of a planned discharge would drastically increase the workload. However, many patients did not want a variety of professionals probing their social and economic circumstances, and

Table 2.2

Discharge standard using Maxwell's dimensions

Access to service

1 All patients will have access to a fully planned discharge service, as defined in the multidisciplinary discharge procedure.

2 Patients requiring transport on discharge, or for follow-up appointments, will have this arranged by nursing staff, and will be informed of arrival and departure times.

3 Patients requiring community services will have these arranged before discharge.

Relevance to need

1 All members of the multidisciplinary team will assess the patient's social, medical and physical needs on discharge.

2 The multidisciplinary team will discuss with the patient their perceived needs on discharge.

3 Patients will be offered the components of a planned discharge to meet their individual needs.

Effectiveness of the service

1 The multidisciplinary team will audit the discharge procedure every 6 months to ensure that component criteria are met.

2 The multidisciplinary team will audit circumstances relating to readmission of patients to hospital within one week of discharge.

3 A postdischarge survey will be undertaken to establish patient satisfaction with their discharge plan.

Equity

1 All patients, regardless of sex, creed or colour, will be offered a planned discharge that takes account of their individual needs and the organization's ability to meet these needs. This may necessitate prioritization for the most needy.

2 Non-English-speaking patients requiring an interpreter will be supplied with one.

Acceptability of service

1 The nurse will obtain feedback from the patient and relatives to ascertain the suitability of the discharge plan in meeting the individual needs of the patient.

2 A cost benefit analysis will be completed to establish the impact of early discharge from hospital, and to identify any necessary increase in community resources.

3 A 'cost of non-compliance' will be measured for this process, and actions taken to improve this cost.

many were content to go home and be left to their own devices. The role of the team was to ensure that those who required this service received it.

This model could be particularly useful on a macro scale, such as when planning a new hospital or department. Its use on a smaller scale can also be helpful. Disadvantages found in using this approach were that many of the dimensions tended to overlap, and similar criteria appeared in different dimensions. Developing audit methods for many of the criteria was markedly more difficult than for the other two approaches. Evaluating 'fairness' and 'acceptability' tended to be very subjective.

Criteria listing

This final method for writing standards is mentioned here because we are aware that, in spite of relatively little being published on this approach, many areas are using criteria listing as a way of defining standards.

Using the discharge standard as an example, the following criteria list was compiled:

- All members of the multidisciplinary team will follow the discharge procedure.
- Members of the multidisciplinary team will assess the patient's social, medical and physical needs before discharge.
- Members of the multidisciplinary team will offer the patient information and advice as outlined in the discharge procedure.
- Members of the multidisciplinary team will formulate a written discharge plan, based on the patient's individual needs, before discharge.
- The members of the multidisciplinary team will audit the discharge standard (using the audit method), at six-monthly intervals.

The main advantage of this approach is that it is easy to use and easy to understand. This can benefit staff, who find it time-consuming trying to fit criteria into the three frameworks outlined above. It is also relatively easy to audit such criteria. The main problem with this approach is that it is only a superficial examination of a number of criteria that may or may not be important in meeting certain standards. The relationship with other criteria is never explored. In the event of criteria not being met, no insight is given as to why this may be the case. Conversely, the use of the Donabedian framework or process model worksheet offers greater potential to identify all the elements necessary to meet the standard or requirements.

In conclusion, it can be appreciated that the use of the four different methods for documenting standards, namely Donabedian, Maxwell, Crosby and criteria listing, led in each case to a slightly different focus, each highlighting different factors for consideration. Maxwell's approach seemed to lend itself better to a macro perspective, while Crosby's method forced us to consider dimensions such as training and knowledge and also to think specifically about who defines and provides certain elements of the process.

In practice, there were specific factors that were important regardless of the method selected, namely:

- ownership of the standard by the multidisciplinary team;
- education of the team in the use and application of the theoretical method for documenting the practice selected;
- a good facilitator;
- an ongoing commitment to audit.

Conclusions and observations from using different standard-setting frameworks

In choosing a framework for setting standards, it is important to consider what the selected framework is to be used for. It can be seen from using the discharge standard as a case study that different frameworks can identify a number of different criteria, although all relate to the same process. Some organizations have attempted to educate staff in the use of only one framework (e.g. Donabedian). This creates two problems. First, staff may become blinkered in the one approach, and fail to consider some of the equally relevant components of others. Second, it is our experience that some frameworks may be more appropriate in some situations than others. For example, Maxwell's six dimensions are helpful in A&E and outpatient departments, but less useful for inpatient case standards. The Donabedian framework is useful for standards that have clearly defined structural, process and outcome criteria. However, criteria listing may be more appropriate for relatively simple standards. For example, the standard for changing an oxygen cylinder cited earlier in this chapter, when all that was needed was a verbal agreement between the staff concerned that they will observe the cylinder whilst it is in use and change it when empty. Conversely, the difficulty with many of the criteria lists in the commonly used quality assurance tools is that they only inform staff what is going wrong, not why. If a more detailed examination of the components is required, one of the other frameworks would be a more appropriate choice.

The process model worksheet is useful for analysing work processes that are causing problems, through the use of identifying and agreeing requirements. We found that, for many work processes, the requirements were absent or poorly defined. This commonly led to a breakdown in the process due to lack of understanding by individuals of what was expected of them.

Maxwell (1984) adds some new dimensions that are particularly useful when examining organizational standards, such as for a new unit or service. Another common mistake is to attempt to write a standard when what is really required is a procedure, a policy or a protocol.

In examining the benefits of one framework over another for setting standards, comparisons can be drawn with the chequered history of the introduction of nursing models. There is a variety to choose from. Some are better validated than others; some lend themselves more easily to certain settings than others and some are more easily understood than others. Given these factors, it would seem sensible to develop an eclectic approach to setting standards. Now we have examined standard setting as one method, the next section will examine other methods for documenting best practice, namely procedures, guidelines and protocols, and patient care pathways.

PROCEDURES

We have identified the following characteristics of a procedure which we find helpful in making the distinction between these and other methods of documenting best practice.

Table 2.3 *Example of a procedure:* *fire procedure*	**On discovering a fire:** • Operate the nearest fire alarm. • Attempt to extinguish the fire, but without taking risks. • Proceed to the assembly point at ... • Await roll call. **On hearing the fire alarm:** • Proceed to the assembly point quickly but without panic or running. • Leave without stopping to collect belongings. • Close doors to isolate the fire. • Remain outside the building until told by a senior fire officer that it is safe to re-enter.

- Procedures are a set of criteria that are generally non-negotiable. Anyone following the procedure would not be expected to deviate from it.
- They do not generally require any element of expertise or judgement to follow.
- They document a series of steps, in chronological order, to be taken in response to a given situation (e.g. fire procedure; major incident procedure; sharps injury procedure).

An example of a procedure is shown in Table 2.3.

Uses

Procedures have an important part to play in setting out clear instructions for people under a given set of circumstances. Unfortunately, in our experience they are often the most unpopular of all the methods described in this chapter. This is perhaps because although there is a recognition they are important, especially in nurse education centres, they tend to be tedious to write, boring to read and referred to only when things go wrong, rather than a proactive tool to ensure that things go right.

There are some ways in which the weaknesses of this method can be addressed. These include:

- Get the document presented in a more visually striking layout. If key points can be summarized on a poster for staff to see, they are more likely to learn it than if it is filed in a procedure file. An example is shown in Figure 2.3.
- Think up a strategy for dissemination. If you have a hospital newsletter, include a short article on key points explaining why staff should read the procedure.
- Develop education for the staff who need to be familiar with the procedure. We have found workshops to be the best forum. The key points of the procedure can be presented, followed by a question-and-answer session with staff identifying their own action plans for this procedure.

STAFFORDSHIRE
UNIVERSITY
LIBRARY

Brighton Health Care NHS Trust
CODE OF PRACTICE
MANUAL HANDLING OF LOADS

DO

1. Follow BHC 'manual handling of loads' policy
2. Carry out and follow manual handling assessment
3. Weigh the load as far as is reasonably practical
4. Follow principle of safe movement and handling
5. Use an ergonomic approach
6. Participate in available training
7. Make full and proper use of safe systems of work
8. Slide/glide the load rather than lift it
9. Inform your line manager of potential handling hazards
10. Be aware of your responsibilities to yourself and to others
11. Contact your key trainer for more information
12. Know your limitations

DON'T

1. Don't do anything outside your own capabilities
2. Don't handle a load without carrying out a manual handling assessment
3. Don't use equipment that is unfit for the purpose for which it is intended
4. Don't use equipment without prior training
5. Don't use the 'drag lift'
6. Don't use the 'orthodox lift' (otherwise known as the 'cradle' or 'bucket')
7. Don't use canvas and poles to lift patients for patient transfers after new measures have been implemented
8. Don't let patients put their hands/arms around your neck/waist whilst carrying out a patient manoeuvre
9. Don't manually lift a patient taking the full body weight

WHEN IN DOUBT DON'T

Figure 2.3

An example of a procedure: Brighton Health Care NHS Trust Lifting & Handling poster (reproduced with the permission of Brighton Health Care NHS Trust)

- Holding a practice session can be useful for some procedures – one we use with good effect for fire and major incident. Getting people to apply their knowledge is the most effective way of getting them to internalize the procedure. In many workshops we use case studies for this purpose, e.g. discharge planning and drug error procedures.
- Have link workers and use them to disseminate information about the

procedure to other staff. For example, we provide link workers with specific training in lifting and handling and infection control.
- Audit to ensure that procedures are complied with; don't wait until something goes wrong!

GUIDELINES AND PROTOCOLS

The *Chambers English Dictionary* defines a guideline as 'an indicator of a course that should be followed, or of what future policy will be'.

In the health service we have come across a number of different terms that tend to be used synonymously or ambiguously, including:

- protocols
- algorithms
- clinical policies
- practice parameters
- clinical guidelines
- practice policies

The Institute of Medicine offers a more helpful health-related definition (Field and Lohr, 1992), describing them as 'systematically developed statements to assist practitioner and patient decisions about appropriate health care for specific clinical circumstances'.

In the literature, the terms 'guideline', 'protocol' and 'algorithm' are used interchangeably. Essentially, all of these fall with the definition offered above. We draw the distinctions between them as one of presentation and format. Unlike (for example) in Donabedian's framework, there is no set format for documenting guidelines, protocols or algorithms. This can be both a strength and a weakness. It is a strength because it allows more flexibility: the practitioner does not feel constrained to make the criteria fit into the format, rather than choosing a format that best suits the information that needs to be documented. It is a weakness because, for the novice faced with a plethora of information and a blank sheet of paper, sometimes a set framework or format can be helpful in systematically producing a user-friendly document.

Algorithms and protocols are terms that tend to be used to describe a flow-chart that sets out in an explicit and logical fashion the guidelines for the practitioner to follow. An example is shown below in Figure 2.4.

There are a number of useful points to consider when developing guidelines using the above format (referred to from now on as a flowchart, rather than an algorithm or protocol).

Points to consider in developing flowcharts

Define the scope of the clinical practice you are describing, i.e. where does it start and finish, and what elements of the care do you wish to include?

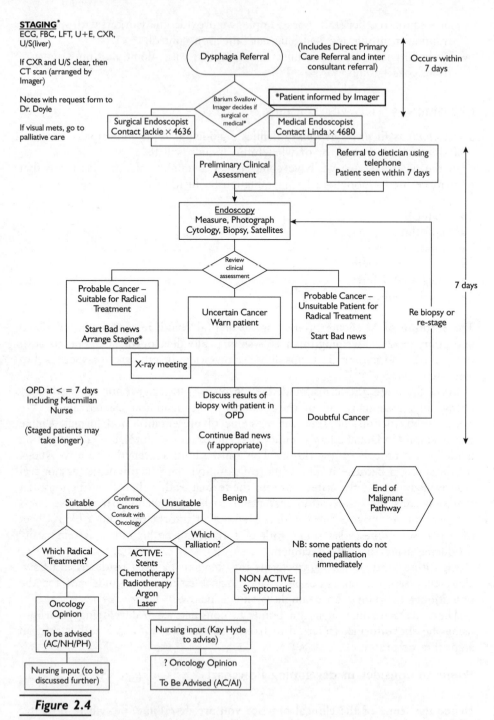

STAGING*
ECG, FBC, LFT, U+E, CXR, U/S(liver)

If CXR and U/S clear, then CT scan (arranged by Imager)

Notes with request form to Dr. Doyle

If visual mets, go to palliative care

Dysphagia Referral

(Includes Direct Primary Care Referral and inter consultant referral)

Occurs within 7 days

Barium Swallow Imager decides if surgical or medical*

*Patient informed by Imager

Surgical Endoscopist Contact Jackie × 4636

Medical Endoscopist Contact Linda × 4680

Preliminary Clinical Assessment

Referral to dietician using telephone Patient seen within 7 days

Endoscopy Measure, Photograph Cytology, Biopsy, Satellites

Review clinical assessment

Probable Cancer – Suitable for Radical Treatment

Start Bad news Arrange Staging*

Uncertain Cancer Warn patient

Probable Cancer – Unsuitable Patient for Radical Treatment

Start Bad news

7 days

Re biopsy or re-stage

X-ray meeting

OPD at < = 7 days Including Macmillan Nurse

(Staged patients may take longer)

Discuss results of biopsy with patient in OPD

Continue Bad news (if appropriate)

Doubtful Cancer

Suitable

Confirmed Cancers Consult with Oncology

Unsuitable

Benign

End of Malignant Pathway

Which Radical Treatment?

ACTIVE: Stents Chemotherapy Radiotherapy Argon Laser

Which Palliation?

NON ACTIVE: Symptomatic

NB: some patients do not need palliation immediately

Oncology Opinion

To be advised (AC/NH/PH)

Nursing input (Kay Hyde to advise)

Nursing input (to be discussed further)

? Oncology Opinion

To Be Advised (AC/AI)

Figure 2.4

Flowchart for the management of oesophageal cancer (reproduced with the permission of Brighton Health Care NHS Trust)

Our experience has been that it is easy to define the start; the difficulty is knowing where to stop, and what can be excluded. Our advice is to keep the scope as simple and specific as possible. For example, in developing the above flowchart for oesophageal cancer, the multidisciplinary team started to think about all the possible types of pain relief that may be appropriate at different stages, and got into debates on what to include with regard to palliation. In fact, these two elements warranted flowcharts of their own. It is important to remember that the purpose of a guideline (in whatever format) is to provide information on best practice to the practitioner at the point of delivery. Anything that runs to more than a few pages defeats this objective.

Ensure the flowchart runs in a logical and chronological order

This sounds obvious, but can be difficult if the multidisciplinary team is compiling a group flowchart for a given condition. We found it easiest to work with each of the professional groups involved in the above example in unidisciplinary forums in the first instance to gain consensus on the agreed process of care. Each group developed a flowchart for their own discipline, as shown in some of the examples reproduced in Figure 2.5.

Once this was agreed, we brought the whole multidisciplinary team together to decide how all the different parts of the respective processes would fit together. This allowed an agreement to be reached when, for example, it was most appropriate to refer the patient to the dietitian. It also initiated some interesting discussions around organizational process as well as clinical practice. For example, the booking systems for endoscopy and referrals from the outpatients department came under scrutiny and were changed when team members identified problems with the present system. It raised an important point for consideration: that for genuine improvements in the quality of the patient's experience, it is not enough to look at clinical practice in isolation. The organizational systems to support clinicians in carrying out their practice also need to be effective. Insufficient theatre sessions or lack of intensive therapy unit (ITU) beds can have as profound an impact on patient outcomes as poor clinical practice. Documenting these processes is as important as documenting clinical practice.

Challenge the evidence base of each of the steps in the flowchart

In developing the example in Figure 2.4 we faced a chicken-and-egg dilemma: do we start from scratch, review all the evidence and construct a flowchart – or document current practice? The problem with the former was that the evidence is often inconsistent or missing. It is also quite a challenging approach to use, since there is a danger that clinicians involved in the work will view it as a challenge to their competence. In the event, we found the most useful approach was to work with the clinicians to document current practice. This in itself caused useful debate and challenge within the team as they rationalized the need for each of the steps in the process.

This process alone led to clarification of current practice, and also helped to achieve a consensus within each of the professional groups about what constituted

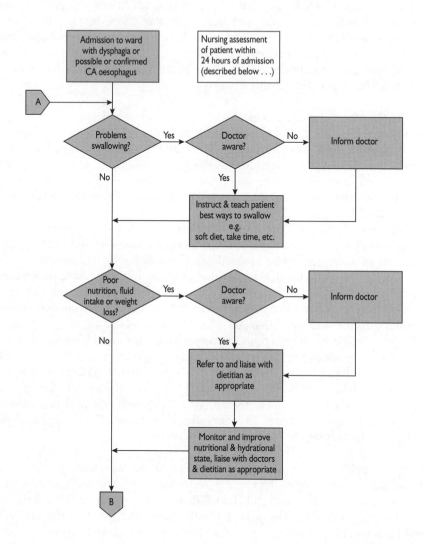

Figure 2.5a

Example of nursing flowchart (reproduced with the permission of Brighton Health Care NHS Trust)

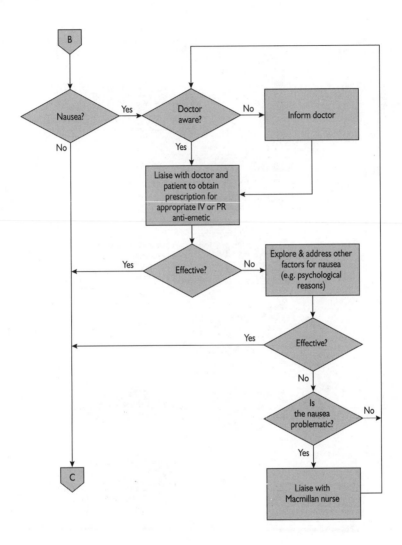

Figure 2.5b

Example of nursing flowchart (cont.)

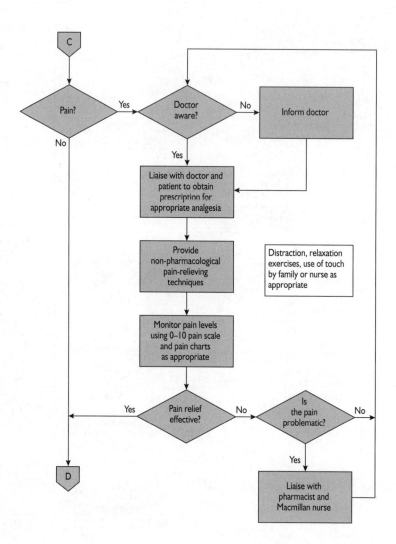

Figure 2.5c

Example of nursing flowchart (cont.)

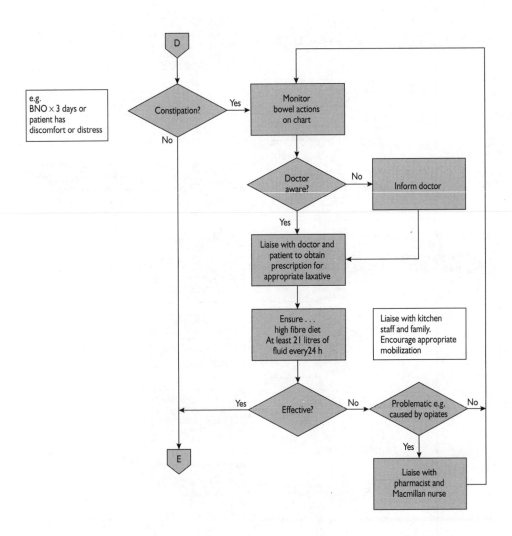

e.g.
BNO × 3 days or
patient has
discomfort or distress

D

Constipation? — Yes → Monitor bowel actions on chart

No

Doctor aware? — No → Inform doctor

Yes

Liaise with doctor and patient to obtain prescription for appropriate laxative

Ensure . . .
high fibre diet
At least 2 l litres of fluid every24 h

Liaise with kitchen staff and family. Encourage appropriate mobilization

Effective? — Yes / No → Problematic e.g. caused by opiates — No

Yes

Liaise with pharmacist and Macmillan nurse

E

Figure 2.5d

Example of nursing flowchart (cont.)

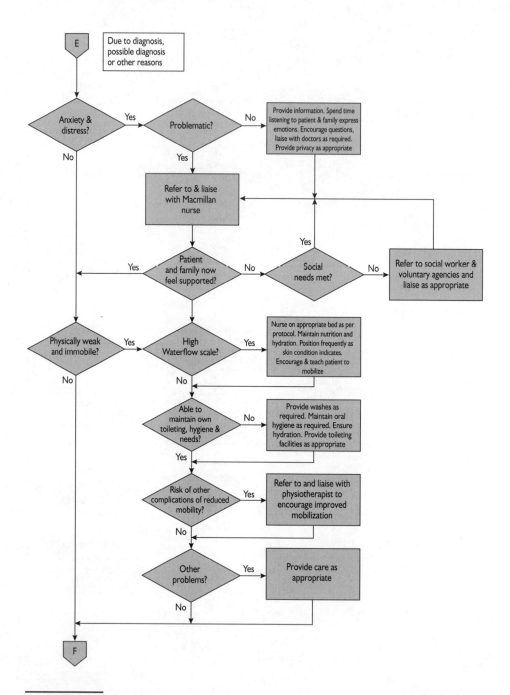

Figure 2.5e

Example of nursing flowchart (cont.)

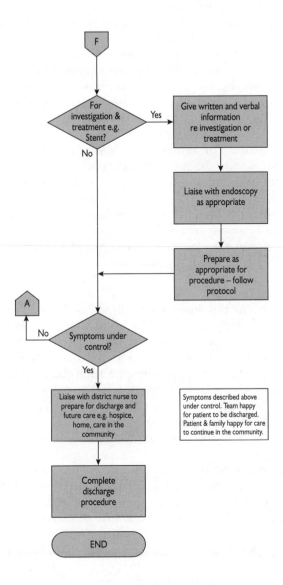

Figure 2.5f

Example of nursing flowchart (cont.)

best practice. In examples of professionals doing the same things but in different ways (all seemingly reasonable and logical and well within the boundaries of safe and dependable practice), some consistency in the process could be negotiated. This was essential for a concise flowchart to be developed. We have had problems in other areas where professionals have not been able to reach consensus and there is insufficient research to favour one way of doing things over another. Here the flowchart has to break into different strands depending on the steps required by the different doctors or nurses. This makes it confusing for the junior staff who are the main users of the guidelines; makes audit difficult and time consuming; and defeats the whole point of documenting practice, i.e. to have a consistent standard for care delivery. Careful selection of areas for documentation of practice is advised. For newcomers to this approach, we suggest picking a few early winners! Tackle the more difficult ones when the multidisciplinary team is used to documenting and auditing the work and has a few successes under its belt.

On a practical note, we found it easiest to keep all the associated literature and rationale for the flowchart criteria in a separate file for reference. Attempting to incorporate these into the document itself proved impractical. The file can also be pulled and updated when the flowchart is due for review.

Create a user-friendly layout

It is important to present the flowchart in an easy-to-follow format. We found it helpful to distinguish decision points (the diamonds on the example in Figure 2.5) from steps in the process (the boxes in Figure 2.5). The flow and direction of each step need to be clearly marked with an arrow. Endpoints need to be marked, and it can be helpful to cross-reference with other guidelines, standards or protocols (as in the above example which refers to guidelines for feeding this group of patients). All criteria statements should follow the SMARTER criteria outlined earlier in the chapter. Where we were able to achieve this, the process of auditing compliance with the flowchart was much easier.

So is there a difference between a guideline and a flowchart?

The only difference we can determine from literature reviewed is that guidelines tend to contain more free text and are often lists of process steps and actions to be taken. Hence the difference is in the format and layout, rather than in the definitions given earlier in this section.

Finally, the points made elsewhere in the chapter about having a skilled facilitator; educating team members in how to undertake this process; generating ownership and commitment to the work; dissemination of the document; education of staff in the new practice; and auditing compliance with the documented practice are equally relevant for flowcharts and guidelines. These points were also made in a useful article explaining how to ensure that guidelines are effective, along with some useful questions for those approaching this for the first time to help choose the topic, get the team together and develop, present and disseminate guidelines (Thomson, Lavender and Madhok, 1995).

It can be appreciated that the development, dissemination, implementation and evaluation of clinical guidelines is a challenging and complex task. The case study outlined in Figure 2.4 took over a year to get the draft ready to pilot. However, there is a growing body of literature suggesting that guidelines encourage effective clinical practice (Thomson, Lavender and Madhok, 1995). There is also an increasing body of knowledge concerning the factors that will influence the effectiveness of clinical guidelines in practice (Grimshaw and Russell, 1994). These principles are equally applicable to any method of documenting best practice.

PATIENT CARE PATHWAYS

Patient care pathways (PCPs) have been defined as 'a multidisciplinary process of patient-focused care which specifies key events and assessments, occurring in a timely fashion, to produce the best prescribed outcomes within the resources and activities available, for an episode of care'.

Potential benefits of this method of documenting best practice have been cited (Brown, 1995) as:

- promoting both intradisciplinary and interdisciplinary collaborative practice;
- enhancing multidisciplinary understanding of each others' roles and contributions;
- promoting consistency in clinical practice across sites between practitioners;
- building best practice into everyday care;
- clarifying processes of care;
- clarifying outcomes of care;
- reducing duplications in care activities;
- managing risk;
- demystifying healthcare and empowering patients.

The 12 stages of pathway development, as observed on a study tour of Australia

The introductory section of this chapter set out the key characteristics of patient care pathways. A number of sites in the UK have been involved in developing and implementing patient pathways. Pathways have also been developed extensively in the United States and in Australia. In 1998, one of the authors was fortunate in securing a scholarship to visit 20 healthcare organizations in Brisbane, Perth, Melbourne and Sydney in Australia. The full study tour findings are set out elsewhere (Parsley, 1998a, b). From the experiences of these organizations, two key findings were noted. First, the organizational infrastructure to support the development, implementation and evaluation of pathways was as, if not more, important than the actual format and design of the pathways themselves. Hence, if critical success factors (including, for example, ownership by clinician; ownership by management; adequate deployment of resources; education and facilitation) are not present, even the best designed evidence-based pathway has limited chance of succeeding in practice. Second, the author was able to identify 12 key stages to developing and implementing patient pathways. These are outlined below, and offer a pragmatic approach for those who may wish to take patient care pathways forward.

Stage 1. Prioritize which pathways to develop

Five key factors can be helpful in prioritizing which pathways to develop:

- **Clinician preference.** Many hospitals in Australia stated the importance of choosing pathways that were of particular interest to the clinician. This had the advantage of securing their involvement and ownership.
- **High volume procedures.** Many areas identified common conditions/procedures and used these as the basis for prioritizing which clinical pathways to develop. This ensures the most significant impact, as it affects the highest number of patients.
- **High cost.** Similarly, some areas identified high-cost procedures/conditions and used these as the mechanism for prioritizing which pathways to develop.
- **Commonly agreed guidelines for which there is a strong evidence base.** It can be easier to start with pathways for which there is already a strong research base, or for which guidelines are already developed that are well supported by evidence. This has the advantage of reducing the amount of time needed to review and critique the literature. Furthermore, clinicians may be more ready to adopt pathways if their evidence base can be demonstrated unequivocally.
- **Areas of high clinical risk or risk of litigation.** Some areas had taken into account clinical risk issues and reviewed their litigation claims as a method for prioritizing which pathways to address first.

Stage 2. Forming the multidisciplinary pathways team

Once the patient path has been prioritized, the next stage is to convene the multidisciplinary team to contribute to the development of a pathway. Many cited the following critical success factors to ensure the correct constitution of this team:

- ensuring all key stakeholders are represented;
- identifying those with relevant expertise for the condition;
- considering how to involve patients and at what stage.

There were huge variations in the numbers of staff who were involved in such multidisciplinary pathway teams. Some areas preferred a small-team, tightly focused approach. This required those in the group to be truly representative of their professional colleagues and to liaise with them outside the meeting to seek their input into the work. This approach had certain advantages. First, because the group was smaller, pathways were drafted more quickly and consensus was often reached more speedily. Second, it reduced the amount of time and number of clinicians who needed to take time out from clinical work to come to meetings. Areas that used such an approach appeared to have a high degree of clinician commitment to the development of pathways, and a culture for strong team-working where staff were happy to be represented by their colleagues. Many areas using this approach acknowledged they had started originally with much larger groups. As understanding of the pathways process increased, staff began to see the potential benefits. This was coupled with the improved multidisciplinary teamwork that arose as a result of the large group meetings. In many instances this had naturally evolved into clinicians recommending a more tightly focused approach once they understood the process and had worked within the larger group. Hence, although the small group approach would appear to have greater benefit, it must be recognized that this is the product of a learning curve, and working initially as a large group may be necessary until trust and understanding are secured.

Stage 3. Educate clinicians in the principles of drafting clinical pathways and variance analysis

As identified earlier, understanding and experience of using clinical pathways are essential. Many educators stated the importance of working through clinicians' reservations about the approach, particularly with respect to 'cookbook' medicine. A favoured approach was to use clinicians who had already successfully implemented pathways and to provide case studies on how these had impacted on patient outcomes and clinical practice.

Stage 4. Map out the current care path

This stage was often combined with stage 3. Although each area used a different approach, by far the most common was to use flowcharting as a technique. The team developed a chronological flowchart, based on the experience of one patient with the specific condition for which the pathway was being developed, and mapping this patient's care and treatment. This would usually incorporate referral from the GP through the outpatients department as a starting point and tended to finish either with discharge from hospital or with follow-up in the outpatients department or the community. For most of the acute hospitals visited, they tended to focus on a pathway mainly for the inpatient stay. Many areas were now broadening the scope of this pathway, with a number of centres interested in developing paths that transcended organizational boundaries. Identifying the scope of the path was essential before the flowcharting exercise in order to determine the start and finish points.

Flowcharting the process
For some conditions it was easy to map out the patient flow on a day-by-day basis (especially for surgery). For others it was comparatively easy to identify the chronological sequence of events that occurred once the diagnosis had been made.

Most facilitators used a highly participative approach, with clinicians adding information to huge flipchart maps and building up a complete picture of patient care.

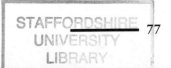
STAFFORDSHIRE
UNIVERSITY
LIBRARY

As the team mapped out the process, many facilitators recognized the need for significant discussion and debate about elements of clinical practice. The facilitator's role was to challenge clinicians about each of the stages in the flowchart so that they would reflect on the evidence base that supported the approach under consideration.

Once the process had been flowcharted, the facilitator was then usually the person responsible for pulling all the information together into a flowchart document. Some used software packages to map the process out. There was then usually an interim stage when it was sent out to the group for validation and checking, and in some organizations the representatives were responsible for circulating this to a wider cohort of their colleagues for comments and amendments. The facilitator then incorporated these amendments into the final draft.

The number of times this process was repeated varied considerably among the organizations I visited. One or two took the pragmatic view that any changes needed to be agreed in the first or second draft, and any further amendments could be ironed out after the pilot stage. Others felt that there needed to be complete agreement on all elements of the pathway, and repeated the dissemination and amendment several times until this consensus was reached.

Once the process had been flowcharted, it was then presented in the format of a care pathway (some examples of which are shown later). This could be done either by the clinicians or by the facilitator. Many felt the facilitator could do this more speedily, especially as many facilitators had developed software to simplify the formatting process. This also reduced the amount of time that clinicians needed to spend on such tasks. Not surprisingly, this approach was popular with clinicians. In some areas the ward manager had become quite expert at formatting pathways and so had taken on this role. This was advantageous, as more and more pathways were being developed and a single facilitator could not accommodate them all.

Some places visited were using the blank pathway format with the multidisciplinary team to chart the patient process directly. However, this had evolved once clinicians became more familiar with the process and format.

At the end of this stage, a draft of the clinical pathway in the agreed format was completed.

Stage 5. Retrospective audit
This stage was used in some, but by no means all, of the organizations visited. Those who used it felt it was extremely beneficial.

An agreed number of casenotes (ranging between 10 and 60 in the places visited) for the condition or diagnosis that was covered by the pathway were pulled. Using the multidisciplinary notes, a retrospective audit was carried out against the stages on the draft pathway to identify compliance of current practice against the proposed path. The results of this audit were then fed back to the multidisciplinary team for discussion and review. The value of this exercise was that clinicians believed certain things were happening in practice, but what happened in reality often differed from their assumptions. For example, they may believe that the referral time from the outpatients department to endoscopy is seven days. Yet reviewing the sample of patients demonstrated wide variations in referral times. This then offers the pathway development team two choices: either to adapt the path to meet what is happening in practice, or to adapt practice to enable the standard indicated on the path to be met. This stage therefore often led to significant improvement in clinical processes and also identified possible changes in support services to expedite the pathway. For example, availability of discharge medications, waiting time for test results, and waiting time for procedures were often cited as 'roadblocks' in the system. These could be addressed and resolved before the implementation of the pathway. This ensured that when the pathway was implemented the goals and outcomes identified on the path were more likely to be achievable in practice because the processes required to meet these standards were in place.

Some places visited that had not used this approach found that clinicians quickly became despondent about the use of the path when they consistently reported variances against the pathway. In some areas this led to them perceiving pathways to be unrealistic and they quickly stopped using them. Seeing good compliance rates against the pathway was cited by many as a strong motivational force for clinicians to use them. It would therefore seem important to undertake a retrospective audit to ensure that any barriers to achieving the goals on the pathway are eradicated before the formal pilot.

Stage 6. Pilot the pathway

Once the pathway is complete, the next stage is to pilot it in practice. There are a number of different approaches to doing this. Some areas agreed to pilot it over an agreed timeframe (either one week or one month). Others sought a sample size of patients from as broad an area as possible. Yet others targeted a discrete ward or department for a pilot and used it on all appropriate patients for a given period of time. There were differing views on the respective benefits of these approaches. Many noted that any glaring problems with the pathway were picked up almost immediately. Some therefore had a 'short, sharp' pilot approach. Others pointed out that it took staff time to become familiar with the pathway and that unless a reasonable amount of time was allowed to elapse it was difficult to identify whether difficulties were the result of user unfamiliarity or derived from the pathway itself.

There were a number of practical problems that emerged from people piloting pathways. The first was that staff often found it difficult when some but not all patients were on pathways. This led to them forgetting to complete the documentation (particularly with regard to variance analysis). Pulling notes to audit the pathways was also a problem if a careful record of patients who had been using them was not kept. Some areas used stickers on the front of the notes to indicate which patients were on a pathway.

At the end of the pilot phase, someone (usually the facilitator) compiled a report and made recommendations for final amendments. This was then fed back to the multidisciplinary team.

Stage 7. Formal approval of the pathway

Different organizations had different approaches to this. Those with a supportive infrastructure would submit pathways to their pathways committee, which would formally approve them and endorse them as Trust policy. Many areas also required the pathway to be sent to the most senior consultant for that specific condition, who would formally sign it off. In many places the consultant would attach a letter of authorization to the pathway, and some would write to all doctors stating this should be followed where appropriate. This seemed to be key in seeking junior doctor compliance with the pathway.

Stage 8. Educating staff about the pathway

Many areas stressed the importance of proper education for staff on its use once the pathway has been formally endorsed by the organization. This is particularly important in the early stages of pathway development, when staff may never have seen such a format or know how to complete variance analysis. The time spent on education on the specific pathways reduces as staff become more familiar with the format and documentation.

The other focus of education is on the clinical treatment required as indicated on the pathway. Since the information on the path is necessarily brief, it is essential to ensure staff have the skills and knowledge necessary to care for patients with each of the conditions covered. The pathway was, as many identified, a very helpful teaching tool. Some areas had left it to the individual lead clinician to educate their professional group on the parts of the path that applied to them. In others, the facilitator or the ward manager was responsible for ensuring all of the multidisciplinary team were familiar with both the format of the pathway and the clinical care involved.

Many areas stated that the education had significant impact on the quality of patient care, as it often highlighted skills or knowledge deficiencies of individual staff. Some areas used the clinical nurse specialist very proactively in the educational process.

Stage 9. Review and update the pathway

Most areas did this on an annual basis. Some reconvened the original multidisciplinary team to do an in-depth review. One area circulated the pathway once more, asking for suggested amendments. If these numbered less than three, these were incorporated and the pathway was reissued without another meeting being considered necessary. The review needed to include practical suggestions for improvement and also to take account of recent literature reviews to ensure new research findings were incorporated into the pathway.

Stage 10. Check the evidence base

Making sure the pathway is evidence-based is inevitably an ongoing process. Although there may be specific review times stated on the pathway, clearly if new research emerges in the meantime the pathway will need to be updated. With respect to the evidence base for the original pathway, as stated earlier, there were widely differing approaches. Some made this an integral part of the first draft and pilot. Others waited until the first cycle had been completed and then did a more rigorous review of the literature to present back to clinicians once they had become familiar with and committed to the pathway.

Stage 11. Incorporate variance analysis

This stage is discussed more fully in the next chapter. However, it is relevant to mention it here since there were differing approaches as to when variance recording and analysis should be introduced and at what stage of the pathway development. Many areas visited had not incorporated variance analysis at all in the early stages of pathway development. This had evolved later, once staff had become familiar with the process of drafting pathways and also using them in practice. Others incorporated development of the variance analysis at the same time as drafting the tool. Although this made the process more complex, even areas that had not adopted variance analysis in the early stages identified that this was fundamental if one was to really measure the impact of the pathway. It is strongly recommended that the variance analysis is incorporated in the design of the pathway and tested as part of the pilot.

Stage 12. Evaluate the impact of the pathway

Many areas visited had identified a final stage which sought to evaluate the impact of the clinical pathway. This was done by using variance analysis reports for both departmental and corporate areas to highlight where variances were occurring. This proved to be a very powerful quality assurance tool and gave clinicians immediate feedback about their compliance with the pathway. It also identified support service failures that could be addressed. This then fed into an audit cycle which enabled improvements to be made and a review of variance at a later stage to ensure that the corrective action had been effective.

Clinical outcomes and patient goals

A few places visited were beginning to experiment with the incorporation of clinical outcomes into the clinical pathway. This needed to be incorporated into the initial session to flowchart current practice. Clinicians were helped to identify anticipated patient outcomes and to include these on the path.

Looking at an example of an outcomes sheet from Western Australia (Figure 2.6), it can be seen that the patient outcomes are identified on the Gantt chart. What was useful about this particular format was that it allowed for some variance around the mean for when these goals should be achieved. Other examples collected as part of the tour limited the achievement of the outcomes to a specific day. This causes problems when recording variance, since inevitably there will be a standard distribution curve for patients around the mean.

Figure 2.6 shows an example of a patient care pathway. This example was selected from many collected, as the format and layout were felt by the clinicians to be user friendly. The approach in this organization had also begun to tackle an issue raised in many organizations visited, namely that the patient pathway

SURNAME		UMRN	

ST JOHN OF GOD HOSPITAL
SUBIACO

CARE PATH FOR
TOTAL HIP REPLACEMENT

SURNAME	UMRN
GIVEN NAMES	
D.O.B.	SEX
DOCTOR'S NAME	

Use patient Identification Label when available

WARD_____

Operation_____   Operation Date_____

COMORBIDITY   (Refer also Discharge Summary)

☐ Rheumatoid Arthritis   ☐ Diabetes Mellitus
☐ Peripheral Vascular Disease ☐ Altered Mental State
☐ Thrombosis   ☐ Asthma
☐ Cardiovascular Disease   ☐ Other_____

TYPE OF ANALGESIA

Please circle type of post-op pain management
1. PCA   3. IM/SC/PR/ORAL
2. Epidural (Infusion/topup/PCEA)   4. Other_____

OBJECTIVE

To improve mobility
To promote optimal dignity, fullness of life for each patient

NURSING CARE

Unless otherwise indicated, nursing care is given as per
the following St. John of God Hospital Nursing standards.
☐ General Standards
☐ Patient undergoing Arterial Surgery
☐ Management of the Coronary Care Patient
☐ Care of the Ventilated Patient
☐ Diabetic Patient
☐ Oncology / Haematology Patient
☐ Patient undergoing Orthopaedic and Neurosurgery
☐ Patient with Plaster Cast
☐ Patient in Balanced Traction
☐ Patient under Fourteen (14) years of age
☐ Patient undergoing Urological Surgery

PROGRESS CHART   (See next page)

EDUCATION PROGRAM : CHECKLIST	SIGNATURE
PART ONE	
1. Pre-op education	
2. Post-op education	
3. Education book given to patient	
4. 'Log Rolling'	
5. Measure equipment, e.g. over toilet seat, crutches,	
walking stick, high back chair, Zimmer Frame	
6. Assess discharge requirements	
PART TWO	
6. First time getting up out of bed	
7. Use of Zimmer Frame	
PART THREE	
8. Use of elbow crutches	
9. Going up & down steps/stairs	
10. Getting into/out of motor vehicle	
PART FOUR	
11. Discharge plan completed on discharge, days 8–12	

0467H

Jan '98

This Care Path is based on the average experience of this case type. It is intended as a guide only, and does not replace clinical judgement.

CARE PATH FOR TOTAL HIP REPLACEMENT

MR420 (08-02)

Figure 2.6a

Example of care path for total hip replacement (reproduced by permission of
St John of God Hospital, Subiaco, Western Australia)

CARE PATH FOR
TOTAL HIP REPLACEMENT
No 08:02

SURNAME	UMRN
GIVEN NAMES	
D.O.B.	SEX
DOCTOR'S NAME	

Use patient Identification Label when available

PROGRESS CHART

WHEN PROGRESS MILESTONES ARE REACHED, INITIAL AND RECORD TIME IN CORRESPONDING COLUMN / MILESTONE ROW

V = Variance for items 7, 8 & 9   D = Indicator not achieved on discharge

Path day	Admins Day	Pre-op	Post-op	Day 1	2	3	4	5	6	7	8	9	10	11	12
Date															
1 Placed on Care path															
2 Investigations Completed															
3 Education check list completed															
4 Operation															
5 Anticoagulants ceased															
6 Haemodynamically stable															
7 Pain score <5 on movement each day															
8 Neurovascular stability maintained each day															
9 Correct Limb Alignment each day															
10 Diet Tolerated															
11 Normal Bladder / Bowel Function															
12 Incision healed															
13 Discharge arrangements commenced / completed															
14 Able to mobilise using crutches															
15 Discharge Date															

Figure 2.6b

PRINT NAME	DESIG	INITIAL	PRINT NAME	DESIG	INITIAL

RG3903_PMS

Figure 2.6c

CARE PATH FOR TOTAL HIP REPLACEMENT

V = Variance (record variation to planned care on variance record) n/a = Not Applicable
Unless otherwise indicated, care activities are the responsibility of the nurse.

SURNAME | UMRN
GIVEN NAMES
D.O.B. | SEX
DOCTOR'S NAME

Use patient Identification Label when available

PATH DAY / DATE:	Admission	Initials	Pre-Op / Op Day	Initials	Post-Op / Op Day	Initials	Day 1	Initials	Day 2	Initials
TESTS / INVESTIGATIONS	If not done pre-admission, arrange for: • Bloods • FBP • X Match • CXR • MSU • ECG as indicated by Dr's preferences						• Bloods • HB as indicated by Dr's preferences		• Post-op check X-Ray	
CONSULTS	• Consent signed • Anaesthetic review and pre-med • Physio • OT									
PAIN MANAGEMENT & COMFORT	• Discuss/reconfirm Pain Control options and devices • Explain pain assessment including pain scoring		• Pre-op -clarify understanding & reassure		• PCA, Epidural or IV analgesia • Assess pain using pain scale				• Remove PCA / Epidural as per Dr's orders. • Commence M / Oral analgesia • Assess pain using pain scale	
TREATMENTS / MEDICATIONS	• Pre-med ordered • Dr to consider anticoagulants • Clarify / order existing medications • Order TEDS as per Dr's preferences • Shave limb		• Administer pre-med • TED stockings • AV impulse or sequential compression device (SCD) • Abduction pillow		• Operation. Dr to insert -IV -Epidural -wound drains • Med chart review by Clinical Pharmacist		• Check Dr's orders for removal of drains and record on care path		• Reduce Dressing	
DISCHARGE PLANNING • If discharge/risk assessment score is 11 or more, take appropriate action	• Assess home equipment needs • Refer to Silver Chain and / or Social Worker if needed • Assess the need for Medication List		Ongoing							

RG0904 PMS

Figure 2.6d

PATHWAY DAY	Admission	Initials	Pre-Op / Op Day	Initials	Post-Op / Op Day	Initials	Day 1	Initials	Day 2	Initials
ADL'S MOBILITY & SAFETY • If injury risk score > 11 blue dot protocol	• Self caring with ADL's or assist as needed.		• Pre-op shower • Rest in bed following pre-med		• Rest in bed • Wash in bed • Pressure area care		• Stand with assistance (Mr Forwards patients only) • Sling exercise (Balkan frame)		• Mainly rest in bed • Stand with physio • Shower with assistance • Gently mobilise with Zimmer Frame • Sling exercises	
ASSESSMENT & OBSERVATION	• Complete nursing assessment form including discharge/risk assessment • Baseline TPR, B/P, Weight, Urinalysis, Neurovascular status, 0₂ Saturation. • Assess skin integrity • Risk Score ☐		• TPR, B/P, Neurovascular status & pedal pulses		• TPR, B/P, Neurovascular status as per hospital policy • Check drain site each shift • Check IV site each shift • Check wound dressing		• Risk Score ☐		• Risk Score ☐	
NUTRITION & HYDRATION • If nutrition risk 3 or 4 - Dietician consult	• Patients Normal Diet • Fast from food • Fast from fluids		• Fast from _____		• Ice to suck / sip H20 • IV therapy		• Free Fluids • Light Diet		• Diet & fluids as tolerated • Remove IV as per Dr's orders	
ELIMINATION • If continence score is 3 or 4 refer to continent resource manual	• Give aperient if necessary				• IDC post-op FBC • Assess bowel sounds				• Remove IDC as per Dr's orders • Monitor urine output	
EDUCATION	• Introduce / explain Care Path • Part one of checklist completed		• Ongoing • Reinforce						• Part two of check list complete	
INDIVIDUAL NEEDS	• Offer Pastoral Care Services • Refer to other services if needed • Listen, support & encourage									
PRINT NAME DESIGNATION AND INITIALS	AM									
	PM									
	ND									

RG0904 PMS

Figure 2.6e

CARE PATH FOR TOTAL HIP REPLACEMENT

V = Variance (record variation to planned care on variance record) n/a = Not Applicable
Unless otherwise indicated, care activities are the responsibility of the nurse.

SURNAME		UMRN
GIVEN NAMES		
D.O.B.		SEX
DOCTOR'S NAME		

Use patient Identification Label when available

PATH DAY	Day 3		Day 4		Day 5		Day 6		Day 7	
DATE:		Initials		Initials		Initials		Initials		Initials
TESTS / INVESTIGATIONS										
CONSULTS	• OT Consult day 3–6						• Ensure OT Consult Completed			
PAIN MANAGEMENT & COMFORT	• IM / oral analgesia • Assess pain using pain scale								• Oral Analgesia	
TREATMENTS / MEDICATIONS	• Dressings as per Drs preferences • Anticoagulants • TED Stockings • Abduction pillow in situ • AV impulse in situ until Day 5 - 7 • Existing medication				• Cease anticoagulants as per Dr's preferences • Commence oral anticoagulants as indicated • Cease AV impulse as per Dr's preference				• Cease AV impulse as per Dr's preferences	
DISCHARGE PLANNING	• Review Daily • Assess the need for Medication List				• Confirm discharge needs • Check equipment arranged		• Check OT consult attended			

RG0904, PMS

Figure 2.6f

PATH DAY	Day 3	Initials	Day 4	Initials	Day 5	Initials	Day 6	Initials	Day 7	Initials
ADL'S MOBILITY & SAFETY	• Sling exercises • Shower with assistance		• Sit out of bed for meals • Increase mobilisation		• Encourage independence - offer assistance • Commence hydro if indicated					
ASSESSMENT & OBSERVATION	• 4/24 TPR, B/P neurovascular status • Risk Score ☐		• Risk Score ☐		• BD, TPR, B/P neurovascular status • Risk Score ☐		• Risk Score ☐		• Risk Score ☐	
NUTRITION & HYDRATION	• Patients Normal diet									
ELIMINATION	• Give aperients as required • Cease FBC if voiding spontaneously									
EDUCATION	• Reinforce part 2 of education checklist & encourage						• Reinforce part 3 of education checklist & encourage			
INDIVIDUAL NEEDS	• Listen, support & encourage									
PRINT NAME	AM									
DESIGNATION	PM									
AND INITIALS	ND									

PtG0904 PM5

Figure 2.6g

Care Path For Total Hip Replacement

v = Variance (record variation to planned care on variance record) n/a = Not Applicable
Unless otherwise indicated, care activities are the responsibility of the nurse.

SURNAME | UMRN

GIVEN NAMES

D.O.B. | SEX

DOCTOR'S NAME

Use patient Identification Label when available

PATH DAY	Day 8	Initials	Day 9	Initials	Day 10	Initials	Day 11	Initials	Day 12	Initials
DATE:										
TESTS / INVESTIGATIONS										
CONSULTS	• Ongoing									
PAIN MANAGEMENT & COMFORT	• Oral Analgesia • Assess pain using pain scale									
TREATMENTS / MEDICATIONS	• Check incision daily • TEDS • Existing medication • Normal pillow between legs				• Check Dr's orders for removal of clips and record on Care Path.					
DISCHARGE PLANNING	• Ongoing • Assess the need for Medication List						• Commence discharge arrangement checklist			

RG0904_PMS

Figure 2.6h

PATHWAY DAY	Day 8		Day 9		DAy 11		Day 12	
		Initials		Initials		Initials		Initials
ADL'S MOBILITY & SAFETY	• Minimal assistance with ADL's • Encourage independence • Mobilise on crutches • Attend hydro							
ASSESSMENT & OBSERVATION	• Daily TPR & BP neurovascular status							
NUTRITION & HYDRATION	• Patients Normal Diet							
ELIMINATION	• Check bowels daily							
EDUCATION	• Part 3 of check list completed days 8 - 12 • Part 4 of check list completed on discharge							
INDIVIDUAL NEEDS	• Listen, support and encourage							
PRINT NAME	AM							
DESIGNATION	PM							
AND INITIALS	ND							

RG0904 PM5

Figure 2.6i

DISCHARGE ARRANGEMENTS

To be completed by all caregivers
eg. Nurses, Allied Health & Resident Medical Officers

SURNAME		UMRN
GIVEN NAMES		
D.O.B.		SEX
DOCTOR'S NAME		

Use patient Identification Label when available

COMMUNITY RESOURCES

REQUIRED   NO ☐   YES ☐   (SPECIFY)

Service	Date Arranged	Sign

INFORMATION GIVEN TO PATIENT

	Yes / No	Date	Sign
Follow up Appointments arranged and given to patient			
X-Rays given to patient			
Discharge/Transfer Letter (if applicable)			

DISCHARGE MEDICATIONS

	Yes / No	Date	Sign (Nurse/ Pharmacist)
Medication list provided			
Patient / Carer counselled			
Patient / Carer understands instruction			
Current medication returned to patient			

EQUIPMENT

REQUIRED   NO ☐   YES ☐   (SPECIFY)

Type	Date Arranged	Date Given	Sign

EXIT FROM HOSPITAL

Yes / No

Transport Arranged [ ]   Mode _____

Identification Check [ ]   Signature _____

Destination Address (if different to addressograph above)

_____

_____

Phone _____

Date of Discharge [ ]   Time of Discharge [ ]

ALL CAREGIVERS/CONSULTANTS PLEASE PRINT NAME AND SIGN WITH INITIALS

PRINT NAME	DESIG	INITIAL	PRINT NAME	DESIG	INITIAL

RG0903 PMS

Figure 2.6j

is only one part of a multidisciplinary patient care record. The whole record consisted of:

- an assessment of the patient's problems and diagnosis;
- patient goals and clinical outcomes;
- the patient care pathway;
- clinician notes on how the patient is progressing against the agreed plan of care – which will incorporate additions to the care plan where required (e.g. if the patient develops postoperative complications);
- variance analysis.

A key recommendation of the report (Parsley, 1998a, 1998b) was the need to review all five components listed above.

Features in Figure 2.6 worth noting are as follows.

Page 1 of the pathway sets out co-morbidities that may preclude the patient from following the preset path according to plan. An individual care plan would need to be developed either instead of the total hip replacement pathway or to complement it to ensure all care needs are met. Other features on this page include:

- Nursing care is cross-referenced to relevant guidelines and standards which are set out elsewhere. This illustrates the point earlier that pathways do not replace guidelines or standards – the two are mutually supportive. Hence the pathway explains *what* to do and *when* to do it. The more detailed guidelines and standards give clinicians information on *how* to do it.
- An educational programme checklist which is signed off when complete.
- The date the pathway was completed.
- A footnote stressing that this is a guide only and does not replace clinical judgement.

Page 3 of the pathway provides space for specimen signatures, designation and initials. This is completed by all who initial the care pathways, so a full record is kept of all care givers, enabling initials on the path to be identified should medico-legal claims be made in subsequent years.

Pages 4 and 5 of the pathway follow an often used format, with the days of the pathway numbered across the top of the page (i.e. Admission day/Pre-op day/Op day/Post-op/Op day/Days 1, 2, 3, etc.). Down the left-hand side of the page are the key elements that make up the framework for care planning, namely:

- tests/investigations
- consultations
- pain management and comfort
- treatments/medications
- discharge planning
- ADL's mobility and safety
- assessment and observation

- nutrition and hydration
- elimination
- education
- individual needs

These two axes then make up a matrix which is completed for each day of the patient care pathway. The above 11 elements were common in many of the pathway examples collected in Australia. As each element of the care was delivered, it was initialled for in the box provided. In addition to this, the main care giver (usually the nurse) is required to print their name, designation and initials at the end of the shift so a record is kept of who they were.

Pages 6, 7, 8 and 9 continue the care path for the rest of the anticipated length of stay. Page 10 sets out the discharge arrangements and prescribed plan of care for completion by all care givers.

Care path variance record (Figure 2.7)

This document is for use by all multidisciplinary team members to note any variation from the care path. The date and pathway day (i.e. pre-op day 1) are noted, along with a description and reason for the variance. The variance typed is coded as either S (a system variance, e.g. service not available; bed not available; or appointment schedule fully booked); P (a patient reason, e.g. complications, unforeseen family problems impacting upon care or discharge); or C (clinician or care-giver reason, e.g. consultations, assessments, treatments, interventions performed that were not ordered or not done as ordered). The variances can then be coded, analysed, and action taken where appropriate.

It can be seen that further details of assessment, action plan and response should be documented in the multidisciplinary notes. Hence it is not sufficient merely to note a variance (e.g. wound not healed): a subsequent plan of action to manage the variance, and of evaluation to note whether the action was effective, is required.

Nursing assessment form (Figure 2.8)

This form shows the nursing assessment record. Nurses at this hospital identified that it would be helpful to develop this further into a full multidisciplinary assessment of the patient – as in all organizations visited, each healthcare professional group completed an independent patient assessment and there was a significant amount of duplication. The discharge and hospital risk assessment score appeared comprehensive and worked well in practice.

Patient care plan (Figure 2.9)

This document is a blank care pathway that can be used either as a template for drafting new pathways, or for developing individual care pathways for patients for whom a standardized care plan is either not yet developed or not appropriate because of complex care needs.

This proved particularly useful, since it meant all documentation had a similar format and layout with which clinicians soon became familiar. This overcame the

St. John of God Hospital Subiaco	SURNAME		UMRN	
	FORENAMES			
CARE PATH VARIANCE RECORD	D.O.B.		SEX	
	DOCTOR'S NAME			
	Use Patient I.D. When Available			

For details of assessment, action plan and response, see multidisciplinary notes

No	Date	Pathway Day	Description of Variance	Reason for Variance (if known)	Variance Type *

* Variance Type Code

S = System reason - eg. service not available, equipment problems, bed not available, appointment schedule fully booked.

P = Patient reason - eg. complications, unforeseen family problems impacting care or discharge.

C = Clinician / Care giver reason - eg. Consults, Assessments, Treatments, Interventions performed that were not ordered, or not done as ordered.

CARE PATH VARIANCE RECORD

MR421

Figure 2.7

Example of care path variance record (reproduced by permission of St John of God Hospital, Subiaco, Western Australia)

problem in many other places visited that the layout of patient documentation using a traditional format was very different from that of patient pathways. This proved confusing, particularly for agency nurses and junior doctors as they moved between wards. The added advantage was that it meant variances could also be tracked against the personalized care path. It also encouraged clinicians to identify goals and outcomes for care in a systematic way.

In conclusion, it can be seen that patient care pathways can offer an alternative method for documenting best practice which is accessible to the clinician at the point of healthcare delivery. Integrating these as part of the patient documentation has additional advantages, namely that they act as a trigger for best practice, as clinicians are given a timely reminder of care and treatment required. They can cut down on documentation time, as common elements of care are on a preprinted pathway, rather than needing to be written in full for each patient with the same procedure or condition.

They are an adjunct to, not a replacement for, guidelines, procedures and standards. Pathways advise the user what to do and when to do it. Guidelines, procedures, protocols and standards are needed to explain in more detail how to do it.

Pathways are a guide to treatment only – they cannot replace clinical autonomy and judgement, since the clinician needs to use their professional knowledge and judgement to assess the patient and decide whether or not the patient pathway is appropriate for their health needs.

Now we have examined patient care pathways and stressed the importance of evidence-based guidelines in supporting them, the next section will examine a case study in an acute Trust which concerns the development of an evidence-based guideline for the management of malignant pain.

The management of malignant pain

Previous case studies in this chapter have focused on specific examples to illustrate different methods for documenting best practice. It can be seen from many of these that rather than pursuing one method in isolation it is often necessary to underpin one method with another. Hence a discharge procedure necessitates the development of a discharge policy.

For ease of presentation, the examples illustrated (with the exception of the oesophageal cancer flowchart) were comparatively straightforward. The purpose of this final case study is to provide an example of how our attempts to document best practice have followed the principles of applying evidence-based practice, namely:

- Formulate a clear clinical question.
- Search the literature for relevant clinical articles.
- Critically appraise the evidence.
- Implement useful findings.

This specific clinical example also demonstrates the importance of cross-referencing standards and guidelines.

NO DRUG ALERT/ADVERSE REACTIONS ☐ SIGNATURE.............................	DRUG OR OTHER ADVERSE REACTION	DATE OF REACTION	DETAILS OF REACTION	SIGN
DRUG ALERT ATTACH LABEL ENTER DETAILS				

SOCIAL

Age .... Primary Language .... Interpreter required Yes ☐   No ☐

CONTACT PERSONS

1. Name...Relationship to Patient. ....

Telephone Numbers; (H) .... (W) .... (Mobile)...........................

2. Name...Relationship to Patient. ....

Telephone Numbers; (H) .... (W) .... (Mobile)...........................

GP Name and Address ....

Current Support Network - Formal e.g. Silver Chain...

            - Informal e.g. Family ....

Discharge Destination..

REASON FOR ADMISSION

PATIENT'S STATED REASON FOR ADMISSION

MEDICAL HISTORY	SURGICAL HISTORY

Have you been hospitalised or worked in any hospital outside of W.A. in the past 12 months?   Yes ☐   No ☐

ADMITTING NURSE NAME(S) ....DESIGNATION..................................

Figure 2.8a

Example of nursing assessment form (reproduced by permission of
St John of God Hospital, Subiaco, Western Australia)

NURSING ASSESSMENT - All sections must be completed by Nursing Staff

RESPIRATION (eg. rate, rhythm, cough, smoking habits, relevant family/work history)

CIRCULATION (eg. rate, rhythm, warmth, peripheral pulses, oedema)

NUTRITION/HYDRATION (eg:Alcohol consumption, usual intake, dentures)

Recent Weight Loss/Gain   Y ❑   N ❑

Special Dietary Requirements

WEIGHT ....Kg   HEIGHT ....CM   *SEE RISK ASSESSMENT SCALE*

ELIMINATION
Urinary: (eg. Incontinence, frequency, burning, stoma)
Ward Urinalysis results:

Bowel: (eg. usual habits, laxative use, stoma)
                                      SEE RISK ASSESSMENT SCALE

GENITO/REPRODUCTION (eg. Discharge, itch, abnormal bleeding)

Date of LMP ....
(if applicable)

MUSCULOSKELETAL (eg. Use of aids, gait, degree of assistance and ADLs)
Significant Falls History   Y ❑   N ❑

                                        SEE RISK ASSESSMENT SCALE

CONSCIOUS STATE (eg. level of consciousness, orientation to time, person and place)

                                        SEE RISK ASSESSMENT SCALE

SENSORY (eg. speech, hearing, vision, use of aids)

REST/SLEEP (eg. sedation, any difficulties/special requirements)

Figure 2.8b

St. John of God Hospital
Subiaco

NURSING ASSESSMENT FORM

ADMISSION DATE: _____

WARD: _____ ROOM _____

SURNAME	UMRN
GIVEN NAMES	
D.O.B.	SEX
DOCTOR'S NAME	

Please use I.D. label or block print

Pain History (Identify location, occurrence, intensity)
Include history of current complaint and other painful conditions.

On admission establish patient's preferred scale for ongoing assessment of pain.

Verbal Numerical Rating Scale (VNRS)

0 1 2 3 4 5 6 7 8 9 10

Verbal Descriptor Scale (VDS)

no pain   mild   moderate   severe   v.severe   worst pain possible

Shade affected areas

FRONT   BACK

SKIN (eg. colour, turgor, lesions, oral mucosa)
DESCRIBE ANY ALTERATION IN SKIN INTEGRITY

Anticipated nursing care explained to patient?	Y ☐	N ☐
Does the patient have: x-rays / scans?	Y ☐	N ☐
test results?	Y ☐	N ☐
electrical devices to be tested?	Y ☐	N ☐
Has the patient been shown the patient compendium?	Y ☐	N ☐
Has the patient been oriented to the ward?	Y ☐	N ☐
Does the patient have any concerns relating to this hospitalisation?	Y ☐	N ☐

Would the patient like to receive pastoral care/religious services?   Y ☐ Referred on ....N ☐

OTHER RELEVANT INFORMATION

MR 400   NURSING ASSESSMENT FORM

Figure 2.8c

DISCHARGE AND HOSPITAL RISK ASSESSMENT SCALE

AGE	Score	CONSCIOUSNESS AND ORIENTATION	Score	ACTIVITIES OF DAILY LIVING	Score	MOBILITY	Score	CONTINENCE	Score	APPETITE AND NUTRITION	Score	OTHER RELEVANT FACTORS
<50	1	Alert and oriented to Time, Place & Person	1	Self Caring	1	Ambulant with or without aids	1	Always continent	1	'GOOD'	1	eg. 1) Medical conditions such as Diabetes, Epilepsy, PVD 2) Sensory Deficit 3) Falls History (+1 per Risk Factor) • Risk Assessment Scale to be completed on admission and reviewed as required.
<60	2	Disoriented to time or place or person	2	Minimal assistance required i.e. assist with occasional hygiene needs	2	Walk with nurse or orderly assistance	2	Usually Continent (incont 1-2 times / 24 hrs idc/spc/ urodrome in situ)	2	'FAIR'	2	* Any patient with a significant history of falls will be commenced on the blue dot protocol regardless of score.
<70	3	Disoriented to time and place and person	3	Moderate assistance required i.e. assist with meals and most hygiene needs	3	Confined to chair	3	Often incontinent (incont 3 or more times/24 hrs)	3	'POOR' and/or recent unintentional weight loss	3	* Patients with altered skin integrity must be assessed for & receive pressure area care where appropriate, regardless of score.
>70	4	Unresponsive	4	Full Assistance required	4	Confined to bed	4	Always incontinent	4	Parental feeds, Nil By Mouth, Clear fluids, Intravenous Infusion only for 3 days or more	4	

Date	Score	Initials

SCORING:

Continence: If score is 3 or 4 refer to Continent Resource Manual

Pressure Risk: 11 or less (Low) Review as required. Implement measures as required.
12 or more (High) Implement use of pressure relieving devices.

Nutrition Risk: If nutrition score is 3 or 4, contact dietitian.

Injury Risk: 11 or less (Low) Review as required. Implement measures as required.
12 or more (High) Blue dot protocol. Patient transfer aids as required. Orderly transfer. Consider use of hoist.

Discharge Planning: 10 or more (High) At risk for home care resources, take appropriate actions as required - eg. organise home appliances, contact OT/ Discharge Planning Nurse.

Document score and care provided on patient care path / patient care plan

© St. John of God Health care System

Figure 2.8d

St. John of God Hospital Subiaco

PATIENT CARE PLAN

SURNAME		UMRN
FORENAMES		
D.O.B.		SEX
DOCTOR'S NAME		

Use Patient Identification Label when available.

WARD: .... ROOM:..............................

Admission date _____ Operation date _____

Diagnosis / Operation _____

OBJECTIVES

To promote optimal dignity and fullness of life for each patient.

NURSING CARE

Unless otherwise indicated, nursing care is given as per the following St. John of God Hospital Nursing standards.

☐ General Standards
☐ Patient undergoing Arterial Surgery
☐ Management of the Coronary Care Patient
☐ Care of the Ventilated Patient
☐ Diabetic Patient
☐ Oncology / Haematology Patient
☐ Patient undergoing Cranial Surgery
☐ Patient undergoing Orthopaedic and Neurosurgery
☐ Patient with a Plaster Cast
☐ Patient in Balanced Traction
☐ Patient undergoing Abdominal Surgery
☐ Patient undergoing Surgical diversion of Bowel or Urinary System to Abdominal Wall
☐ Patient undergoing Ophthalmic Surgery
☐ Patient under Fourteen (14) years of age
☐ Patient undergoing Urological Surgery

PROGRESS CHART

	Day of Care (Eg Pre-op, op day, 1 post op)	Expected Date of Achievement							
	Date								
1									
2									
3									
4									
5									
6									
7									
8									
9									
10									
11									
12									
13									
14									

Instructions
1. Identify and record important patient milestones (in collaboration with doctor, patient and care team).
2. Fill in day of care and corresponding date row.
3. When progress milestones are reached, initial and record time in corresponding date column / milestone row.

0208X

PATIENT CARE PLAN

MR420

Figure 2.9a

Example of a patient care plan (reproduced by permission of St John of God Hospital, Subiaco, Western Australia)

PATIENT CARE PLAN

v = Variance (record variation to planned care in multidisciplinary notes)

Unless otherwise indicated, care activities are the responsibility of the nurse.

SURNAME	UMRN
FORENAMES	
D.O.B.	SEX
DOCTOR'S NAME	

Use Patient Identification Label when available.

DAY OF CARE	Initials Time	Initials Time	Initials Time	Initials Time	Initials Time
DATE:					
TESTS / INVESTIGATIONS					
CONSULTS.					
PAIN MANAGEMENT & COMFORT					
TREATMENTS / MEDICATIONS					
DISCHARGE PLANNING	• If Discharge/Risk Assessment score is 11 or more, take appropriate action.				

Figure 2.9b

DAY OF CARE		Initials Time		Initials Time		Initials Time		Initials Time	
DATE:									
ADL's, MOBILITY AND SAFETY	• If falls score is 12 or more, implement Blue Dot Protocol • If pressure score is 12 or more, implement appropriate pressure relieving devices								
ASSESSMENT & OBSERVATION	• Nursing Assessment form including Discharge/Risk Assessment scale								
NUTRITION & HYDRATION	• If nutrition score is 3 or 4, contact dietican								
ELIMINATION	• If continence score is 3 or 4, refer to Continence Resource Manual								
EDUCATION									
INDIVIDUAL NEEDS	• Offer Pastoral Care Services								
Nurses to print name, designation and initials	AM								
	PM								
	ND								

Figure 2.9c

DISCHARGE ARRANGEMENTS

SURNAME		UMRN
FORENAMES		
D.O.B.		SEX
DOCTOR'S NAME		

Use Patient Identification Label when available.

COMMUNITY RESOURCES

Required   No ☐   Yes ☐   (Specify)

Service	Date Arranged	Sign

INFORMATION GIVEN TO PATIENT

	Yes/No	Date	Sign
Follow up Appointments			
X-Rays			
Discharge Letter			
Medications			

DISCHARGE MEDICATIONS

	Yes/No
Required	
Supplied	
Prescription	

EQUIPMENT

Specify	Date Arranged	Signed

EXIT FROM HOSPITAL

	Yes/No	
Transport Arranged		Mode _____
Identification Check		Signature _____

Destination Address (if different to addressograph above)

_____

_____

Phone _____

Date of Discharge [_____]   Time of Discharge [_____]

ALL CAREGIVERS/CONSULTANTS PLEASE PRINT NAME AND SIGN WITH INITIALS

PRINT NAME	DESIG	INITIAL	PRINT NAME	DESIG	INITIAL

Figure 2.9d

STAFFORDSHIRE UNIVERSITY LIBRARY

Background to the pain review

The roots of this project lay in the Trust's Strategy for Nursing & Midwifery. Quality was one of eight key areas identified by the strategy for the development of professional practice (outlined in Chapter 7).

The group wanted to take the lead by developing Trust-wide written documentation for areas of high volume or cost where it was felt that evidence of best practice existed yet actual practice varied between wards. Although at the outset the evidence was anecdotal, the group felt the management of pain might fall into this category. The challenge for the group was to assess whether this intuitive (gut) feeling was an actual reflection of the current situation and, if so, to apply the theory of evidence-based practice in order to document and implement best practice for the management of pain.

Moving from theory to practice can often be problematic. As we highlighted earlier, the first stage in carrying out an evidence-based review is to formulate a focused clinical question. This was difficult given the broad nature of the subject – pain. In formulating a clear clinical question it is often helpful to consider the following:

- population
- intervention
- outcome

With our question on pain, we narrowed our *population* down to adult patients, our *intervention* was pain relief and our *outcome* was the patient having their pain relieved to their satisfaction. The question that the Quality Nursing Focus Group (QNFG) finally opted for was, 'What evidence currently exists to support the management of pain in adults by nursing staff in an acute hospital setting?'

The second stage of our evidence-based review involved searching the Medline, CINAHL, British Nursing Index, Cochrane and Best Evidence databases. The initial results were disappointing. For example, the Medline search for English articles pertaining to adults for the period 1966–1997, produced the following results:

	PAIN	92,069	articles
and	MANAGE*	1141	articles
and	NURS*	64	articles
and	HOSPITAL	21	articles

None of the 21 articles identified was helpful in answering our original question. However, some of the articles identified made reference to pain guidelines. Therefore in the second series of searches the strategy remained the same but was modified to:

	PAIN
and	MANAGE*
and	GUIDELINE*

This approach produced much improved results. For example the Medline database identified 156 articles when searching all fields and 22 when searching the title alone. Additional clinical guidelines were identified by a search of the Internet. In total this second search identified six pain guidelines.

Our original search, in which we attempted to apply the theory of evidence-based medicine to the management of a whole population of patients, was misguided. What the QNFG was looking for was not evidence to manage an individual patient, but rather evidence to manage a whole population. As Gray and Donald (1997, p. 2) observe, 'Unlike 'evidence-based medicine', which concentrates on using evidence to make decisions about individual patients, evidence-based health care uses the best available evidence to make decisions about the health and health services of whole populations or groups of patients.'

The third stage in carrying out an evidence-based review is to appraise the evidence. Whether the search identifies individual papers or clinical guidelines, it is still necessary to appraise the evidence critically. If you have individual papers, be they quantitative (Oxman, Sachet and Guyatt, 1993) or qualitative (Cobb and Hagemaster, 1987), you may wish to consider some of the following questions:

- Was the problem or question clearly defined?
- Was the correct approach used?
- Is the sample size appropriate to address the question?
- Does the researcher state how data were collected and transcribed?
- Is there a statement of steps to minimize bias?
- Were all results considered?
- Are interpretations relevant to the results and the questions?
- Are the recommendations consistent with the findings?

As a result of our literature review, and following the ward audit on pain discussed in Chapter 3, a multidisciplinary group was established to review the management of cancer pain using the guideline produced by the Agency for Health Care Policy and Research (AHCPR) (Jacox et al., 1994). Malignant pain certainly met our original criterion of high volume. In England and Wales in 1992 (the last date for which figures were available), almost a quarter of a million new cases of cancer were diagnosed; in 1995, cancer was the underlying cause of death in one in four cases (figures provided by the Office for National Statistics); whilst at a local level the Trust admitted over 1800 patients with cancer during the previous calendar year.

Despite the prevalence of malignant disease, the literature on pain management is replete with reports of poor assessment of pain by nursing staff and the under-treatment of patients' pain by medical staff. Experts claim that as many as 25% of cancer patients die without receiving adequate pain relief (Von Roenn et al., 1993; Bonica, 1990). This is despite the fact that studies have indicated that pain can be controlled in 90% of patients (Ventafridda, Caraceni and Gamba, 1990). In addition to undertreatment by medical staff (Marks and Sachar, 1973), many studies have highlighted how nursing staff consistently underassess patients' pain. Camp and O'Sullivan's study of documentation and assessment of pain (1987) suggests that nurses record significantly less than 50% of what patients describe.

Notwithstanding advances in empirical knowledge and available resources for the management of pain, Browne (1996, p.552) argues that the incidence of 'moderate to severe unmanaged pain . . . continues to be the norm among hospitalised patients', and Dufault *et al.* (1995, p.635) suggests 'the relief of pain is awaiting no scientific breakthroughs' but rather the application of best evidence into practice. For this to happen it has been argued that there is a need to shift away from the tradition of practice where 'intuition and historical precedent have dominated clinical decision making' (Hicks, 1997, p.38) towards an evidence-based culture.

Because our search had identified a cancer pain guideline, we used the framework developed by Cluzeau *et al.* (1997) to assess the quality of this guideline. Just as individual papers are reviewed, guidelines too should be appraised with due consideration being given to their rigour and evidence base. The guideline scored well against the framework developed by Cluzeau and colleagues. The QNFG decided to adopt the guideline as the basis for further work because each of its recommendations is graded according to the strength and consistency of the evidence. For example, 'Patients should be encouraged to remain active and to participate in self care when possible' (Jacox *et al.*, 1994, p.75).

The strength of evidence for this recommendation is grade A. The grading A or B means that the consistency of the evidence is high and that the recommendation is based on evidence either from meta-analysis of multiple well-designed controlled studies or from experimental studies. When the recommendation is C or D this means that the panel used the available empirical evidence but based their recommendation primarily on expert opinion.

Auditing practice against the guideline

The AHCPR cancer guideline having been adopted, the next stage was to audit current practice against recommendations made in the guideline. This approach was similar to that adopted by a community hospital in the United States in their implementation of the AHCPR guideline on acute pain. As Bach (1995, p. 516) suggests, the 'first step' in the implementation process should be an 'evaluation of the hospital's current pain management practices to determine if there [are] . . . existing problems'.

The original ward audit essentially reviewed what Donabedian would class as the structural components to the way wards manage pain. The second audit aimed to assess staff attitudes to malignant pain management and their receptiveness to the cancer pain guideline. As Campese (1996) suggests, the first question that needs to be addressed when implementing guidelines is 'Are physicians supportive of such an initiative?'

The original plan was to review the 66 recommendations made in the cancer pain guideline, select those pertinent to nurses and create a new document based on the original guideline. However, the process of allocating a recommendation to a specific profession proved to be a futile operation, as the group decided that all but three recommendations were multiprofessional. Despite the group's belief that nurses perform a pivotal role in the management of patients' pain, it was also recognized that the successful implementation of the recommendations 'requires collaboration across disciplines' (Jacox *et al.*, 1994, p. 144). Therefore a senior registrar from oncology and a pharmacist were co-opted onto the working group, joining the head of nursing from the outpatients department and a ward sister from oncology.

The main aim of this second audit was to:

- review staff attitudes to the assessment of cancer patients' pain;
- assess attitudes on the issue of patient–staff communication;
- evaluate the level of staff knowledge in relation to managing pain caused by cancer;
- assess attitudes to the use of drugs for managing cancer pain;
- identify who staff feel is responsible for the management of cancer patients' pain;
- review staff's overall evaluation of how cancer pain is managed;
- determine how enthusiastic staff are about using the guidelines for cancer pain management.

The questionnaire used to assess staff opinions was based on published work (see, for example, Scott, 1992; Hunt, 1995). Following a pilot, 433 doctors and nurses were sent a copy of the questionnaire, of which 199 were completed and returned.

Some of the findings of this audit are as follows:

- 81% of staff felt that using a pain assessment chart would improve the management of pain.
- 98% of staff felt that the patient was best placed to determine the extent of their pain.
- 91% of staff were in favour of using a pain assessment tool – although our earlier ward audit identified that few clinical areas systematically use one.
- 88% of staff did not feel that patients would spontaneously report pain. This was despite most staff believing that good communication is a vital component of effective pain management.
- 99% of staff felt that each individual has a different pain tolerance level; however, 41% of staff believed that some ethnic groups can tolerate a greater intensity of pain than others.
- 26% of staff were using the 'analgesic ladder' which is recommended as the foundation for the pharmacological management of pain.
- The majority of staff felt that responsibility for assessing, documenting, informing and reviewing the effectiveness of pain management should be shared by doctors and nurses.
- 94% of staff did not use a guideline to manage cancer patients' pain,

although 86% of respondents felt that the development of such a guideline would improve the management of cancer pain.
- Overall 42% of staff said they find managing cancer pain difficult, and
  31% of staff said that cancer pain in their area was poorly managed.

Implementing the guideline

Having identified that most staff were in favour of the cancer pain guideline, our
next stage was to implement guidelines. In reviewing our implementation strategy
we will highlight how this fits in with the fourth stage of an evidence-based
review of implementing useful findings. In this section we also highlight the benefits of using literature reviews to inform how findings are implemented.

One of the questions that staff were asked was what suggestions they would
make for ensuring the successful implementation of the guideline. Sixty-three per
cent of staff proposed using educational sessions. In addition a number of respondents suggested multiple approaches to the guideline dissemination; for example,
a registered nurse proposed 'teaching sessions initially, followed up by a leaflet
with continued leaflets to remind people'.

In reviewing the literature, it is easy to understand the appeal of an approach
based upon continuing education. Hunt's (1995) study identified a training requirement around various aspects of pain and analgesia, whilst Carr (1997) highlights
the lack of formal teaching in medical schools on pain management.

Although educational sessions are perhaps the most obvious approach to disseminating best practice, Max is sceptical of this method, remarking that 'perhaps
the formula of 'educate and change attitudes' is insufficient'. He argues that the
process of providing information alone 'may have little effect on behaviour, which
is largely determined by established patterns of practice and tradition' (Max,
1990, p. 886).

Because of some commentators' reservations about the low impact that educational programmes may have on achieving behavioural change, we reviewed the
literature in order to inform our guideline implementation process.

The most apparent feature of our review on implementing guidelines is the
lack of robust evidence for the effectiveness of many implementation strategies.
Indeed, Cheater and Closs (1997), in their review of implementation and dissemination strategies for nursing guidelines, conclude that there is an 'urgent' need
for evaluative research in this subject. They suggest, however, that the mere
dissemination of guidelines does not result in 'substantial changes'. Grimshaw
and Russell (1993) argue that guidelines are more likely to be successful if there
is an active implementation strategy rather than a passive dissemination. Oxman,
Sachet and Guyatt (1993), however, suggest that no one implementation strategy
is more effective than another and therefore the way forward may be to employ
multiple strategies with repeated exposure.

The effectiveness of multiple strategies was assessed in a study by McNaull
et al. (1992) that sought to identify which educational approach was the most
effective in teaching nurses to assess pain systematically. They used several educational techniques for examining the impact that these had on nurses' practice.

Although the sample size for this study was small – only 39 nurses – they found that the group of nurses exposed to multiple education techniques performed a greater proportion of pain assessments than those who had received only an explanatory letter.

In reviewing the literature, we identified a number of case studies from the United States addressing the implementation stage of the AHCPR pain guidelines. One of these case studies has in many respects been the blueprint for this work (Clarke *et al.*, 1996). Clarke and colleagues examined nurses' knowledge and attitudes towards pain management as part of the process for implementing both the acute and cancer pain guidelines. Based on their findings they made the following recommendations:

- Incorporate a pain assessment sheet into the patient's records.
- Distribute an abbreviated version of the appropriate guideline to nursing staff.
- Introduce regular patient satisfaction monitoring of pain management.
- Include pain management information in the Trust's induction programme.
- Initiate pain bulletins, to provide news and updates on pain-related topics.
- Set up 'pain practice groups' of nurses to establish and promote non-pharmacological pain interventions.
- Develop a periodic ongoing evaluation programme to assess the effectiveness of pain control.

In the second case study, a group from Utah developed a number of additional tools for the guideline to facilitate its implementation. These included a series of pocket cards entitled 'Managing cancer pain for physicians and nurses', 'About cancer pain treatment', and 'First step cards'. These tools paralleled staff suggestions made in our audit for 'inserts in the house officer's handbook' ($n = 4$) and additions to the 'prescribing guidelines filofax' ($n = 3$).

One of the surprising factors in the review of staff suggestions was the number of proposals that already existed in the Trust. For example, there are pages on cancer pain management already in the house officer's handbook and in the prescribing guidelines.

It has therefore been decided that the *Pain Bulletin* initiated by the QNFG to provide staff with a an update of the group's progress should set one edition aside for focusing on resources for pain management that are already available within the Trust.

Proposals of staff audit

As a result of our literature review and staff suggestions, a multiple implementation strategy for the guideline will include:

- sending a copy of the guideline to each clinical area;
- sending a concise version of the guideline to individual members of staff;
- producing leaflets for staff on the various aspects of pain management;

- designing posters for the ward on various aspects of pain management;
- adapting the Utah flowcharts and reminder cards.

In addition, it is planned to:

- incorporate pain management into the nurses' and doctors' induction programmes;
- establish educational sessions that are ongoing and compulsory for junior doctors;
- devise a series of ward workshops for nurses on how to use the assessment chart;
- encourage each clinical area to clarify who is responsible for the initial assessment, documentation and evaluation of the effectiveness of patients' pain management;
- hold a launch day for the guideline, at which the results of both audits and a forthcoming patient satisfaction audit will be presented.

Summary

The main aim of the QNFG review of pain was to develop an evidence-based standard on pain management for use by nurses in the Trust. What seemed a relatively simple task was much more complex than anticipated. Although the AHCPR guidelines have made the process of identifying the evidence simpler, it would have helped if these guidelines had also addressed the question of their implementation. Indeed, the cancer pain guideline scored badly against the implementation criteria in the recently released guidelines appraisal instrument produced by Cluzeau *et al.* (1997). The cancer pain guideline also scored badly against the appraisal instrument criteria on likely costs and benefits of introducing the guideline. However, these shortcomings probably reflect the pace of change in the development of clinical guidelines, rather than a criticism of the cancer pain guideline itself.

The last part of the review of cancer pain management involves looking at this issue from the patient's perspective. A patient questionnaire based on the work of the American Pain Society has recently been completed (see Miaskowski *et al.*, 1994).

Because we now have written documentation on best practice to manage pain, it will be possible to develop a policy statement for the Trust. For example, 'each patient entering Hospital ... will have his or her pain managed in such a way that it remains at or below a level of three ... or is at a level acceptable to the patient' (Campese, 1996). Using specific recommendations from the guideline, it will also be possible to set standards of care against which performance can be measured; for example, '95% of patients will have their pain assessed and documented while awake for the first 24 hours following surgery' (Agency for Health Care Policy and Research, 1995, p. 13).

Looking at the long-term development of this work over the next 6–18 months, there are number of issues to address. The QNFG anticipates that the wards will include a pain audit in their annual audit programme. The assessment of pain by nurses will probably be the first area to be reviewed. The structure for this assessment tool will be similar to the AHCPR (1995) example of a clinical practice guideline-derived evaluation tool for determining quality of care for postoperative pain control.

Another option for the group may be to develop a critical pathway as a way of instituting pain management. Gordon (1996, p. 258) argues that the development of critical pathways is an effective way of incorporating pain guidelines into everyday practice; she suggests that pathways provide an excellent opportunity to 'increase the visibility of pain and accountability of healthcare professionals' .

Although there are a number of potentially interesting areas that may develop out of this work the greatest challenge will no doubt be to encourage other staff not involved with originating this work to feel ownership of it. Whilst we can provide evidence of best practice in the form of the guideline, it is clear from our review that evidence alone does not change practice. The challenge for the group will not necessarily be to provide staff with details of the guideline, but rather to motivate those individuals to use it. Unfortunately it is here that other less tangible factors, like the culture of the organization and its flexibility and ability to adapt, will come into play.

A re-audit of both audits is scheduled for late 1998 and this will give the first indication as to whether patient care has started to improve. Von Roenn and colleagues' study (1993) suggests that 'patients need to be assured that pain management is an integral part of their total management and good pain control can be achieved throughout the course of the disease'. However, before the patient can be assured of good pain control, a demonstrable improvement in pain management may be necessary.

FINAL SUMMARY AND CONCLUSIONS

This chapter has defined and given examples of a variety of methods that can be used to document best practice; namely policies, standards, guidelines, protocols, procedures and care pathways. For each of these we have identified that it can be helpful to follow the SMARTER criteria to ensure that the documents are easy to understand and apply.

Through the final case study we have worked through the complexities of finding, documenting, implementing and evaluating evidence in clinical practice. This has demonstrated that careful consideration needs to be given to all of these steps if genuine and lasting improvements to patient care are to be made. Indeed, in many respects it was the implementation phase – with the need to work across professional boundaries and ensure that the methods of implementation also had a sound evidence base – that was the most challenging.

Another lesson learned as part of this exercise was that the amount of time and resources needed can be significant if we are to avoid merely documenting current practice, rather than best practice. The two may of course be exactly the same, but challenging this assumption is an important part of the process. The resource issues need to be addressed if policy makers are serious about clinicians devoting time and effort to this kind of rigorous approach to their work.

The last chapter highlighted the difficulty for most clinicians to find time out from their clinical work to participate in projects such as this. Without the resources of the clinical audit department, it is unlikely the pain guidelines work would have been carried out with such rigour. Most of the time spent by the multidisciplinary team on the work was carried out in their own time.

In summary, there are a number of important steps when attempting to document best practice. These are:

- Ensure you pick the right method or framework for the task in hand.
- Identify who else needs to be involved, and involve them.
- Use the SMARTER criteria.
- Follow the steps for implementing evidence into practice outlined in this chapter .
- Pilot the document.
- Develop an evidence-based implementation strategy.

Finally, as identified in this chapter, an evaluation of the impact the documentation has had is fundamental to the process. As the documents are developed, the team needs to be simultaneously considering how they are going to measure the criteria they have set. The next two chapters therefore address different approaches to measuring clinical practice.

REFERENCES

Agency for Health Care Policy and Research (1995) *Using Clinical Practice Guidelines to Evaluate Quality of Care*, Vol. 1, US Department of Health and Human Services, Rockville MD.

Bach, D. (1995) Implementation of the Agency for Health Care Policy and Research postoperative pain management guideline. *Nursing Clinics of North America*, 30(3), 515–27.

Bonica, J. (1990) Cancer pain, in *The Management of Cancer Pain*, 2nd edn (ed. J. Bonica), Vol. 1, Lea and Febinger, Philadelphia, pp. 400–60.

Brown, S. (1995) *Examining the Nursing Contribution to Multidisciplinary Clinical Protocols*. Florence Nightingale Foundation Scholarship Report, Florence Nightingale Foundation, London.

Browne, R. (1996) Accepting the challenge of pain management. *British Journal of Nursing*, 5(9), 552–5.

Camp, L. and O'Sullivan, P. (1987) Comparison of medical, surgical and oncology patients' descriptions of pain and nurses' documentation of pain assessments. *Journal of Advanced Nursing*, 12(5), 593–8.

Campese, C. (1996) Development and implementation of a pain management program. *Official Journal of the Association of Operating Room Nurses*, 64, 931–40.

Carr, E. (1997) How to achieve effective pain management. *Nursing Times*, 93(37), 52–3.

Cheater, F. and Closs, S. (1997) The effectiveness of methods of dissemination and implementation of clinical guidelines for nursing practice: a selective review. *Clinical Effectiveness in Nursing*, **1**, 4–15.

Clarke, E., French, B., Bilodeau, M. *et al.* (1996) Pain management knowledge, attitudes and clinical practice: the impact of nurses' characteristics and education. *Journal of Pain and Symptom Management*, **1**, 18–31.

Cluzeau, F., Littlejohns, P., Grimshaw, J. and Feder, G. (1997) *Appraisal Instrument for Clinical Guideline Version 1*, St George's Hospital Medical School, London.

Cobb, A. and Hagemaster, J. (1987) Ten criteria for evaluating qualitative research proposals. *Journal of Nursing Education*, **26**(4), 138–43.

Crosby, P. (1989) *Quality Education System for the Individual*, The Creative Factory, Crosby Quality College, London.

Donabedian, A. (1969) Evaluating the quality of medical care. *Millbank Memorial Fund Quarterly*, **4**, 166–203.

Dufault, M., Bielecky, C., Collins, E. and Willy, C. (1995) Changing nurses' pain assessment practice – a collaborative research utilisation approach. *Journal of Advanced Nursing*, **21**, 634–45.

Field, M.J. and Lohr, K.N. (eds) (1992) *Guidelines for Clinical Practice: From Development to Use*, National Academy Press, Washington.

Goldstone, L. (1991) A very pe'QA'liar practice. *Nursing Times*, **87**(20), 41–3.

Gordon, D. (1996) Critical pathways: a road to institutionalising pain management. *Journal of Pain Symptom Management*, **11**, 252–9.

Gray, M. and Donald, A. (1997) Policy and quality standards. *Evidence-Based Health Policy and Management*, **1**(1), 1–5.

Grimshaw, J.N. and Russell, I.T. (1993) Effect of clinical guidelines on medical practice: a systematic review of rigorous evaluations. *Lancet*, **342**, 1317–22.

Grimshaw, J.N. and Russell, I.T. (1994) Achieving health gain through clinical outcomes. II Ensuring that guidelines change medical practice. *Quality In Health Care*, **3**, 45–52.

Hicks, C. (1997) Individual responsibility or corporate culture. *Nursing Times*, **93**(39), 38–9.

Howell, J. and Marr, H. (1988) Visible improvements. *Nursing Times*, **84**(25), 33–4.

Hunt, K. (1995) Perceptions of patients' pain: a study assessing nurses' attitudes. *Nursing Standard*, **10**(4), 32–5.

Jacox, A., Carr, D.B. and Payne, R. *et al* (1994) *Management of Cancer Pain*, Clinical Practice Guideline No. 9, Agency for Health Care Policy and Research, US Department of Health and Human Services, Rockville MD.

Kendall, H. (1988) The West Berkshire approach. *Nursing Times*, **84**(27), 334.

Kennedy, M. (1995) Ten strategies for making clinical guidelines and pathways work. *Quality Letter*, October, 2.

Kitson, A. (1988a) Raising the standards. *Nursing Times*, **84** (25), 29–32.

Kitson, A. (1988b) Caring standards. *Nursing Standard*, 5 November.

McNaull, F., McLees, J., Belyeh, M. and Clipp, E. (1992) Comparison of educational methods to enhance nursing performance in pain assessment. *Journal of Continuing Education in Nursing*, **23**(26), 267–71.

Marks, R. and Sachar, D. (1973) Undertreatment of medical inpatients with narcotic analgesia. *Annals of Internal Medicine*, **78**, 172–81.

Max, M. (1990) Improving outcomes of analgesic treatment: is education enough? *Annals of Internal Medicine*, **113**, 885–9.

Maxwell, R.J. (1984) Quality assessment in health. *British Medical Journal*, **288**(5), 1470–2.

Miaskowski, C., Nicols, R., Brody, R. and Synold, T. (1994) Assessment of patient satisfaction utilising the American Pain Society's Quality Assurance Standards on acute and cancer related pain. *Journal of Pain and Symptom Management*, **9**(1), 5–11.

NHS Executive (1997) *Review of Cervical Screening Services at Kent & Canterbury Hospitals NHS Trust*, Department of Health, London.

NHS Executive (1998) *A First Class Service : Quality in the New NHS*, consultation document, Department of Health, London.

Overton, P. and Stinson, S. (1977) *Journal of Advanced Nursing*, **2**(137), 46.

Oxman, A., Sachet, D. and Guyatt, G. (1993) Users' guides to the medical literature. *Journal of American Medical Association*, **270**(17), 2093–5.

Parsley, K. (1998a) Study tour report: exploring the development, implementation and evaluation of patient pathways in Australia, Brighton Health Care internal publication.

Parsley, K. (1998b) In search of pathways. *Nursing Times*, **94**(32), 40–41.

Royal College of Nursing Standards of Care Project Team (1990) *Quality Patient Care, The Dynamic Standard Setting System*, Scutari, London.

Scott, I. (1992) Nurses' attitudes to pain control and use of pain scales. *British Journal of Nursing*, **2**(1), 11–16.

Thomson, R., Lavender, M. and Madhok, R. (1995) How to ensure that guidelines are effective. *British Medical Journal*, **311**(22), 237–42.

Tingle, J. (1992) Legal implications of standard setting in nursing. *British Journal of Nursing*, **1**(14), 728–31.

Ventafridda, V., Caraceni, A. and Gamba, A. (1990) Field-testing of the WHO guidelines for cancer pain relief: summary report of demonstration projects, in *Proceedings of the Second International Congress on Pain: Vol. 16 Advances in Pain Research and Therapy* (eds K. Foley, J. Bonica and V. Ventafridda), Raven Press, New York, pp. 451–64.

Von Roenn, J., Cleeland, C., Gonin, R. *et al.* (1993) Physician attitudes and practice in cancer pain management. *Annals of Internal Medicine*, **119**, 121–6.

Waterlow, J. (1988) Prevention is cheaper than cure. *Nursing Times*, **84**(25), 69–70.

3 MEASURING BEST PRACTICE: AN INTRODUCTION TO CLINICAL AUDIT

INTRODUCTION

The measurement of professional practice against known best practice is not new to the health professions. The founding charter of the Royal College of Physicians, written in 1517, refers to the need for members to set and maintain standards of practice 'for their own honour and for the public benefit'. Florence Nightingale was responsible for collecting statistics which underpinned her work to improve the standards of hygiene in the field hospitals at Scutari and the Crimea in 1855.

More recently, the professions have adopted the clinical audit framework as a method for introducing a systematic approach to measuring their practice. Audit was incorporated into National Health Service policy with the inclusion of medical audit in the Government White Paper, *Working for Patients* (Department of Health 1989). Medical audit involves only doctors. Other health professionals have developed their own unidisciplinary audit programmes. Since 1993, the Department of Health (DoH) have proposed a move towards clinical audit, which involves multi-professional groups rather than just doctors. This has a number of advantages. Primarily, most of the professional groups involved in unidisciplinary audit recognized that improving patient care was reliant on *all* carers adopting and measuring best practice if genuine benefits were to be realized by the patient. This was formally recognized by the DoH in 1994 with proposals that clinical audit should be patient focused, develop a culture of continuous evaluation and improve clinical effectiveness by examining patient outcomes. The DoH document (1994) identified the following features of a successful clinical audit programme:

- undertaken at healthcare team level;
- links made between health and social services, particularly with respect to vulnerable adults and children living in the community;
- contribution encouraged from individual healthcare professionals.

The National Audit office defines clinical audit as:

> *a process in which doctors, nurses and other healthcare professionals systematically review and where necessary make changes to the care and treatment they provide to patients. (1995)*

Norman and Redern (1995) propose that clinical audit can be categorized into:

- **Generic audit** – which involves addressing the overall quality in a ward or unit (examples of such audits are given in the following chapter).
- **Problem-specific audit** – measuring quality related to a clinical topic.

- **Activity-specific audit** – measuring the quality of care provided by a person or group of people.

Berwick and Knappe (1990) identify that audit can be further categorized into:

- **An implicit view** – where only the professional can recognize good care.
- **An explicit view** – where care is evaluated against expert-generated criteria.
- **Sentinels** – where events spark off incidents such as a suddenly increasing number of people who, for example, experience deep vein thrombosis post-operatively.

Hunt and Legg (1994) define the hallmarks of clinical audit as having:

- an appropriate design
- valid measures of quality of care
- reliable data
- a clear review of findings
- problem identification
- effective action to eliminate or minimize problems
- evidence of improvement through re-audit

Gillies (1997) proposes that clinical audit follows a cycle of activity (Figure 3.1). Gillies notes the similarities of this cycle to the classical process improvement techniques pioneered by Deming (1986). The cycle illustrated in Figure 3.1 shows the key stages of audit, which are well defined in the literature.

The audit process can also be visualised as a spiral, rather than a cycle, shown in Figure 3.2. The audit spiral is described as the process passes through four stages, namely:

- **Selection.** Problems are identified and prioritized and, when they are selected, specific audit objectives are developed for them. The most suitable methodology is then chosen.

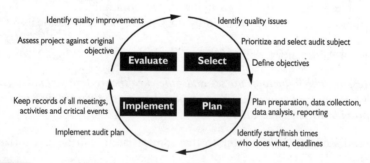

Figure 3.1

The clinical audit cycle (reproduced with the permission of Brighton Health Care NHS Trust)

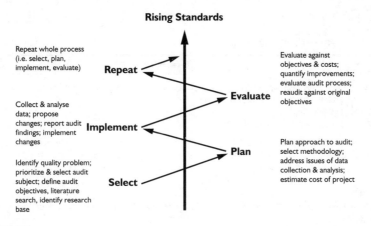

Rising Standards

Repeat whole process
(i.e. select, plan,
implement, evaluate) **Repeat**

Evaluate against
objectives & costs;
quantify improvements;
evaluate audit process;
reaudit against original
objectives

Evaluate

Collect & analyse
data; propose
changes; report audit **Implement**
findings; implement
changes

Plan

Plan approach to audit;
select methodology;
address issues of data
collection & analysis;
estimate cost of project

Identify quality problem;
prioritize & select audit
subject; define audit **Select**
objectives, literature
search, identify research
base

Figure 3.2

The clinical audit spiral (reproduced with the permission of Brighton Health Care NHS Trust)

- **Planning.** A data collection strategy is developed. At this stage any resource implications are identified.
- **Implementation.** Data are collected and analysed, and any changes required are implemented. The findings are reported to those involved and distributed throughout the organization.
- **Evaluation.** The audit project is then evaluated to determine whether the objectives were met and to identify what auditors learned about each stage of the process. Evaluation is important to ascertain what improvements resulted and what factors prevented their success. Understanding what was done well, and what did not work so well, enables participants to appreciate the components of a successful audit project.

The whole process is then repeated. The spiral demonstrates that, as each series of steps is repeated, there will be an incremental increase in the quality of the service being audited. Hence, the spiral is an iterative process of continuous improvement.

The application of clinical audit into practice is diverse. Gillies (1997) suggested three 'views' of clinical audit to resolve inconsistencies of application.

The 'process' view

This involves measuring not only existing performance, but any improvement of performance. Therefore, once activities have been measured, results need to be fed back to change practice. This brings together both quality improvement and quality assurance activities.

The 'research' view

The boundaries between audit and research are often confused. It is helpful at this point to clarify the distinctions between them (see Table 3.1). Audit and

Table 3.1

The differences between audit and research

Audit	Research
Is a systematic approach to peer review of clinical care to identify possible improvements and provide a mechanism for bringing them about.	Is a systematic investigation that aims to increase the sum of knowledge. It usually involves hypothesis testing.
Raises questions to be answered by research.	Generates the knowledge used by audit.
Is a test of whether things are being done the way it has been agreed they should be done: it compares care provided against agreed standards in order to identify whether best practice is being applied locally.	Is concerned with discovering the right thing to do, identifying the most effective form of treatment and establishing what constitutes best clinical practice.
Never involves allocating patients randomly to different treatment groups.	May involve allocating patients randomly to different treatment groups.
Never involves a placebo treatment.	May involve administration of a placebo.
Never involves a completely new treatment, and usually focuses on treatments where there is some consensus about what constitutes best clinical practice.	May involve a completely new treatment, and usually focuses on treatments where knowledge about what is best clinical practice does not exist.
Examines particular types of care given over a particular period of time, in a particular location, and the results apply only to the population examined.	Results can be generalized.
Involves the voluntary participation of specialities and departments; data recorded and analysed relate to the participating clinician's own work.	Chooses clinicians and patients to participate because they are representative so that results can be generalized.
Is an ongoing, continuous process.	Usually has an endpoint, which is often when an adequate sample size has been obtained.
Changes indicated by the audit are made at a local level. Audits are published to educate others and publicize how best practice is being achieved.	Results are usually published so that all relevant clinicians can learn from the research.

Reproduced with the permission of Brighton Health Care NHS Trust.

research have much in common. In particular, they share a rigorous approach to methodology in terms of design, procedure, analysis and interpretation of data. However, the primary differences between them are:

- Research asks the question: 'What is best practice?'
- Audit asks the question: 'Are we actually following best practice?'

The 'defect analysis' view

This view incorporates activities that identify critical incidents or adverse events, which are then investigated. This is similar to identifying sentinels as suggested previously by Berwick and Knappe (1990).

Gillies believes this latter approach is resisted by clinicians in the UK because they believe the focus should be on identifying positive improvements rather than identifying defects (1997). However, a balance needs to be achieved. Focusing all attention on positive improvements avoids identification of the defects within a healthcare system that cause significant problems and distress for patients, for example, a sudden rise in wound infections postoperatively, or an increase in urinary tract infections linked with a change in suppliers or brand of catheter. It is important that these incidents are investigated and resolved, and that this is recognized as an important part of clinical audit activity.

The next section will examine the stages clinicians need to follow when carrying out an audit.

The process of audit

The stages of the audit cycle or spiral are shown in Figures 3.1 and 3.2. Each of these stages will now be described in more detail to outline how to approach them.

The audit process can be used to address issues and problems within any setting in an organization. It is not exclusive to clinical areas and can also be used for non-clinical services such as hotel services and management.

There are four key stages to the audit cycle: selection, planning, implementation and evaluation.

STAGES OF THE AUDIT CYCLE

Stage 1. Selection

This stage involves identifying quality issues and prioritizing potential projects.

Identifying quality issues

This can be achieved through brainstorming ideas with the team. At this stage all ideas should simply be recorded, not prioritized or discounted. When considering the prioritization of audit topics, we have found the following categories helpful in prompting ideas for projects:

- **An area where there are problems already identified** – either by staff or through patient complaints; e.g. the team may be able to recognize current problems that need attention and it is obvious to all in the group what they are.
- **An area that is important to either the team or the organization** – e.g. it may be due to the high numbers of patients involved, or a clinical priority that needs addressing.
- **A national priority** – e.g. team members may be aware of issues that will receive regional or national attention in the forthcoming months and may want to concentrate on those.

Prioritizing potential projects

Agreeing audit priorities may be difficult. In our experience, an audit has more chance of being successful if the project ensures the multidisciplinary team is supportive of the topic chosen. All members should be involved in the design, the data collection and the analysis of results.

Once the project has been chosen, it is then important to decide who should be involved and to obtain their cooperation for the next stage: planning the audit.

Stage 2. Planning

Once you have decided on a topic, drafting a plan of how the project will progress is important to give some structure and direction to your project. The following questions are helpful pointers:

- **What:** do you want to know and what are the objectives of the project?
- **Why:** do you want this information?
- **Who:** should be included in the project?
- **When:** is the audit going to take place and for how long?
- **How:** is the audit going to be developed and what is the data collection strategy?

Planning the project properly is crucial in order to ensure that all aspects of the project are considered and that time is not wasted by unforeseen problems. It is important to decide who should participate and what skills the team require to make the project successful. You may want to include those with authority for the budget or others who can directly influence the change process in the future.

The key aspects to consider at this stage are:

- developing the audit objectives
- specifying time periods, events and a strategy for data collection and analysis
- involvement of patients
- costing the project

Each of these will now be examined.

Developing audit objectives
To develop audit objectives, the following principles are helpful:

- Write down clear aims and objectives and specify the anticipated outcomes of the project.
- Use verbs, for example 'determine, confirm, demonstrate'. This makes it easier to evaluate at the end of the project whether or not the objectives were met.
- Before embarking on the project, confirm with the team that they are committed to take action on the results. If this is not agreed, determine why they want the audit undertaken.

Specifying time periods, events and the data collection strategy
Weekly, daily, monthly and seasonal variations may need to be considered when planning the audit. Recent changes in staffing or training and rotations of staffing

also need to be taken into account. In acute hospitals, undertaking an audit related to workload on wards will be affected by the rotation of medical staff in February and August.

Sampling
The sample size is the number of cases (whether they are patients, respondents to a survey, events, or whatever) that you need. People involved in audit and quality improvement are often unsure of the sample size they need and sometimes confuse the needs of audit with the needs of research. In research, results need to be applicable to the population as a whole in order to establish best practice. So the sample size must be sufficiently large to be both statistically significant and to allow results to be generalized. In audit or quality improvement projects, results do not need to be generalized to the population and will not be used to develop new theories or knowledge. In audit, results are mostly used to show to what extent the current practice of a particular department adheres to known best practice. Audit and quality improvement make use of mostly descriptive statistics and the issues of statistical significance are not usually relevant. It is still helpful to consult someone with a knowledge of statistics in choosing your sample size.

The set of criteria that are used to choose the sample in an audit project also needs to be discussed and agreed within the team who are carrying out the project. Usually the sample is identified as a specified number of patients in a particular patient group (such as those undergoing hip replacements, or those admitted to a specific ward). The most important point is that the patients in the sample should not be systematically different in any way from the group of patients from whom they were picked. For example, if you want a sample of inpatients undergoing elective surgery and you pick your sample by taking case notes from one surgical ward when patients are discharged, your sample will probably not be representative of the whole group. Patients admitted to that ward might be mostly those of one consultant, or those with a particular surgical condition. The sample will not give you a true picture of the standard of care given to all patients.

Audit sample
Helpful questions to consider include:

- Are all patients/events to be included or excluded from the project?
- Are the patients/events representative of the service?
- How will patients be identified?

For example, if an audit was taking place on patients' pain assessment scores and analgesia dosage, it may be decided to include only emergency patients or preoperative patients. Therefore, to prevent unnecessary data collection the criteria for inclusion must be decided and the sample size agreed.

Data collection strategy
This can be either retrospective or concurrent. Specific issues need to be considered in relation to validity for either method. If the data are to be collected retrospectively, you need to confirm how representative the client group was at that time in comparison with the current client group. For valid conclusions to be drawn, the team also needs to be aware of any specific events that may affect the usefulness of retrospective data; for example, a change in consultant, a change in community practice, or epidemiological factors.

Sources of data
When seeking to measure clinical practice and determine whether standards, guidelines or expectations are being met, there are a number of commonly used sources of data which are available for clinicians to use, namely:

- National databases (such as the *National Confidential Enquiry into Peri-Operative Deaths* (NCEPOD) and the *National Confidential Enquiry into Sudden Deaths in Infants* (NCESDI), and national comparative audits like the *Major Trauma Outcome Study* (MTOS)).
- Regional databases (like the *South Thames Cancer Registry*).
- Hospital information systems (such as your Patient Administration System (PAS), or management systems like Casemix or Management Information Systems (MIS)).
- Departmental information systems in individual clinical or service departments (such as clinical information systems like ABIES or Metabase, A&E nursing workload and care-planning systems, and laboratory or radiology systems and systems in other departments).
- Routine paper records (such as theatre lists and registers, referral or request forms, letters and all the many other paper information transfers that take place).
- Patient records (the medical, nursing and paramedical patient record should generally be kept in one place, with all the information about an individual patient's care in it).
- People themselves (their attitudes, knowledge or opinions, gathered through surveys, interviews, meetings and other forms of data collection).

Each of these data sources has some advantages and disadvantages. Different quality problems will demand a different kind of data. Some examples of the ways in which you might use them are given below.

National databases
If you want to learn about how your hospital or clinical area compares with others around the country, then national databases can be a useful source of information. The data are usually retrieved by contacting the professional body that collects and/or collates that data. For example, the Royal College of Surgeons of England collates NCEPOD data.

Regional databases

Regional databases can be used to see how your hospital or clinical area compares with others around your region, but they can also be used to identify a sample of patients or cases. For example, if you wanted to study patients with a certain type of cancer then you could use the regional cancer registry to establish how many patients have that cancer not only in your region but also in your catchment area. These data can be retrieved by contacting the body collecting and/or collating them.

Hospital information systems

If you need to gather information from a large number of patients or cases, or from all patients admitted, then hospital information systems will probably be the source to use. Data includes facts about:

- the patient (hospital number, name, date of birth, address, GP, marital status and so on);
- the latest episode of care (inpatient or outpatient, admitting consultant, dates of appointments, dates of admission and discharge, clinical coding of diagnoses and procedures);
- the history of contacts with the hospital (past inpatient and outpatient episodes, with the same sort of data as for the latest episode).

The data can be retrieved by running reports on the computer system, although the exact mechanism varies from system to system. When you have collected this type of data together, it can be used to provide counts of the numbers of patients or episodes (such as the number of patients admitted under a particular consultant in a specified time period). It can also be used to identify a group of patients that you want to study further using some other data source like their patient records (such as all patients who underwent a total hip replacement).

Departmental information systems

In much the same way as hospital information systems, departmental systems are designed to store data about patients which is relevant to a particular department. However, there are a number of departmental systems that hold data pertinent to the work of the whole hospital, such as the complaints database, accident and incident reporting system, and staff sickness, absence and turnover information held on the personnel system. In general, departmental systems collect more detailed information about patients than do hospital information systems and the nature of the data will vary greatly from system to system. Data collected might include information on GP referrals to a department; details of the investigations or procedures undergone by patients and their results; text describing patients' admissions, treatments and complications; and other clinical details. As with hospital information systems, this data can be used to generate numbers of certain events relevant to the department (such as the number of a type of investigation or procedure, and to identify groups of cases or patients for further study).

Routine paper records

Computer-based information systems can be very useful for gathering data together for a quality improvement project, but when computer data are not available or not accessible, you often need to use the many routine paper records kept in departments. These include registers, ledgers, books, files, forms and others. For example, theatre lists are ideal sources for identifying the sample of patients to be included in an audit concerning a particular operation. Appointment books can be used to start an audit of missed appointments. Although using routine paper records can be laborious, they are often the only available source for the data you need.

Patient records

The patient's individual records are generally the most complete and comprehensive source of information about his or her care and treatment, with information from all the professions involved recorded in one or more case record files. Data that are typically collected from this source include: staff groups involved in the care of a patient; drugs prescribed; tests and investigations carried out; and patterns of management for particular conditions. Patient records are one of the richest sources of data available, but they can be difficult both to find and to use as a data source once they have been found. The data they contain is largely unstructured, so data extraction can be time-consuming.

People

For information that is rich in detail, written records are not always the best source. Patients, carers and staff groups involved in providing care often need to be approached to obtain information about their experiences, opinions and attitudes relating to the quality problem being studied. There are, of course, other people to consider too, such as general practitioners, purchasers and relatives. Often information is collected from people to measure their satisfaction with care. Data can be collected through questionnaires that are filled in or through interviews, meetings, focus groups and user panels.

Collecting data using questionnaires

In many audit or quality improvement projects, data are collected using some sort of questionnaire format – a carefully thought-out, highly structured list of questions, designed to gather specific items of information. This next section will outline how to collect data using questionnaires.

Questionnaires can be used when screening or reviewing patient records, when distributing self-completion questionnaires to staff or patients, or when carrying out semi-structured interviews with patients. The same rules that govern the construction of a questionnaire given to people to fill in also apply to the development of an interview schedule and to the creation of a data collection form for you to use yourself in gathering data from patient records and other sources.

Who collects the data?
The main difference between a data collection form (used to gather data from patient records), a questionnaire and an interview schedule lies in who completes them.

- **Data collection forms** – usually completed by trained staff who are accustomed to patient records and who have often been involved in the design of the data collection form. The information is usually abstracted from patient records or some other source, and each member of staff will fill in many data collection forms (indeed, all the data may be collected by one person). Any problems encountered in the use of the forms can be discussed between the staff and solved as they occur.
- **Questionnaires** – completed individually by staff or patients, each interpreting the questions in their own way and without discussing the questionnaire with the other people who are completing it. This means that the only way to ensure that each question is understood in the same way by everyone filling in the questionnaire is to construct it in an unambiguous, user-friendly format. For this reason, the development of a data collection form for use by trained staff is usually far easier than the development of a questionnaire for use in a survey.
- **An interview schedule** – administered by a person trained to interview people. They ask questions of the participants either in a face-to-face meeting or over the telephone. The interview schedule guides the interviewer in terms of both the phrasing of the questions and the noting of the responses, which can be recorded by hand or on tape.

Table 3.2 indicates some of the characteristics of each of these methods which you might like to consider before deciding how to collect data for your project. For example, although the response rate for face-to-face interviews is high, the cost of carrying out such a survey is also high, compared with a high response rate for telephone interviews, at only a moderate cost. Alternatively, if you want to carry out a survey that guarantees anonymity and does not have an interviewer bias, then you would probably choose to send out a questionnaire by post.

Designing your questionnaire
There are some simple rules which can help produce a well-designed, unambiguous and easily understandable questionnaire. Some of the important issues for consideration include what subjects to include in the questionnaire, how to structure questions and how questions will be worded. In the next section, some guidance is given on how to address each of these issues when designing a questionnaire.

The subjects you need to include in the questionnaire can be identified by carrying out a literature search, by looking at established questionnaires on the topic that other people have used, by looking at questionnaires used by other departments in your organization, and by getting a team of people together to produce a list of the key areas they think need to be addressed.

Table 3.2

Comparison of various characteristics in postal, telephone and face-to-face data collection

Characteristic	Survey type		
	Postal	Telephone	Face to face
Data collection costs	Moderate	Moderate	High
Time for data collection	Long	Short	Long
Control over respondent selection	Low/moderate	High	High
Response rate	Moderate	High	High
Length of questionnaire	Moderate/long	Short	Long
Complexity of questionnaire	Moderate	Simple	Complex
Completion of tedious questions	Moderate	Moderate	High
Completion of sensitive questions	Moderate	Moderate	High
Interviewer bias and error	None	Moderate	Moderate/high
Number of open responses	Moderate	Low	High
Perceived respondent anonymity	Moderate/high	Moderate/high	Low

Reproduced with the permission of Brighton Health Care NHS Trust.

- **Literature search.** A literature search, which can usually be done for you by library staff, will produce a list of journal articles written on and around the subject area in question. A number of the articles will be studies in which questionnaires were used, and these questionnaires are often included in an appendix to the article. You can learn from the problems and issues that the authors of the articles encountered and you can use their questionnaires as a guide when constructing your own.
- **Established questionnaires.** There are many long-established questionnaires which have been rigorously tested by their designers for their reliability and validity and which you might want to use. Many of these ready-made questionnaires cover a range of subjects and have subsets of questions which can be used to address a particular topic.
- **Questionnaires used in your organization.** You may also find your colleagues in other departments have already administered questionnaires in related, or even the same, subject areas as yours. You therefore need to find out what others have done already and whether you can use or amend the questionnaire that they administered.
- **Key issues.** By drawing up a list of the key issues for your audit project, you can identify the main areas on which your questions need to focus. If you produce this list of issues with a team that involves everyone participating in the project, then you should be able to identify all the issues your questionnaire needs to address.

The sort of information you will get from your questionnaire depends on the type of question you use. There is no point in collecting data for the sake of it. You need to be able to do something with them and they should be relevant to the project's objectives. The main sorts of information that you can gather using a questionnaire are:

- **Facts.** Information about the respondent and people known to them (such as their age, sex, education, medical history, eating habits, attendance at screening programmes, procedures undergone and so on). In this category, it can be tempting to collect too much data that which will never be analysed, simply because 'it would be interesting to know *x*, *y* or *z*'.
- **Opinions and attitudes.** The respondent's opinions on or attitudes to various subjects (such as staff attitudes towards caring for dying patients, or patients' opinions about the quality of care experienced during an inpatient stay).
- **Knowledge base.** An assessment of the level of knowledge that the respondent has on any subject (such as the knowledge among nursing staff about hospital acquired infections, or diabetic patients' understanding of their condition).
- **Beliefs.** Respondents' beliefs about a given situation or set of circumstances (such as what they expect to happen when they see the doctor at an outpatient clinic, or what they believe will happen during their admission).
- **Intentions.** Respondents' intentions in areas such as their future actions or behaviour (such as patients' plans to give up smoking or change their diet, or mothers' preferences for analgesia during labour).

Types of question
Once the type of information required has been agreed, the next step is to write the questions. There are two main forms of question: closed and open. They produce very different forms of response:

- **Closed questions.** Closed questions are formatted in such a way that they can only be answered by using one of a number of given options. For example, you might give respondents a choice of Yes or No, or ask them to select Male or Female, or you might give them a list of choices from which they can choose one option (such as marital status, where they choose between the options Single, Married, Separated, Divorced or Widowed). Another kind of closed question is one where you give the respondent a numbered scale each end of which has a meaning. For example, you might ask people to rate the pain felt from 1 (meaning no pain) to 5 (meaning a great deal of pain). This kind of scale is called a Likert scale and is often used in questionnaires. Data collected in this way is perfect for statistical analysis, since all responses can be allocated a certain value and can be coded accordingly. The main disadvantage of closed questions is that response options are predetermined by the group who construct the questionnaire. This means that respondents may feel forced to give an answer that does not truly reflect their opinions.

- **Open questions.** Open questions ask for a free text response (answers in the respondent's own words). Examples include 'Why?' 'Please explain?' and 'How?' They may produce simple one-word answers, but can produce paragraphs of text. There is little doubt that open questions yield far richer information than closed questions but it is advisable to think carefully about when and where to use them. Be sure that you do want more information than can be generated from a series of closed questions, and use open questions sparingly. When it is time to analyse the responses, free text gathered from open questions is not easy to deal with. One approach used in large studies is called content analysis. It involves identifying themes within people's free text answers which are then used to develop closed questions in place of those open questions.
- **Combining closed and open questions.** This is where closed and open questions are used in combination. For example, a closed question may be used to determine whether the subject matter applies to the respondent and if it does then an open question can be used to gauge their opinion in more depth.

Wording the questions

If you are intending to distribute a set of questions to a wide-ranging group of people and expect those questions to have the same meaning to all of them, the wording of the questions is of great importance. There are a number of rules that can help you to make sure questions are clear, unambiguous and understandable:

- **Use simple language.** Avoid flowery prose and long sentences. In most cases, the shorter your questions the better. Questions should be written using clear, simple and unambiguous language and you should avoid the use of jargon and abbreviations. In healthcare we use many jargon words, technical terms and acronyms which to members of the public are often either meaningless or mean very different things. The safest course to take is not to use such terms in your questions and to use ordinary language instead, even if it means making the questions longer. Of course, you should also beware of making the wording too simple and patronizing. A good way to check your wording is to get people from other departments to read the questions to see if they understand them.
- **Be consistent.** Once you have decided on which words you will use to refer to particular procedures, conditions and people, make sure that they are used in the same way throughout the questionnaire. For example, if you say 'doctor' do you mean consultant, senior house officer, registrar or general practitioner?
- **Do not assume common knowledge.** Do not assume that respondents will know everything that you know. Try not to make assumptions about respondents' knowledge and remember that you need to make things explicit in your questions which you would not need to when talking to colleagues. For example, not everyone knows what a 'biopsy' is.
- **Avoid leading questions.** Do not be tempted to put words into the mouths of respondents, by asking questions that presuppose or encourage a particular

answer; for example, 'Don't you agree that nurses play an indispensable role in the multidisciplinary team?' If you ask such a question, your results may well be skewed and not a true reflection of the situation that you are trying to measure.

- **Avoid double-barrelled questions.** It is a common mistake in questionnaire design to combine two questions into one. For example, 'Have you experienced any pain or nausea since your operation?' asks two questions in one. If the respondent answers Yes, all you will know is that they had pain, or had nausea, or had both, but you will not know which. Instead, break the question into its two parts, each of which can then be answered with a Yes or No response.

- **Be aware of the social desirability effect.** Some questions may involve issues that are affected by notions of prestige, self-image or wanting to say the right thing. For example, when you ask whether people have understood what the doctor told them about their condition, experience shows that many people who have not understood will say that they have because they do not want to appear stupid. In this kind of situation it is better to ask questions that will allow you to assess their level of understanding directly, or to find a way of asking the question which is free of any stigma.

- **Use care with questions referring to time.** Many questions ask respondents to recall information from memory, such as what pain they felt or how long they waited in clinic. However, people's memories are distorted over the course of time and their responses to questions about time should be treated with caution. It is also important that the time period to which the question refers is described in precise terms. For example, when asking the question 'What happened during the last week?', do you mean in the last seven days, or from Sunday to Saturday, or from Monday to Sunday or from Monday to Friday?

- **Collect only essential data.** The line between what data are necessary and what data would be interesting is very easily crossed. For most people involved in audit or quality improvement, both time and money are issues. For this reason (and to reduce the risk that respondents are put off by the length of the questionnaire), it is best to stick to the essential information that is directly related to the project's objectives.

- **Think carefully about the type of question to use.** Closed questions, which were discussed earlier, are quicker to answer and the data from such questions are simpler to analyse. Open questions are much more difficult to handle in a consistent way. For this reason, they should be used sparingly and reserved for issues about which you really need more information than would be obtained from closed questions.

- **Collect data only on subjects that you can do something about.** It may seem obvious, but even though the length of time someone waited for a bus may affect their attendance at an outpatient clinic, unless you plan to take over the bus company there is nothing that you can do about it. It is therefore questionable whether you should collect this information in the first place.

Getting responses to questionnaires

You also need to consider the point of contact for your study (how the questionnaire is to be distributed to the people in your sample). Usually, there are two options. You can hand questionnaires out to people and then collect them, or you can send them out and have them returned by post.

- **Postal questionnaire surveys.** In this type of survey, the questionnaires are either posted or handed out to the sample and a stamped addressed envelope is enclosed for the return of the completed questionnaire. Postal questionnaires can easily reach a large sample of people and they give a degree of anonymity to respondents. However, the response rate is likely to be lower than for questionnaires that are handed out, the postage costs can be high, and if respondents are anonymous it is not possible to identify and chase non-responders. Postal surveys generally produce a return rate of 65–75%. Failure to include a stamped addressed envelope or Freepost address will further reduce the response rate.
- **Handout questionnaire surveys.** Questionnaires in this type of survey are handed out directly to the respondents, completed and returned to an identified collection point more or less immediately. They can also be posted back to the audit team with a stamped addressed envelope. If handed out and collected in person, they have the advantages that response rates tend to be higher and it is easy to identify non-respondents. However, respondents may not have time to fill in the questionnaire on the spot and this approach does not allow them any time to reflect on the questions and give considered answers. Respondents may also be less willing to be critical when they are filling in their questionnaire in the hospital or clinic rather than in their own home.

There are many other factors that can affect the response rate to questionnaires:

- its layout (clarity helps);
- the subject itself (sensitive subjects can get very low or very high response rates);
- its length (the longer it is, the lower the response);
- the content and complexity of the questions;
- whether or not respondents feel it is anonymous (most respondents prefer anonymity).

A covering letter should go out with the questionnaire explaining about the audit and what is required of the respondent. The letter needs to include information on who you are, what the aim of the survey is, why the person has been chosen, what they are being asked to do, how long you think it will take them and an assurance that the process is confidential and anonymous.

If the response rate is low, the suspicion will arise that the people who have returned their questionnaires might be different, in some way, from those who have not. For example, people who were not satisfied with their care might be more inclined to respond than those who were. To try to avoid this, you can code or number questionnaires before they are sent out so that you can identify people who have not responded and send them a reminder.

Piloting the questionnaire
When you are going to use a questionnaire to collect information from patients and/or staff, it is always advisable to carry out a small pilot study first. This involves giving the questionnaire to a small number of people (usually just five or ten) to test out how they fill it in and what problems they encounter. In this way, questions that are not clear or that are misunderstood by the pilot sample can be readily identified. Other problems such as duplication of question content in more than one question can also be highlighted by the pilot study. Even experienced questionnaire designers usually find they need to make significant changes to their questionnaire after the pilot study.

If you do not pilot your questionnaire first, you may find when your data are analysed that one of the questions has been consistently misinterpreted and so that item of data is of little or no use. A short pilot study is often effective in preventing this kind of wasted effort.

Data analysis
The team may be clear about the data collection strategy, but it is also important to determine how the data are going to be analysed and by whom. If staff have access to additional organizational resources, such as an IT or clinical audit department, it is worth finding out how they can assist, such as with statistical packages, developing spreadsheets or other data analysis.

Analysing and presenting data
Following the design of the questionnaire and/or collection of data, the next task is to analyse and present the results. Consideration therefore needs to be given on how to present the results in a way that is clear and understandable.

How to analyse the data
In some small-scale projects, analysing the data by hand may be the quickest way. To most people, however, spending several hours face-to-face with pages of numbers and a calculator is an onerous task. There are many computer software packages that incorporate both data input and data analysis in their facilities. There are some quite complex packages (such as SPSS, the Statistics Package for Social Sciences) that perform sophisticated statistical analyses, but most audit and quality improvement projects do not require that level of sophistication. Simple databases (like Epi Info) offer all the facilities that are commonly used in the analysis of data collected in audit and quality improvement projects. Many organizations have audit, information or computing departments that can help.

STAFFORDSHIRE
UNIVERSITY
LIBRARY

Table 3.3	Value label	Value	Frequency	%	Cumulative %
Example of descriptive data produced from a questionnaire regarding methods of transport	Car	1	18	25.7	25.7
	Public transport	2	27	38.5	64.2
	On foot	3	9	12.9	77.1
	Hospital transport	4	15	21.4	98.5
	Missing cases		1	1.5	100.0
	Total		70	100.0	
	Valid cases		69		

Reproduced with the permission of Brighton Health Care NHS Trust.

What to look for in the data

A good starting point is to produce a description of the data. This means looking at the average response and the extremes for each question or data item. A description of the data would include the minimum and maximum values given as a response and the value most commonly given as a response. Another way to look at the description of the data is to produce a frequency table for each question which lists each possible response and how often it was given (like Table 3.3). As Table 3.3 illustrates, it is inappropriate to produce an 'average' method of transport and so in this instance describing data involves listing frequencies.

Reading through the descriptions of the data will help you to identify where to look for relationships among the data. Observe which questions are producing responses that are associated with responses to other questions. For example, did those patients who reported a high level of pain on the first day postoperatively tend to be those who had undergone one particular procedure? Also note any interesting differences between groups. For example, did those who were treated as day cases require less medication than those who were inpatients? Whatever the particular questions you want to answer, it is advisable to:

- produce descriptive statistics such as the minimum, maximum, median, and frequency counts for all questions or data items;
- use these to guide the cross-tabulations you carry out if you decide you need to look for associations within and differences between groups.

How to present the results

There are basically two ways in which you can present your results – a written report, or a series of charts and graphics that you use to make a presentation. Usually a combination of the two (a visual presentation backed up by a written report that contains detailed explanations of the project and resulting data) will be the most effective. The audience will understand and remember much more about the findings if you combine the visual power of charts and graphics, your verbal description of the results, and the written materials in a report.

Data can be presented graphically in the form of tables, pie charts, bar charts and histograms. Each has its own strengths and weaknesses, which you should be aware

Table 3.4	Consultant referred to	Patients referred				
Example of a table (good example)		Males		Females		Total
		(n)	(%)	(n)	(%)	(n)
	A	83	33	41	40	124
	B	67	27	24	24	91
	C	98	40	36	36	134
	Total	248	100	101	100	349

Reproduced with the permission of Brighton Health Care NHS Trust.

of when choosing how to illustrate your results. In the next section, we offer some ideas on how you should and should not use these ways of presenting data.

Tables

Tables are most useful for showing the relationships between different factors. For example, you might show mean length of stay (factor 1) according to procedure (factor 2).

In the example in Table 3.4 it can be seen that:

- the table has a title;
- the sample size is indicated;
- all the rows and columns are labelled;
- the frequency counts add up to the sample size total;
- the figures in the column showing percentages add up to 100%;
- each row can be tracked through the table.

In the example in Table 3.5, there is a portion of a table that was not constructed using any of the above rules.

The table in Table 3.5 does not have a title and there is no indication of either where the sample was drawn from or the sample size. To make matters worse, the number of patients for whom there is information reported changes from one column to the next. The rows are not labelled and the labels given to the columns are meaningless because we don't know where the sample has come from. Far too many factors (variables) have been included in the table.

The rows are not used in a consistent way throughout the table. In two columns there are only two rows of information, while in others there are as many as four.

Table 3.5	No. of patients	Diagnosis category	Age of patient	Sex of patient
Example of a table (poor example)	12 of 60	8 definite 13%	Under 65 = 3	Male = 8
	20%	2 query 16%	Over 65 = 9	Female = 4
		1 unrelated	Over 80 = 4	
		1 no information	Average = 74	

Reproduced with the permission of Brighton Health Care NHS Trust.

Finally, cumulative totals have been used within the table without any indication that they are not frequency counts. A much better way is to report the frequency counts in the table and the actual totals at the ends of rows and columns. If cumulative totals are required, they should be in a separate column that is clearly labelled as the cumulative totals column.

Pie charts

Pie charts are often used to show the contrasts or differences within a data set. Differences in proportions (such as the percentage of patients who underwent one of three procedures) are far clearer if displayed as a pie chart rather than in a table. In the example in Figure 3.3,

- the pie chart has a title;
- the sample size is indicated;
- each segment is labelled;
- the labels do not overlap (it is advisable to limit the number of segments in any pie chart to a maximum of five or six).

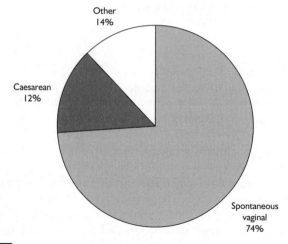

Figure 3.3

Example of a pie chart (good example) (reproduced with the permission of Brighton Health Care NHS Trust)

There are also times when pie charts are not suitable and can be very hard to understand; an example is shown in Figure 3.4. The immediate impact of differences in the sizes of segments (the most powerful function of a pie chart) is lost because of the sheer number of segments. If the results you are trying to portray with a pie chart involve a large number of response values, as in this example, there is something that you can do to make the chart work. By combining those responses that have low frequency counts into a category called 'Other', you can

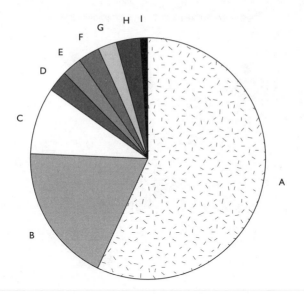

Figure 3.4

Example of a pie chart (poor example) (reproduced with the permission of Brighton Health Care NHS Trust)

produce a chart more like that shown in Figure 3.3. It is now much easier to compare the relative proportions of each segment.

Another problem that arises when you have too many segments is that the labels begin to overlap, or are printed in a font size so small that they are difficult to read on an overhead slide. One final hint is to include the percentages by each segment. Even if the actual number of responses is reported next to each segment, the percentage makes it much easier to see the pattern of responses of the whole sample.

Bar charts and histograms

Bar charts and histograms are different, although people sometimes use the two names interchangeably. Essentially, bar charts are used to display data from discrete categories whereas histograms (or frequency polygons) are used to show grouped data (like the daily temperature ranges in Figure 3.5). Both are used to illustrate the distribution of values across a sample. They provide a visual way of presenting the frequency counts produced in a frequency table in a description of a data set. In the example of a bar chart in Figure 3.6,

- the chart has a title;
- the sample size is indicated;
- the axes are clearly and properly labelled.

With the increased availability of software packages to produce graphics, it is tempting to produce impressive but confusing charts. Many people find three-dimensional

STAFFORDSHIRE
UNIVERSITY
LIBRARY

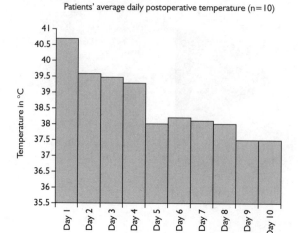

Figure 3.5

Example of a histogram (reproduced with the permission of Brighton Health
Care NHS Trust)

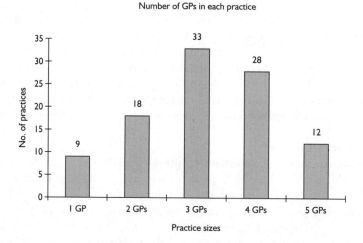

Figure 3.6

Example of a bar chart (reproduced with the permission of Brighton Health
Care NHS Trust)

bar charts almost irresistible and they are encouraged by the common use of such
graphics on television and in journals. However, such bar charts can be difficult
to read and can be very misleading. Figure 3.7 shows a three-dimensional bar chart.
Its visual impact is strong, but, if you look at the actual data values you can see that

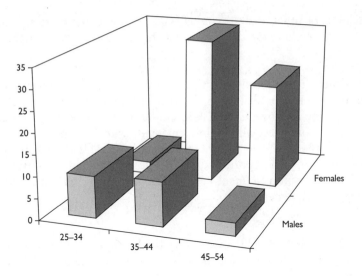

Figure 3.7

Example of a 3D bar chart (reproduced with the permission of Brighton Health Care NHS Trust)

the chart is actually highly misleading, because it is very hard to know how far up the vertical axis each bar comes.

Report writing

Writing a comprehensive and interesting project report at the end of the work is important if findings are to be disseminated. It is often helpful to base the report around the project objectives that you set out earlier in the planning stage. Some suggestions for sections to include follow.

Introduction

Use this section to set the scene, report any relevant research findings or other work, highlight anything of importance from your literature review, explain the reasons for undertaking the audit project and set out the project's aims and objectives.

Method

Explain how the project was undertaken. Include things like how and why the sample was chosen, what measurement tools were used and how they were found or developed and anything else that people will need to know about what you have done.

Results and discussion

Report the results of your data collection, including both the facts and figures from tables, charts and diagrams, together with some commentary on the results and their meaning. This would also be where you would include any statistics, cross-tabulations or other analysis you have done. In a large report you may want to have separate sections for the results and the discussion of what they mean.

Proposals
These should not be produced until the team involved in the project has met to discuss the results. It should include the specific proposals made for changes in practice and quality improvements. There should be details of any resources those changes require, how they will be implemented, who is responsible for taking action and what the timescale for the changes will be. This is probably the most important section of your report, and the whole area of finding solutions to the quality problem once measurement has been carried out is dealt with in the next section (Stage 3, Implementation).

Conclusions
Your report conclusions should cover a very brief summary of the key findings of the project and its implications for the service or process involved. There should also be an indication in the conclusions of when you plan to return to this quality problem to check that the changes set out in your proposals have actually been effected. As part of Stage 2, planning the audit cycle, it can be appreciated that careful planning of the data collection, analysis and presentation of results is fundamental in achieving a worthwhile audit project. Many clinical audit projects will need to involve patients or service users in the data collection process. Consideration for their involvement is given in the section below.

The role of the patient in audit
Anderson (1989) is quoted as stating,

> *the difference between the provider of health services and the patient resembles that between the hen and the pig in the preparation of eggs and bacon. The hen is involved but the pig is committed.*

It would seem obvious that patients who use the services of the NHS should have a legitimate voice in the planning, delivery and evolution of these services. However, very often the voices of the patients are only ever sought when auditing how effective services are and eliciting patient satisfaction responses.

Cooke (1994) suggests there are three broad approaches underlying research on patients' views. These are:

- **The consumer approach** – which has emphasized the role of the patient as a consumer of the service. The tendency here has been to concentrate on the public image of the services and to involve patients in deciding on, for example, the curtains and wallpaper. Although patients complain about poor environmental facilities, there is an assumption that they do this because these issues are of most importance to them. However, they are rarely given the opportunity to comment on their satisfaction with the clinical content of care, since professionals may feel that patients are incapable of forming a judgement on these issues.

- **The paternalistic approach.** Cooke (1994) suggests this stems from nurses believing that dissatisfaction with care is a failure of the nurse–patient relationship. Buckenham (1986) supports this view and suggests this is because nurses do not believe that patients can make judgements about quality of nursing care based on interpersonal aspects. This view has been confirmed by other authors (Jennings, 1981; Van Essen, 1991) who suggest that this is 'an ideological denial of legitimacy' by professionals who are anxious to retain power.
- **The democratic approach.** Groups predominantly outside the NHS believe decisions by patients represent a legitimate factor in developing health services. Patients appear to be asked to validate professional views of quality, but are not invited to define their own view of quality (Kelman, 1976).

In conclusion, other methods of involving patients in audit need to be sought. These must involve processes that are not predetermined standardized questionnaires based on the values and assumptions of professionals. Forms, interviews and open-ended questions that enable patients to make honest responses about their care and experiences will more likely provide an accurate reflection of what the service really is and provide the basis for change.

However, although many health professionals agree with this concept, there are still limitations to its application within an NHS organization. Standardized survey techniques are often based on the assumptions and values of the professionals within an organization and not on the genuine views of patients.

Costing the project

It is important at the planning stage to identify any resources required. Such costs typically include:

- training individuals to undertake the audit;
- staff time from other departments, e.g. finance, clinical audit;
- costs of producing and sending questionnaires;
- expenses for participants.

In conclusion, the principles of constructing questionnaires are invaluable for the data collection stage of the audit cycle, hence the detail on this important issue outlined above.

Once all of the components of the project have been agreed, a summary of the project should be pulled together in the form of a project plan. Table 3.6 shows an example of a simple audit project plan. The plan can be used as a bid for funding audit projects or as a basis for renewing potential costs and amending the audit if the costs exceed the budget allowed.

Stage 3. Implementation

This stage involves implementing the audit plan. It will incorporate data collection and analysis, dissemination of results, and managing any changes that may be required.

Table 3.6

Simple audit project plan

Audit topic:	Patients admitted to the Medical Admissions Unit
Objectives:	1 To determine whether they receive a full assessment of physical, psychological and social needs. 2 To determine whether the multidisciplinary team receive relevant referrals following assessment. 3 To confirm that the discharge plan is instigated within 2 h.
Involvement:	• Medical Admissions Unit. • Social Work Department.
Patients:	All patients admitted to the unit.
Time period:	Over the next three months.
Data collection strategy:	Concurrent using patients' medical records.

Although members of the audit team may feel it unnecessary to meet until this stage has been completed, it is worth addressing how to keep records of the meeting to monitor progress. Notes of audit meetings should include:

• the outcomes of the meetings and achievements to date
• correspondence sent/received
• incidents and events crucial to the project
• how long each phase has taken

This can provide information to other clinical audit teams which is useful at the re-audit stage or if they should ever undertake a similar project in the future.

Once all the data have been collected, analysed and written up, the team needs to discuss its dissemination strategy. This will depend on what the project is and who would value the information. Ways of achieving this include:

• e-mail
• focus groups
• in-house presentations
• reports
• Internet

. . . or a mixture of the above, depending whether the results are to be used internally, for the board, to purchasers, to regions, to GPs, or nationally. The evidence base for effective dissemination strategies was outlined in more detail in the case study at the end of chapter 2.

Making changes

The results will need thorough discussion. It is important to identify what changes need to be made and how they will be achieved. Chapter 5 will address ways in which changes can be successfully managed. It is important that the audit project team all agree with the changes and are involved in planning these.

Stage 4. Evaluation

The purpose of evaluating audit is to determine which elements of the project contributed to a successful outcome and which factors may have inhibited the full potential of the project. Questions to ask include:

- Did we achieve our objectives? If not, why not?
- If problems did arise, was it due to unforeseen events, interpersonal problems with colleagues, or incidents that were beyond the control of the audit team? The project team need to know if problems arose because of lack of planning, or unpredictable events. This should be a constructive, rather than critical, process.
- What changes or improvements have been made?
- Does the project either entirely or in part need revisiting in order to test whether the changes have had an impact?

Reviewing projects in this way ensures the teams reflect and learn, thus increasing the chance of future projects being more successful.

The above section has covered the four stages of the audit cycle:

- Select.
- Plan.
- Implement.
- Evaluate.

The next section will provide a case study of a local audit project to illustrate the application of these principles.

Clinical audit: a case study – ward audit and pain management

Here we present a baseline audit which looked at how ward-based nurses were managing patients' pain. As we discussed in Chapter 2, the evidence that provided the conceptual foundation for this review was the two pain guidelines published by the US Agency for Healthcare Policy and Research (1995). Each pain guideline makes a number of recommendations. For example, the one on cancer pain makes 66 specific recommendations. To audit all 66 in one go would have been an enormous task. Therefore, it was necessary to prioritize the specific areas that staff felt were the most important to review first. The areas that staff chose to review formed the basis of our objectives. These included:

- to review how pain is documented;

- to identify what assessment tools were being used to manage patients' pain;
- to assess what written protocols are used for managing patients' pain;
- to ascertain what access staff have to pharmacological and non-pharmacological interventions.

As the aim of this audit was to identify current practices on individual wards, it was decided that a ward questionnaire would be the best approach for collecting the necessary data.

The sample size for this audit was relatively straightforward. Twenty-eight of the 30 wards were eligible for the audit, in that they had a quality focus group link worker at the time of the data collection. These 28 wards therefore formed our sample group. Before they were sent a questionnaire, the link workers were invited to attend one or two educational workshops, where the rationale for this audit was explained. We piloted the original questionnaire on four wards, and following some amendments the final questionnaire was sent out to the link worker on each of the 28 wards. The questionnaires were coded so that any link worker who had not returned their questionnaire could be sent a reminder. In total 24 wards responded, giving a response rate of 86%.

Our first objective sought to identify how pain was documented. Both the cancer pain and acute pain guidelines emphasize the importance of documenting pain. Although based on panel consensus, both guidelines stress that 'clinicians should assess pain with easily administered rating scales and should document the efficacy of pain relief at regular intervals after starting or changing treatment. Documentation forms should be readily accessible to all clinicians involved in the patient's care' (Jacox, Carr and Payne, 1994). Lack of documentation is an issue raised by a number of commentators; Max (1990) observes that pain management is not perceived to be important, as it does not justify the provision of a designated patient record: 'unlike "vital signs", pain isn't displayed in a prominent place on the chart or at the bedside or nursing station'. In other words, pain is not 'visible'.

Because we had clearly defined objectives at the start of this audit, this made the construction of the questionnaire much easier. For example, the first question our linkworkers were asked was 'Does your ward use a specially designed document to record patients' pain?' If the respondent said No they were directed to question 3; if they said Yes they were asked to complete question 2, shown in Table 3.7.

Link workers on 13 wards reported using specially designed documentation to record patients' pain. Question 2 was based on a combination of expert opinion (McCaffery and Beebe, 1994; Biallie, 1993; Bourbonnais, 1981) and recommendations based on panel consensus in both pain guidelines. Table 3.8 illustrates that none of the 13 specially designed pain charts meets all the criteria.

The evidence for the use of defined requirements, i.e guidelines, standards, etc., for improving patient management is well documented. It has been suggested that guidelines offer a vehicle by which the latest research findings can be translated into practice; as Humphries comments, they are the 'union of research,

Table 3.7	**Does the specially designed document include space to complete the following:** (please tick all that apply)		
Pain documentation criteria: link worker questions		**Yes**	**No**
	Date and time of onset of pain		
	Duration of pain		
	Information on what increases/decreases pain		
	Space for the patient to include a description of their pain		
	A body chart		

Reproduced with the permission of Brighton Health Care NHS Trust.

Table 3.8	**Criterion**	**Yes**	**No**
Assessment of pain charts against criteria for documenting patient pain	Date and time of onset of pain	12	1
	Duration of pain	8	5
	Information on what increases or decreases pain	10	3
	Space for patients to include a description of pain	11	2
	Body chart used to identify the location of pain	10	3
	A tool to measure the intensity of the patient's pain	12	1

Reproduced with the permission of Brighton Health Care NHS Trust.

experience and expert opinion' (1994). Grimshaw and Russell's 1993 study provides the evidence that guidelines can lead to improvements in patient care. In our audit we found that guidelines and standards for the management of pain existed on only eight wards.

The next question that all the link workers were asked was whether staff on their ward use an assessment tool to measure patients' pain. Once again, this objective was based on sound evidence; as Ferrel and colleagues remark, 'communication among healthcare professionals is paramount in assessing pain and is best facilitated by objective measures of pain' (1991). Fifteen of the 24 link workers said that an assessment tool is used on their ward to measure patients' pain.

The same approach – using questions based on expert opinion or evidence-based recommendations – was used to ask questions about pharmacological approaches to pain management, for example the use of patient-controlled analgesia (PCA) devices and syringe drivers.

Similarly, non-pharmacological interventions were also reviewed, as Ferrel and colleagues observe that 'non-pharmacological management of pain is acknowledged as an important component of pain treatment but is vastly under-used in clinical practice' (1991). Our audit highlighted that heat pads are a most popular non-pharmacological intervention, being used on 13 of the wards. In the cancer pain guideline the strength of evidence for the use of cutaneous stimulation techniques, i.e. heat pads and massage is not strong, being graded at C. This means the recommendation is based on the available empirical evidence but is based primarily on expert opinion. Indeed, the cancer pain guideline highlights how the literature is divided on the use of superficial heat for cancer patients. However, because 'of the lack of research findings that clearly contra-indicate this use of superficial heat, the panel recommends that it be used as a method of pain control in patients with cancer' (Jacox, Carr and Payne, 1994).

The other area reviewed under the heading of non-pharmacological interventions was whether wards have information leaflets for patients on how to manage their pain. Only two link workers said that information leaflets were available on their wards. Access to written information was one of the recommendations made in a consensus statement by the American Pain Society Quality of Care Committee (1995):

> *The patient at risk of pain should be informed verbally and in an electronic or printed format at the time of the initial evaluation that effective pain relief is an important part of their treatment.*

Findings

Having collected and analysed our data, we returned to the original objectives of our audit and summarized our findings as follows:

- 13 of the wards surveyed use a specially designed sheet to document patients' pain.
- None of the 13 specially designed pain charts recorded all the criteria suggested by expert opinion.
- The link workers reported that an assessment tool to measure patients' pain was being used on 15 of the 24 wards.
- Eight link workers reported the existence of standards or guidelines for the management of pain on their wards.
- Ten link workers said that PCAs were used in their ward.
- 19 of the 22 wards that admitted patients with cancer used syringe drivers to manage these patients' pain.
- Heat pads were the most popular non-pharmacological intervention to relieve pain, being used on 13 wards. Massage ($n = 7$), relaxation therapy ($n = 6$) and reflexology ($n = 3$) were the other non-pharmacological approaches that the link workers reported using.
- Two link workers said that their ward had written information for patients about pain management.

Proposals

When we had reviewed the management of pain and identified areas where we felt practice could be improved, the next task was to turn these findings into recommendations for improving the quality of care. In other words, we needed an action plan. An action plan is a simple table that everyone involved in implementing the proposals needs to agree to. The table should include the following:

- what the *proposal* is;
- what *action(s)* needs to be taken;
- who is going to take *responsibility* for the action;
- a *completion date*.

So, for example, one of our proposals was that we needed a pain chart for the management of malignant pain. The action for this proposal was that a chart should be designed. The Head of Nursing in oncology took responsibility for setting up a team, and the team agreed to complete this task within three months.

Similar proposals were made for the production of patient information leaflets on pain management, the development of a pain assessment tool and the introduction of the acute and cancer pain guideline.

Just as we prioritized which areas to review in the audit, so it was with the action plan. Thus, because the evidence for non-pharmacological interventions was not as strong, we will look at the introduction of these techniques after the above proposals have been implemented. The key principles of developing tools for the audit guidelines are therefore:

- Prioritize the specific areas you want to audit and consider how reasonable it would be to audit all the guidelines or in part.
- Ensure there are clearly defined objectives for the purpose of the audit.
- Whatever method of data collection is agreed, e.g. questionnaire, ensure that it is piloted so that any problems can be eliminated.
- Ensure that the data are analysed and an agreed action plan is formulated and disseminated to all those involved in the project.

The criteria outlined earlier relating to undertaking audit apply here. All stages of the audit cycle should be followed to ensure that the audit tool is valid, can be replicated, and will bring about beneficial changes in clinical practice.

A final check must be to evaluate the effectiveness of the audit itself. This is critical if audit is to evolve and develop. Hence auditing audit and assessing its effectiveness has to be integral to any audit project or programme if it is to follow its first principles of 'closing the audit loop'. The next section looks at evaluating the effectiveness of clinical audit projects and programmes.

Assessing the effectiveness of clinical audit projects and programmes

Robinson identified that because clinical audit had not been fully implemented throughout the health service it was difficult to assess the impact of clinical audit (1995). The following questions and issues can be helpful when evaluating audit.

What impact has clinical audit had on the quality of care?
- Have waiting times reduced for patients?
- How have services improved, e.g. better information, communications systems?
- Are appointment systems more effective?
- Have changes been made to the clinical care that patients receive?

What impact on workload does clinical audit have?
- Has the resulting work from the clinical audit topic enhanced the health-care provided or added significantly to the stress of being able to manage effectively?
- Do individual professional groups believe that the effort put into clinical audit is worthwhile?

How has clinical audit affected individual professional groups?
- Has there been a positive increase in morale, or do professionals resent the increased time spent on non-clinical activities?
- Have all multidisciplinary groups benefited equally from the inclusion of clinical audit projects?
- Are professionals more aware of each other's contribution to care problems?

Have ongoing training needs been identified and addressed?
- Are individuals able to receive appropriate training to enable them to participate fully in clinical audit?

What dissemination strategies have been addressed?
- Is there a clear strategy for dissemination of results and findings of clinical audit project work?
- Are all directorates and departments aware of the end results of audit projects within the organization?

Is there a national or local effect on the result?
- Have the networks for local and national dissemination been fully utilized, e.g. e-mail, websites, local discussion groups, national registry of projects?

Factors that enhance or inhibit the development of clinical audit

In our experience, the success of any clinical audit project appears to be dependent upon the following four factors. Understanding and planning for these as part of the project can increase the likelihood of its success.

- **Education and Training.** Participants within any group require certain elements of knowledge which enable them to successfully implement each stage of the audit cycle. Individuals participating in audit can also benefit from developing skills and expertise in obtaining funding, designing projects, data collection and interpretation of results. Clinical audit groups may need to tap into external expertise if these skills are lacking. Without sufficient training and guidance, it is unlikely that sufficient rigour will be applied to the audit processes. Robust findings are essential if the effort invested in audit is to be worthwhile.
- **Time.** It is rare to find multidisciplinary groups who have specific time allocated to undertake audit activities. Generally, individuals will try to fit audit in and around their current work schedule. This can work, although

the following issues can cause problems. First, if individuals cannot attend meetings due to workload demands the project may take an inordinate length of time to complete. Second, enthusiasm may be affected if project work is undertaken in the participants' own time and individuals feel resentful at having to do this. Negotiation with managers is key in ensuring that audit projects have allocated work time ringfenced.

- **Lack of professional or managerial commitment.** If individual professional heads of department or managers are disinterested in the purpose of audit, they can undermine audit projects; first, by not allocating time so that therapists or nurses can participate in the audit process, and second, by preventing changes being implemented afterwards. This can be a particular problem if it is identified that further resources are required to make necessary changes. It is therefore crucially important to ensure from the outset the full commitment of those who may have a stake in either the process or the outcome.
- **Lack of resources/support.** This may be a lack of suitable places to meet, or inadequate information technology (IT) resources. The latter is particularly problematic if large amounts of data need to be managed, or if manual records need to be reviewed to find other information. The necessity for both clerical and IT support will often affect how quickly the project is completed and therefore has an impact on retaining the interest and involvement of other participants.

Although general audit projects differ from clinical audit projects, it is still important to address the effectiveness of audit at both programme and project level. The following framework can help to ensure that the right questions are asked of both processes.

Audit effectiveness

Lessons can often be learned from an audit project by evaluating how effective the project was and the way the whole process was managed. Therefore audit effectiveness can be assessed at two levels:

- the programme level
- the project level

Undertaking a review of programme/project effectiveness can aid in the following:

- identifying whether audit works, and feeding the results into local or national networks;
- assessing what elements of the audit process require improvement or revision;
- assessing what impact the audit has on patient care or service improvement;
- demonstrating whether the resources put into a clinical audit programme are justifiable.

The framework below can be used to evaluate either project or programme assessment, as many of the criteria are relevant to both. The questions could assist the evaluators to develop a clearer picture of what they are trying to achieve in undertaking a systematic review of effectiveness.

Strategic intent
- What is the objective of the evaluation?
- Will the results of the evaluation impact on further changes?
- How will the evaluation results be disseminated?
- Will policy decisions for the organizations be affected by the results?

Method
- Will the programme evaluation include all projects regardless of nature, e.g. service developments, changes in clinical care, etc.?
- Will a cost analysis be required for each project included?
- What factors represent successful audit, e.g. improvements in clinical care, higher patient satisfaction scoring in questionnaires, increased knowledge for audit participants, etc.?
- Will the programme/project evaluation take place at the end of the year or be incorporated into the current cycle in order to influence the outcome of the project/programme?

Bias/validity: who will undertake the evaluation ?
This may affect the results if undertaken by a key stakeholder. Other motives or agendas may affect the perspective of the individual. Therefore it is essential that the views of all representative groups are included within the evaluation.

There is little evidence at present to suggest that either project or programme evaluation techniques are effective, robust or sufficiently well developed for us to draw any significant conclusions as to the overall impact of clinical audit. However, future funding policies may well encourage closer examination of this aspect, in order to ascertain whether the time and effort invested in audit activity is justifiable.

SUMMARY AND CONCLUSIONS

In the 1970s and 1980s, audit was predominantly viewed as a professionally encapsulated activity. A number of factors have transpired which have influenced the focus and purpose of audit. *Working for Patients* (Department of Health, 1989) was published, which sought to shift the audit agenda to a more managerial focus concerned with resources. However in 1991 the DoH stated that audit 'was a matter for the medical profession and primarily an educational activity'. By 1993 the DoH had decided that 'clinical audit should always be clinically led but have some managerial contribution'.

Packwood and Kober (1995) suggest that several factors inhibit the integration of clinical audit with other forms of audit. These include:

- a lack of clear mechanisms on how this can be achieved;
- the underdeveloped nature of clinical audit;
- potential professional rivalry;
- a lack of adequate information systems, which prevents the integration of outcome measures into broader systematic consensus;
- differing professional views as to the purpose and process of clinical audit;
- a lack of a common view of the purpose of audit among managers and professionals.

There is clearly potential for clinical audit to relate to other audit and quality improvement activities. The above issues need to be addressed in order to ensure that clinical audit is recognized as part of a wider framework and not a stand-alone activity. There is the potential that weak links between clinical audit and wider organizational and national priorities may reduce the status and funding of this activity. Conversely, the changes described in the new White Paper (Department of Health, 1998), particularly the concept of clinical governance, lend weight to the argument that the development of clinical audit as a tool for measuring and, importantly, improving clinical practice is an important priority.

This latter point is fundamental in understanding the role and purpose of clinical audit. There is a commonly held misconception that clinical audit is solely about measurement. This is perhaps because of its association with financial audit in the minds of many non-clinicians. It is important to stress that measurement and data collection constitute only one part of the audit cycle. Clinical audit is a process that involves prioritizing quality issues, planning a project, implementing the plan and evaluating the impact of the project. These principles are transferable to a wide range of clinical settings and activities. The next chapter outlines a number of different methods commonly used in healthcare to measure best practice. For each and every one of these, the stages of the audit cycle are applicable. If measurement is seen as an end in itself, rather than a means to an end, it is unlikely that real and lasting improvements in clinical practice will result. Conversely, if it is viewed as part of a cycle which also includes understanding and interpreting the data and working with colleagues to improve practice, then real and lasting benefits can be obtained.

REFERENCES

Agency for Health Care Policy and Research (1995) *Using Clinical Practice Guidelines to Evaluate Quality of Care*, US Department of Health and Human Services, Rockville, MD.

American Pain Society Quality of Care Committee (1995) Quality improvement guidelines for the treatment of acute and cancer pain. *Journal of American Medical Association*, **274**(3), 515–27.

Anderson, J. (1989) Patient power in mental health. *British Medical Journal*, **299**, p. 1477–8.

Berwick, D. and Knappe, M. (1990) Theory and practice for measuring healthcare quality, in *Quality Assurance in Hospitals*, 2nd edn (ed. N. Graham), Aspen, Rockville, MA.

Biallie, L. (1993) A review of pain assessment tools. *Nursing Standard*, 7, 25–9.

Bourbonnais, F. (1981) Pain assessment: development of a tool for the nurse and the patient. *Journal of Advanced Nursing*, 6, 277–82.

Buckenham, M. (1986) Patients' points of view. *Senior Nurse*, 4(3), 26–7.

Cooke, H. (1994) The role of the patient in standard setting and audit. *British Journal of Nursing*, 3(22), 1182–8.

Deming, W. (1986) *Out of the Crisis*, MIT Center for Advanced Engineering Study, Cambridge, MA.

Department of Health (1989) *Working for Patients*, White Paper, HMSO, London.

Department of Health (1991) *Medical Audit in the Hospital and Community Health Services*, Health Circular HC(91)2, HMSO, London.

Department of Health (1993) *Clinical Audit: Meeting and Improving Standards in Healthcare*, Department of Health, London.

Department of Health (1994) *The Evolution of Clinical Audit*, Department of Health, Leeds.

Ferrel, B. Wisdon, C., Rhiner, M. and Alletto, J. (1991) Pain management as a quality of care outcome. *Journal of Nursing Quality Assurance*, 5(2), 50–8.

Gillies, A. (1997) *Improving the Quality of Patient Care*, John Wiley, Chichester.

Grimshaw, J. and Russell, I. (1993) Effect of clinical guidelines on medical practice: a systematic review of rigorous evaluations. *Lancet*, 342, 1317–22.

Humphries, D. (1994) Clinical guidelines: an industry for growth. *Nursing Times*, 90(40), 45–7.

Hunt, V. and Legg, F. (1994) *Clinical Audit: A Basic Introduction*, Oxford University, Oxford.

Jacox, A., Carr, D.B. and Payne, R. (1994) *Management of Cancer Pain*, Clinical Practice Guideline No. 9, Agency for Health Care Policy and Research, US Department of Health and Human Services, Rockville, MD.

Jennings, B.M. (1981) Systematic misperception – oncology patients' self reported affective states and their care givers' perceptions. *Cancer Nurse*, 4, 485–9.

Kelman, H. (1976) Evaluation of health care quality by consumers. *International Journal of Health Services*, 6(3), 431–41.

McCaffery, M. and Beebe, A. (1994) *Pain Clinical Manual for Nursing Practice*, Nursing Mirror International Publishers, Mosby.

Max, M. (1990) Improving outcomes of analgesic treatment: is education enough? *Annals of Internal Medicine*, 78, 171–81.

National Audit Office (1995) *Clinical Audit in England*, National Audit Office, Leeds.

NHS Executive (1997) *The New NHS: Modern, Dependable*, Department of Health, London.

Norman, I. and Redfern, S. (1995) *Making Use of Clinical Audit*, Open University Press, Buckingham.

Packwood, T. and Kober, A. (1995) Clinical audit and its relationships to other forms of quality assurance and knowledge creation, in *Making Use of Clinical Audit* (eds I. Norman and S. Redfern), Open University Press, Buckingham, Philadelphia, PA, pp.21–38.

Robinson, S. (1995) The benefits and constraints of clinical audit, in *Making Use of Clinical Audit* (eds I. Norman & S. Redfern), Open University Press, Buckingham, Philadelphia, PA, pp.81–98.

Van Essen, L. (1991) The importance of nurse caring behaviours as perceived by Swedish hospital patients and nursing staff. *International Journal of Nursing Studies*, 28(3), 267–81.

4 MEASURING BEST PRACTICE: AN OVERVIEW OF APPROACHES COMMONLY USED IN HEALTHCARE

INTRODUCTION

The previous chapter outlined the audit cycle and some general principles for applying this in practice. Underpinning the cycle are the needs to identify what best practice is; to review current activities to make comparisons against these; to identify variations against known best practice, making changes where deficiencies are identified; and to share good practice with colleagues when this is found. The importance of multidisciplinary working, a structured approach to project planning and rigorous evaluation were also noted.

These principles are broadly applicable to all quality improvement efforts, regardless of the theme or speciality. This chapter sets out a number of different approaches for improving clinical practice. When implementing these, one needs to adopt the principles outlined in the previous chapter. Regardless of whether we are looking at the *Patients' Charter* (Department of Health, 1991), accreditation, benchmarking, risk management or off-the-shelf tools for assessing the quality of clinical care, the fundamental principles of the improvement cycle and rigour of project planning still apply.

This chapter will explore a number of different approaches with which to measure practice. These include:

- government-led initiatives such as the new White Paper and the *Patients' Charter*;
- standard assessment tools such as accreditation;
- the Charter Mark;
- benchmarking;
- clinical outcomes;
- off-the-shelf audit tools such as *Monitor*;
- standard-based audit tools;
- criteria-based audit tools;
- Quality Pointers Tool;
- patient care pathways.

We shall start by examining policies introduced at a national level as part of government policy.

MEASURING PRACTICE: POLICY-DRIVEN INITIATIVES

Chapter 1 noted the increasing interest on the part of governments in seeking to ensure that public expenditure on healthcare for their citizens yields a good return on their investment. It is therefore perhaps not surprising that they are reluctant to leave the measurement of the standards of service and clinical practice entirely in the hands of the professionals. Similarly, there is an increasing consumer demand for information about the quality of healthcare to enable them to make an informed choice, both about the care they receive and the competence of individuals providing that care.

In 1997 and 1998, the Labour government published a series of documents setting out policy for the NHS. The elements of the documents which refer to quality are summarized below.

The New NHS: Modern, Dependable

This White Paper (NHS Executive, 1997) seeks to reaffirm the founding principles of the NHS, i.e. access based on need alone and free at the point of delivery. The drivers identified for enhancing quality and improving efficiency are cited as:

- A new evidence-based national service framework to help ensure consistent access to services and quality of care.
- A new National Institute of Clinical Excellence to give a strong lead on clinical and cost effectiveness. This will be achieved principally by disseminating appropriate evidence-based clinical guidelines and producing and disseminating information nationally on good practice related to audit.
- A new commission for health improvement to encourage and monitor the quality of clinical services at a local level.

Locally, there will be:

- teams of GPs and community nurses working together in new primary care groups (PCGs) to shape services for patients;
- explicit quality standards in local service agreements between health authorities, PCGs and Trusts;
- a new system of clinical governance in Trusts and primary care to ensure that standards are met;
- a new statutory duty for quality in NHS Trusts.

A National Framework for Assessing Performance (1998)

The NHS Executive (1998a) published this consultation document shortly after the White Paper. It proposes to adopt a new national performance framework to support the goals identified in the White Paper. Aimed at both national and local services, the framework proposes to cover:

- **Health improvement** – to reflect the overarching aim of improving the general health of the population.
- **Fair access** – regardless of geography, socioeconomic group, ethnicity, age or sex.

- **Effective delivery of healthcare** – which complies with agreed standards and is delivered by appropriately trained staff.
- **Efficiency** – the way in which resources are used.
- **Patient/carer experience** – reflecting their views on the quality of care they receive.
- **Health outcomes of care** – assessing the impact of the NHS on improvement in the overall health status of the population, including reducing risk factors, complications of treatment, and premature deaths.

It is suggested that this information will be useful not only to the government, but also to the public, health authorities, GPs, primary care groups and NHS Trusts who will have access to it. In addition to the above, a set of high-level indicators will be developed to assist health authorities in driving improvements in performance. These include issues such as early detection of cancer rates, conception rates for girls aged 13 to 15 years and discharge from hospital. Information on these 37 indicators is already collected in some form, although new mechanisms for collecting this information will be required.

The 1998 White Paper is explicit about the criteria it would expect to see in a 'quality' organization. These are summarized in Table 4.1. The authors have adapted the list from the White Paper and in the right-hand column have summarized some of the multitude of approaches already in use in healthcare which can be used to measure performance against these criteria. Hence it can be appreciated that many of these components are already well developed. The challenge is how to integrate these into a comprehensive framework, rather than a series of ad hoc and fragmented initiatives which are seldom cross-referenced despite being inherently interlinked. Another priority is how to ensure that clinicians are actively involved in managing the quality of healthcare services. It would seem there is an expectation that the latter issue will be addressed through the concept of clinical governance. This will now be explored.

Controls assurance

What is controls assurance?

Assurance statements were a key recommendation suggested for good business practice proposed by the Cadbury Committee in 1992. A series of standards were recommended with the aim of ensuring an ethical approach for managing business. In the NHS, assurance statements are designed to give the public an assurance that their hospitals and health authorities are being properly managed. Until now, these assurances have been related purely to financial probity. It has long been a mandatory requirement that Trusts and health authorities include a statement in their annual report confirming that they have adequate control systems in place to ensure that the public's money is being spent in an appropriate way. To prove this, they need to demonstrate there are robust financial systems that would make it difficult for dishonest people to misappropriate funds.

Table 4.1

Current initiatives that can help meet the criteria in the White Paper, The New NHS: Modern, Dependable *(NHS Executive, 1997)*

Criteria in White Paper (p. 47)	Current initiatives that can help meet criteria
Quality improvement processes are in place and integrated with the quality programme for the organization as a whole.	Arrangements for clinical audit; benchmarking; accreditation; outcomes data; Patients' Charter data; patient satisfaction; and reporting structures.
Leadership skills are developed at clinical team level.	Evidence of training needs analysis; shared education; consortia commissioning; in-house provision; action learning; multidisciplinary working.
Evidence-based practice is in day-to-day use, with the infrastructure to support it.	Clinical policy, standards, procedures, guidelines, dissemination strategies, implementation programmes and review; access to library and databases.
Good practice, ideas and innovations (which have been evaluated) are systematically disseminated within and outside the organization.	Communication channels internal and external; networks; R&D structures; databases.
Clinical risk reduction programmes of a high standard are in place.	Multidisciplinary involvement; corporate risk management strategy; clinical and non-clinical risk assessment, identification, evaluation and insurance.
Adverse events are detected and openly investigated; the lessons learned promptly applied.	Incident and accident reporting structures; open culture; shared education.
Lessons for clinical practice are systematically learned from complaints made by patients.	Complaints procedures; forums for discussion and lessons learned; staff training; documented changes.
Problems of poor clinical performance are recognized at an early stage, and dealt with to prevent harm to patients.	Supervision; appraisal; preceptorship; performance review; assessment of competence; whistle blowing.
All professional development programmes reflect the principles of clinical governance.	Training needs analysis process; quality monitoring; review patient/service needs; education contracting and commissioning.
The quality of data collected to monitor clinical care is itself of a high standard.	Patient health records; IT; audit data; variance analysis, internal/external controls; costs, activity, waiting lists, length of stay.

From 1999, for the first time in NHS Trusts, we will be required to sign an assurance statement that our clinical care is of a satisfactory standard. The chief executive has overall responsibility for this and (as with the financial assurance) he or she can face prosecution if there is a breakdown of such systems.

Although the chief executive is the accountable officer, all clinicians (doctors, nurses and professions allied to medicine) also have a responsibility and accountability for ensuring good standards for their clinical practice. In the General Medical Council (GMC) document for doctors, *Maintaining Good Medical Practice* (1998), it is stated (p. 3),

> *Doctors are responsible for maintaining their professional competence and standard of performance. Also, if they work in clinical teams, they should be prepared to take some joint, as well as personal, responsibility for their own and their colleagues' work.*

The United Kingdom Central Council for Nursing, Midwifery and Health Visiting (UKCC) outlines similar guidance in its document *Guidelines for Professional Practice* (1996). Nurses, midwives and health visitors are bound by the following key UKCC standards:

- Code of Professional Conduct
- Scope of Professional Practice
- Midwives Code of Practice

They have to comply with these as a condition for their continued registration to practice.

Registered practitioners (doctors, nurses) are therefore professionally accountable to their registering body (namely the General Medical Council and UKCC), as well as having a contractual accountability to their employer and an accountability in law for their actions. Each professional therefore needs to ensure that their practice meets the professional standards set out by their professional body, adheres to the terms and conditions of the contract of their employing organizations (and respects the policies and procedures laid down by their organization) and is consistent with British law.

There is therefore a clear requirement, on the parts of both the individual practitioner and the organization, to be able to demonstrate that the clinical care offered to patients is of a reasonable standard. Essentially, we need to be able to answer the question: 'How do you know your clinical practice is safe?'

To answer this question, organizations providing healthcare will need to identify a systematic approach that, when subject to external scrutiny by professional peers, can demonstrate in a robust way that they are delivering good care.

The NHS consultation document *A First Class Service* (NHS Executive, 1998b) sets out a framework aimed at assuring the quality of clinical care, which it calls 'clinical governance'.

The principles of clinical governance are outlined in the next section.

Clinical governance

Clinical governance is the framework through which NHS organizations are accountable for continuously improving the quality of their services and safeguarding high standards of care by creating an environment in which excellence in clinical care will flourish. (NHS Executive, 1998, p. 33)

At the heart of clinical governance is the requirement for individual practitioners to get involved in local professional self-regulation. Professional self-regulation is a privilege, not a right. In planning for clinical governance, it is important to understand the characteristics that distinguish professionals from other groups of workers. Essential elements of a profession are that it has recognizable ethics and a strong element of self-regulation. Many members of a profession will also have a vocation. The professional accepts several obligations (Royal College of Physicians, 1996):

- to maintain knowledge and proficiency in the professional fields;
- to comply with standards and ethics accepted by the profession;
- to acknowledge that duties and obligations to public and clients transcend those contained in legal contracts of employment;
- to contribute to the education and training of professional aspirants;
- to support the professionalism of others.

Hence the GMC and UKCC need to be able to demonstrate to the public that practitioners they admit onto their registers are fit to practice and fulfil the above obligations. For self-regulation to work, it is dependent on good local self-regulation by the practitioners themselves. They need to ensure that professional standards are adhered to and poor performance is dealt with in an appropriate manner. The Medical (Professional Performance) Act of 1995 gave the GMC additional powers to take action against doctors whose standard of professional performance is found to be 'seriously deficient'. The new powers took effect from 1 July 1997 with the performance procedures being implemented from 1 September 1997. The new procedure allowed for:

- assessing a doctor's professional performance if it appeared to be seriously deficient;
- suspending, or placing conditions on, a doctor whose performance is found to be seriously deficient;
- requiring a doctor whose performance is seriously deficient to take action to remedy the deficiency.

Under the review currently being undertaken of the regulation of nurses, midwives and health visitors, the UKCC is also seeking additional power to deal with poor performance.

The need for strong, local professional self-regulation has been highlighted in a number of high-profile cases, namely in Kent and Canterbury, and Bristol (NHS Executive, 1994). In the latter case, the GMC identified a number of issues that arose during the course of its enquiry which require addressing by the medical profession, namely (*British Medical Journal*, 1998):

- the need for clearly understood clinical standards;
- how clinical competence and technical expertise is assessed;
- who carries the responsibility in team-based care;
- the training of doctors in advanced procedures;
- how to approach the so-called learning curve of doctors undertaking established procedures;
- the reliability and validity of data used to monitor doctors' personal performance;
- the use of medical and clinical audit;
- the appreciation of the importance of factors other than purely clinical ones which can affect clinical judgement, performance and outcome;

- the responsibility of a consultant to take appropriate actions in response to concerns about his or her performance;
- the factors that seem to discourage openness and frankness about doctors' personal performance;
- how doctors explain risk to patients.

The above issues are equally applicable to nursing and other professions allied to medicine.

In an editorial in the *British Medical Journal* (Scally and Donaldson, 1998) it was noted,

> *Regulation of doctors is not all about the GMC. Innumerable groups influence the practice of doctors, and some of them ... have much more influence than the GMC. The Council may control the ultimate sanction of removing a doctor's licence to practice, but its influence is not felt every day: to the average doctor it feels distant. In contrast, teachers and colleagues have both power and everyday influence. Royal colleges and postgraduate deans also have great influence and they must recognise their role in self-regulation. It is this local, everyday self-regulation that has been especially weak; there are now signs that it is being taken seriously.*

Similarly, a covering letter from the Department of Health about the report of the independent enquiry relating to the deaths and injuries on the children's ward at Grantham General Hospital (the Clothier enquiry investigating the crimes of Beverly Allitt), concluded,

> *Although individuals are criticised, the main criticism is a collective one – of the lack of adequate systems. The report also identifies shortcomings in quality ... in the Paediatric ward at the time of the crime. (NHS Executive, 1994)*

Under the proposals in the White Paper *The New NHS: Modern, Dependable* (NHS Executive, 1997), and the consultation document *A First Class Service* (NHS Executive, 1998), there are a number of components that are fundamental to the principles of clinical governance. Central to this is the need to develop strong local systems for professional self-regulation. It is therefore appropriate that the drive for making clinical governance work needs to come from within the professional groups themselves.

Understanding clinical governance

The document *A First Class Service* (NHS Executive, 1998) outlines the key components of the clinical governance framework:

- a comprehensive programme of quality improvement activity (such as clinical audit and evidence-based practice);

- processes for monitoring care, including complaints;
- internal and external scrutiny;
- participation in a national audit programme (a requirement for all hospital doctors from 1999) endorsed by the new Commission for Health Improvement (CHImp);
- ensuring clinical standards of national service frameworks and NICE (National Institute for Clinical Excellence) recommendations are implemented;
- full integration of workforce planning and development within the Trust's service planning;
- continuing professional development;
- clear policies aimed at managing risk and identifying and tackling poor performance;
- clear lines of responsibility and accountability for clinical care;
- clear procedures for reporting concerns about professional conduct and performance, and action to remedy problems.

The government proposes that clinical governance will be implemented by setting clear national standards, with responsibility for their delivery being taken locally. These standards will be set through the National Service Framework (NSF) and through a new National Institute for Clinical Excellence (NICE). The NSF will address the whole system of care, requiring the NHS to organize its services to ensure the best quality and fairest access. NICE has the role of providing the standards based on relevant evidence of clinical and cost effectiveness. Trusts, primary care groups and health authorities will be responsible for implementing these standards in practice through a process of lifelong learning and professional self-regulation. Thus, local clinical governance will ensure the delivery of dependable, quality healthcare.

While the implementation of these standards will be monitored by Trusts themselves, independent scrutiny will be done through the new Commission for Health Improvement. There will also be a National Framework for Assessing Performance and a National Survey of Patient and User Experience which will be conducted annually. Should there be evidence of failure to meet standards, CHImp will have the power to intervene at the government's request and advise remedial action.

Clinical governance: getting the right balance

It is widely accepted that wherever performance is monitored, variations will be identified around the mean (Scally and Donaldson, 1998), with the bulk of those measured falling close to the mean, with smaller proportions above and below the mean.

Scally and Donaldson (1998) identified that a major shift towards improved quality will occur only if health organizations in the middle of the range of performance are transformed, that is if the quality of care is brought up to the level of the exemplars, with those below the mean likewise making incremental improvements.

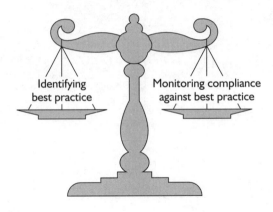

Figure 4.1

Balancing identification and monitoring of best practice

When looking at getting the balance right between these two key components of clinical governance (Figure 4.1), it can be appreciated that one half of the equation is concerned with learning from the exemplar practice, the other in helping to address the performance of all those who fall under the mean in order to improve clinical standards overall. If intransigent problems recur with those below the mean, clearly there is a requirement to ensure these are addressed.

To do this we need a system that creates a culture where we *balance* the identification and adoption of best practice with monitoring compliance against best practice. Essentially, the identification of best practice is about *doing the right things* and monitoring compliance is a way of ensuring we are *doing things right*.

In addressing these two key principles of clinical governance, it can be appreciated that keeping the two components on the scales balanced is critical to create a culture for clinical governance. If the balance is too heavily weighted on monitoring and evaluation, there is a danger that a 'name, shame and blame' culture is created, which is unlikely to inspire and motivate clinicians. It is also conceivable to set up monitoring bureaucracies that lead to no demonstrable benefits to patients, or poorly designed audit tools that monitor known local practice rather than agreed national/international best practice. Conversely, if the scales are weighted too heavily on the side of identifying best practice, there is a danger clinicians will not be able to demonstrate the impact of changes to their practices, nor to make meaningful comparisons with peers elsewhere. Participation may occur only from pockets of motivated teams, with no sanctions available to apply to those who choose not to participate.

For the two components in Figure 4.1 to remain balanced, two other support structures are required. There needs to be a strong foundation based on education of staff, and a clear structure for implementation. These will now be explored.

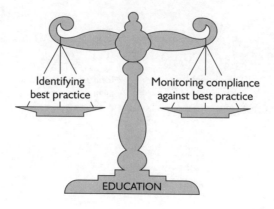

Figure 4.2

Education underpinning the clinical governance agenda

Education

Education is absolutely essential in underpinning the clinical governance agenda, as seen in Figure 4.2. The policy documents make numerous references to life-long learning, and this is a central tenet that distinguishes professional groups, since it is mandatory to their continued licence to practise. As well as the requirements of the individual to take action to ensure they are professionally up to date in their clinical practice, there is a significant educational agenda for all healthcare organizations implementing clinical governance. There is little point in establishing organizational systems to disseminate best practice and evaluate performance if clinicians do not know how to access these, or do not own and understand them. The success of adverse incident reporting systems, clinical audit, policies and procedures, clinical risk management, and other such systems is dependent on creating a culture where these systems are used and owned by clinicians. Clinicians therefore need to be educated in skills such as critical appraisal of the literature, and introduced to policies, procedures and processes and the way local systems work – as a routine part of their induction.

Implementation/use of clinical audit

The previous sections have outlined the importance of getting the balance right between identification of best practice and monitoring for compliance against known best practice. It has also been identified that a strong educational foundation is essential if these concepts are going to be applied in clinical practice. This next section explores preliminary steps for implementing clinical governance based on the model used in one author's organization.

Nine goals were identified from *A First Class Service* (NHS Executive, 1998) to comply with clinical governance; these are shown in Table 4.2. For each of these goals, six key questions were identified to assist in formulating an implementation plan. These are:

Table 4.2	G	oals and actions
Nine goals identified in	O	btaining patients' views
A First Class Service	V	alidating data quality
	E	vidence into practice
	R	isk assessment and reduction
	N	ominate lead responsibilities for clinical governance
	A	ssuring quality of clinical practice
	N	otifying staff/patients about clinical governance systems
	C	linical leadership
	E	ducation and training

Reproduced with the permission of Brighton Health Care NHS Trust.

- What system(s) do we have in place?
- What other system(s) do we need?
- Are staff and patients aware of the system(s)?
- How do we monitor to ensure that the system(s) are effective?
- How will we report progress on the system(s) as part of the controls assurance statement?
- What actions do we need to take to make the system(s) more effective?

These goals and key questions were then drawn together in the clinical assessment framework shown in Table 4.3.

Use of the clinical governance assessment framework

The clinical governance assessment framework can be used at both a corporate and clinical directorate level. Local clinical teams can also use this framework at a micro level, both to identify their achievements against the key goals and as the basis for an action plan for future work.

Having analysed both areas of compliance and areas for further work, NHS Trusts, primary care groups and health authorities will need to develop local structures to ensure that the two components identified in Figure 4.1, i.e. identifying best practice and monitoring compliance with best practice, are evenly balanced.

Hence, local mechanisms will need to be in place for ensuring clinical guidelines and latest research findings generated from the NICE are made accessible to clinicians.

Similarly, robust mechanisms for auditing compliance with best practice will need to be in place and demonstrable for the Commission for Health Improvement.

RISK MANAGEMENT

Risk management for both clinical and non-clinical risk is one element of a quality improvement programme that healthcare organizations throughout the world are increasingly obliged to address. In the face of an increasingly litigious public, the financial penalties of failing to address risk management can be significant. The

Table 4.3

Clinical governance assessment framework

Goals and actions	What systems do we have in place?	What other system(s) do we need?	Are staff and patients aware of the systems?	How do we monitor to ensure that the system(s) are effective?	How will we report progress on the system(s) as part of the Control Assurance Statement?	What actions do we need to make the system(s) more effective?
Obtaining patients' views						
Validate data quality						
Evidence into practice						
Risk assessment and reduction						
Nominate lead responsibilities for clinical governance						
Assuring quality of clinical practice						
Notify staff and patients about clinical governance systems						
Clinical leadership						
Education and training						

Reproduced with the permission of Brighton Health Care NHS Trust (adapted from a report by the British Association of Medical Managers)

controls assurance statement with which healthcare institutions in the UK are now mandated to comply by the turn of the century requires a statement in the annual report on clinical as well as financial assurance. Evidence will need to be provided that robust systems are in place for managing and containing risks. Chief executives have been designated as accountable offices for ensuring compliance.

Risk management is a systematic framework that conducts a broad assessment addressing all aspects of an organization which may give rise to risks, including:

- buildings
- equipment (including any chemicals used)
- people (employees, patients and visitors)
- systems (procedures, policies, practices, etc.)

The risk management process comprises the following three phases.

Risk identification

This involves answering three questions:

- What could go wrong?
- How could it happen
- What would the effect be?

Risk assessment

This involves asking the following for each of the issues identified in response to the above questions:

- How often is it likely to happen?
- How severe would the effect be?
- What would it cost in terms of:
  - cash implications?
  - loss of reputation?
  - adverse publicity?
  - damage to staff morale etc.?
  - effect on individual patient care?

Risk minimization

The final step involves identifying:

- how these risks can be eliminated/avoided or made less likely to occur;
- how the effect, if it does occur, can be minimized.

Vincent (1995) identifies that, to succeed in clinical risk management, doctors must be involved in:

- gathering data and finding problems
- improving their skills in analysing evidence
- communicating with patients

The risk manager needs to:

- control lawsuits within their jurisdiction;
- monitor injured patients and make every effort to minimize their injuries and keep them informed;
- help in data gathering and analysis for preventing injury;
- predict clinical effects of new medical and legal changes in healthcare.

Managing clinical risk is often a difficult and complex process, which originally developed as a means of controlling medical negligence. The focus now is on providing safe care for those who are most vulnerable. Vincent (1997) suggests that targets for audit, clinical effectiveness and other quality initiatives should be selected specifically from areas where patients are at high risk.

The approach to risk management described by the Health and Safety Executive (1997) is to *manage quality in* rather than to *inspect the defects out*. The focus is on designing and implementing a proactive system rather than a reactive system. To achieve this, the Health and Safety Executive (1997) suggest ten steps:

1 Establish standards.
2 Implement plans to achieve standards.
3 Measure compliance with standards.
4 Review and take appropriate action.
5 Address the activity.
6 Identify the risks.
7 Assess the potential frequency.
8 Eliminate those risks that can be eliminated.
9 Reduce the effect on those that cannot be eliminated.
10 Address the financial mechanisms to absorb the consequences of risk.

Risk management should not be viewed as a stand-alone activity, but should be integrated into all organizational structures and activities. The literature shows a growing tendency to link clinical audit and risk management activity. Thus, when a risk issue has been identified, the cycle of clinical audit is instrumental in addressing it.

PATIENTS' CHARTER

The *Patients' Charter* was published in 1991 (Department of Health, 1991) with the purpose of establishing national standards with which service providers were expected to comply. The original standards have been amended and revised since then.

In October 1997 EL(97)60 was published, outlining changes to the existing charter. The new charter would be developed in partnership with service users and those who work in the NHS. The focus was on quality and effectiveness of treatment, and the accessibility and standard of information available to the public. The new charter will also emphasize the responsibilities the public has in using NHS services, as well as their rights. Until the new charter is published, the content and monitoring methods of the current charter will remain valid.

The current *Patients' Charter* involves national monitoring of the following:

- respect for privacy, dignity, and religious and cultural beliefs
- arrangements for equal access to services
- provision of information to relatives and friends
- waiting times for ambulances
- waiting times in A/E for assessment
- waiting times in outpatient departments

- cancellation of operations
- a named nurse, midwife or health visitor
- discharge of patients

Local standards, such as waiting times for first outpatients appointments and sign-posting within the organization, are also agreed with the purchasers.

Stages of monitoring the *Patients' Charter*

As outlined in the previous chapter, it is helpful to implement initiatives such as this within an audit framework. Hence the stages we have adopted for ensuring compliance against charter standards include:

- defining the standard
- determining the data required
- collecting and analysing the data
- defining problem areas
- agreeing an action plan
- implementing the action plan
- returning to defining the standard

The intention of monitoring the charter is to:

- assess performance against nationally agreed standards in order to improve the delivery of care;
- take action when standards are not met;
- provide information to GPs and health authorities so that informed choice can be made on where to refer patients;
- provide data returns to the Department of Health so that a national picture is obtained.

Rigge (1997) suggests that the charter has failed to fulfil many of the standards it sets out. Examples include patients failing to receive prompt replies following a complaint, and operations repeatedly being cancelled. Although standards have been set, patients still complain that the service they have received has fallen short of the ideal. Indeed, many professionals feel that the charter raised the expectations of its users to a level that current resources did not enable the NHS to meet. Others doubt that the charter standards actually measure what is genuinely important for patients, and have concerns that the pressure to comply with standards on waiting times is distracting clinical priorities from those most in need. Hence a difficulty in meeting standards for cancellation of operations is compounded by a rise in throughput of medical emergency patients. This may build perverse incentives into the system, as providers who refuse medical admissions in order to meet this standard may score better statistically.

Criticisms have also been levelled at the method of data collection, which makes genuine comparisons difficult. Local differences are not addressed within the national standards. Therefore local communities often do not have the right information or all the information to judge the effectiveness of their local services meaningfully.

Some targets have proved more difficult to measure; for example, patients having their own named nurse, midwife or health visitor. Ambiguity surrounds interpretation of this standard. The *Patients' Charter* has prompted some improvements in achieving the national standards, particularly in relation to waiting times in outpatient clinics. The charter has undoubtedly led to a number of improvements across a range of targets – in particular, waiting times.

ACCREDITATION

Accreditation of hospital services is used widely within the USA and Australia (Scrivens 1995). The system usually involves external peer review of an agreed set of standards which are applicable across a range of services. The accreditation system is based on the premise that there are certain criteria to be met which, when combined, ensure the delivery of a safe and effective service.

Accreditation is sometimes mistakenly viewed as synonymous with litigation, inspection and regulation. This is possibly because accreditation was initially developed in the USA, where these issues are features of the healthcare system. Outside the USA, accreditation is mainly voluntary. It results in either a pass, fail or some form of graded scale. It can therefore be used for organizations to benchmark against themselves, or to make comparisons with other similar hospitals.

Accreditation began in 1917 in the USA and evolved to establishment of the Joint Commission of Accreditation of Hospital Organisations (JCAHO, 1988). The standards are based on an optimum level of achievement. Critics of this system suggest it is a bureaucratic and complex system to administer. It is a system of self-regulation for the healthcare industry, and, although in theory the JCAHO is independent and participation is voluntary, in practice many hospitals are obliged to comply.

An accreditation approach was suggested by Maxwell (1983) to be beneficial to the NHS in the UK. This has so far been developed and adopted only marginally by hospital organizations. Other forms of accreditation currently exist in the UK – which are outlined below. There are also well developed departmental accreditation systems for radiology, pathology and chiropody.

King's Fund Organisational Audit: whole hospital accreditation

The King's Fund Organisational Audit was developed in 1983. Seventeen people sit on the board, including representatives from nursing and midwifery, medical colleagues, the Independent Association, the National Association of Health Authorities and Trusts, the Health Advisory Services and the NHS Executive. They undertake an organizational audit which has no grading system and focuses on both good practice and deficiencies. The focus is on acute hospitals and originally adapted standards from the USA and Australia.

Hospitals pay a fee to have three surveyors (a nurse, a doctor and a manager) undertake a review of standards. The emphasis of this audit remains on self-improvement. Once the King's Fund accepts a hospital to be accredited, a manual of standards is sent to the hospital and over the next 12 months the hospitals are encouraged to address the standards before a survey visit is undertaken. Once the report is sent to the hospital it is their responsibility to take action on the recommendations. The accreditation will last for three years, after which the hospital needs to apply for reassessment.

Hospital Accreditation Programme

The programme was developed in 1988 and awards accreditation status. The scheme is a derivative of a Canadian system, and the primary clients are community hospitals. The awards are graded to either one or two years' accreditation or non-accreditation. The board is a mix of nursing, medical and management representatives.

The surveys take one day's work by two surveyors who are practitioners in the community or general practice setting. This scheme is purely directed to organizational audit and no clinical standards are addressed.

South East Thames Regional Hospitals Accreditation (SETRHA)

An accreditation system for nursing in South East Thames (SETRHA) is currently being developed. This system is being piloted in 42 wards and units and involves both acute and community Trusts. The process consists of four stages:

- **Standard-setting** – identifying what constitutes good nursing practice.
- **Internal self-assessment** – identifying what needs to be improved.
- **Monitoring** – by independent trained assessors.
- **Reporting** – to both providers and the purchasing health authority.

The standards are formulated internally by the organization in conjunction with the audit tool. The nurses are given the opportunity to address the issues within a three-month period themselves before an independent assessor undertakes a review of the standards. The author (Price, 1997) aims to publicize the project in order to promote a nationally based accreditation system. Whilst the project is useful in promoting locally owned standards of care, one needs to be cautious about the generalization of such findings. One could argue that factors such as poor staffing could lead nurses to develop standards of care which could not be used nationally. Similarly, lack of education opportunities for senior nurses may lead them to develop standards that just reinforce outdated practice. Debating the need for nationally agreed 'expert' standards becomes more pressing.

Scrivens (1995) suggests that professionals feel they should be part of any group that assesses organizational standards and that only they can assess the appropriateness of professional decisions. The complexity of professional decision making often needs advice from professionals to interpret. However, this notion tends to promote introspection and an unwillingness to work with other groups to identify potential improvement.

Health Service Accreditation Scheme

Since 1995, this scheme has been developing from the original work undertaken by SETRHA. It now covers accreditation of 19 services, with ten more being developed.

The standards for these services are developed by a multidisciplinary group with input from social services. The standards are patient-centred and clinically based and incorporate existing standards such as Royal Colleges, *Patients' Charter* and Health of the Nation. The standards are sent out for consultation and field tested before use. An organization wishing to be accredited will undertake an internal review of services and agree a visit to take place in nine months' time. Assessors will require evidence to be provided on the day or will ask to witness the required standard being met. The scheme is not profit making. Its authors cite the benefits of undertaking the scheme as follows:

- The Trust embarks on a process of improving care which can set an agenda for clinical audit and potentially improve teamwork through working towards the required standards.
- Independent endorsement of quality is more prestigious, and all information can be used comparatively between Trusts.
- Standards are thorough and cover the most pertinent aspects of the service.

Health Promoting Hospitals Accreditation

In the south and west region of England, the Wessex Institute for Health Research and Development has a contractual responsibility to develop Health Promoting Hospitals (HPH) throughout the region.

In 1995, using a health promotion model developed by Tannahill (1985), the region sought to develop both an audit framework consisting of eight elements and an accreditation scheme for when the elements were met. The eight elements were:

- management issues
- customer care
- health information and communication
- health at work in the NHS
- hotel services and environmental issues
- community involvement and health alliances
- equal opportunities
- clinical audit and effectiveness

For each element, the organization scores itself against core agenda items which involve:

- an overall statement applicable to the philosophy of the section area, which organizations need to demonstrate they are actively working towards;
- a self-audit process, which, when completed, is peer reviewed;

- guidelines for management at Trust Board level to ensure recommendations for progress will be initiated;
- training being developed to ensure consistency of the review process.

The scheme was piloted in eight NHS Trusts which were both acute and community focused. The project was piloted in 1997 and the audit tool is now available to purchase.

Other schemes such as the Health Advisory Service and the Audit Commission are funded by the Department of Health but do not have agreed standards and cannot award gradings. The process involves:

- informing a hospital – elderly care or mental healthcare – of a visit and asking to meet with relevant staff;
- assessors visiting the wards, asking questions and writing a report. Their views are subjective and not based on any measurable criteria.

Critics of accreditation would argue that periodic inspection produces a halo effect and does little to create innovation or involvement in improving a service. As with any system, however, accreditation should not be viewed as a one-off initiative, but as part of an improvement cycle.

The future of accreditation

At the moment there are a number of accreditation systems, none of which seems to be gaining favour with either purchasers or providers. There are, however, growing pressures to inform the public of grading scores and achievements, as evidenced by the *Patients' Charter* and the move by the government to incorporate quality indicators into the performance management arrangements within each NHS organization. Difficulties with the accreditation approach include the following:

- Different purchasers can have different standards, e.g. a purchaser may say 'hospitals must meet waiting list Charter Standards'. This may be acceptable but could involve closing to all medical emergency admissions in winter. A hospital that stays open and ensures local people receive a local emergency service may fail the charter standard.
- It is difficult to find genuine comparators to benchmark hospitals. Many standards will exist due to a variety of factors. This could be for example due to differences in local service provision, waiting list issues due to the type and needs of the population, etc.
- Organizations need to decide whether they are seeking accreditation for the whole organization or just for a particular service.
- Nationally a question needs to be asked whether the system of accreditation should be voluntary or mandatory and, indeed, whether we need one at all.

At present, accreditation lies predominantly within the acute sector. However, in future, shifting the focus of accreditation to the primary sector and social services will be more appropriate, as combined accreditation across services may enhance the changes required for more effective partnerships.

CHARTER MARK

The Charter Mark is bestowed upon public services, and is aimed at promoting a more customer-service-orientated public sector. Charter Mark began in 1993 and is awarded by the Charter Mark panel of independent assessors, who have a background in public and private services. Application for Charter Mark status is voluntary, and participants need to complete an application which demonstrates how they meet the Charter Mark criteria. The written applications are reviewed by two assessors and a visit is undertaken to the organization to talk with staff and service users.

Charter Mark has been defined as 'a journey, not a destination' (Blythe, 1995). When an organization applies they must then continue with their quality improvement plan and provide evidence throughout the next three years in order to renew the Charter Mark status. The following criteria must be met to achieve Charter Mark recognition:

- **Performance standards.** 'Setting, monitoring and publication of explicit standards for the services that individual users can reasonably expect. Publication of actual performance against those standards.'
- **Information and openness.** 'Full accurate information readily available in plain language about how public services are run, what they cost, how well they perform and who is in charge.'
- **Consultation and choice.** 'The public sector should provide choice wherever possible. There should be regular and systematic consultation with those who use the services. Users' views about services and their priorities for improving them should be taken into account in final decisions about standards.'
- **Courtesy and helpfulness.** 'Courteous and helpful services from public servants who will normally wear name badges. Services available equally to all who are entitled to them and run to suit their convenience.'
- **Putting things right.** 'If things go wrong an apology, a full explanation and a swift and effective remedy. Well-publicised and easy-to-use complaints procedures with independent review wherever possible.'
- **Value for money.** 'Efficient and economical delivery of public services within affordable resources.' 'User satisfaction.'
- **Improvements in service quality.** 'Measurable or demonstrable improvements in quality of service over the last two or three years.'

Planned improvements and innovation

When applying to renew the Charter Mark award, the judges will look for:

- evidence that the organization has maintained a high-quality service;

- evidence that the service has actually improved and that users of the service could identify improvements.

The Charter Mark offers all staff at every level in public services the opportunity to highlight their achievements and share good practice. The criteria for assessment are orientated towards public needs from a user's perspective.

BENCHMARKING

Benchmarking is a process used to compare practices at local, national or international level (Maxwell, Kennedy and Spours, 1996). Benchmarking can be used for comparisons to be made in relation to any of the following:

- approaches to care
- clinical practice
- care delivery settings
- delivery of service
- management practices

The purpose of benchmarking is to make comparisons on data collected for similar activities and services, either within the organization or with comparable institutions elsewhere. Where the data show notable differences, these act as a pointer for further investigation. For example, durations of inpatient hospital stay for a common surgical procedure may differ. This will be a pointer that clinicians can examine further to identify possible reasons. It may be that that one hospital had a patient mix of older, sicker patients undergoing the procedure which will explain the difference. Alternatively, further investigation may identify some elements of good clinical practice and innovation that may be transferable elsewhere.

Undertaking benchmarking

The NHS Benchmarking Reference Centre (1994) suggests four elements for the success of benchmarking projects:

- a commitment to continuous improvement, which ideally would be part of the organization's structure and practice;
- knowledge of the organization to ensure that the issues addressed are worthwhile;
- learning from the best, be they public or private organizations;
- a commitment to achieve measurable improvement and to make any changes required.

It also identifies 12 steps for successful benchmarking:

Formulate a benchplan
1 Identify the subject area.
2 Define the process to be benchmarked.

3 Identify potential benchmarking partners.
4 Identify the data required.

Benchmarking analysis
5 Collect the data and select benchmark partners.
6 Determine the gap and compare.
7 Establish differences in process.
8 Target future performance.

Benchmarking action
9 Communication and commitment.
10 Adjust targets and develop a corrective action plan.
11 Implement the plan.
12 Review progress.

These steps provide a useful framework to guide participants through the whole process.

There are a number of initiatives taking place nationally to coordinate benchmarking activities in relation to services. The National Performance Advisory Group requests information on the following when comparing services such as outpatients clinics:

- **Trust profile** – which includes the number of acute beds, outpatients per annum, and outreach activity.
- **Service profile** – detailing the number of day cases, one-stop clinics, monthly clinics, percentage of patients seen in 30 minutes or non-attendees, number of doctors, nurses and support staff, and the type of computerized system.
- **Departmental profile** – of staffing grades and establishments.
- **Financial profile** – including the total budget.
- **Quality** – any quality measures in use, e.g. Investors in People, Charter Mark, etc.
- **Other measures** – such as patient satisfaction surveys, clinical audit, interpreting service and information booklets.

There are a number of criticisms about the benchmarking process. Bullivant (1996) points out that 'there is limited value in statistical measures as they tend to highlight symptoms rather than causes of problems . . . it was recognised that processes behind the statistics should be defined'.

The same author questions the contribution of benchmarking in achieving genuine improvements, as very often circumstantial differences are emphasized, rather than identifying deficiencies when performance is poor. Maxwell, Kennedy and Spours (1996) suggest that each area is truly unique and therefore that benchmarking cannot be truly comparable.

Other constraints to benchmarking include a lack of willing benchmark partners and the fact that organizations are often unwilling to share practice for fear of being labelled 'poor performers'. Issues such as demography, population wealth, resources and types of setting also need to be considered. Matching a similar organization can be difficult, making it difficult to find truly comparative data.

If senior managers do not act on the information they receive through this process, the momentum for change is lost. A systematic framework is required to guide participants through all the stages of benchmarking to ensure that improvements are made.

In conclusion, some benefits can be derived from using benchmarking. Some hospitals participate in the process through national benchmarking initiatives. Benchmarking has been used with some degree of success in hotel services. Clinical benchmarking is rare in the literature, probably because the principles outlined as benchmarking are those that also apply to clinical audit and clinical outcomes, and as such are better understood by clinicians.

CLINICAL OUTCOMES

Outcomes have been defined as 'the cumulative effect of one or more processes on a patient at a defined point in time, as in patient survival (or death) following a medical intervention'. Shaugnessy (1998) defines outcome measures as 'the change in health status between a baseline time point and a final time point'.

The approaches outlined above, which are used to measure clinical practice and health services, have focused on structural or process issues. A different way of examining the quality of patient care is to focus on the outcome of care as well as on the process. Outcome measures are tools that can be used to do this, by assessing the effect an intervention has on patients' health (quantitative measurement) and the patients' experience of the care they have received (qualitative measurement). Aspects of the patient's health are measured (objectively and subjectively) before and after the intervention. The difference between the two measurements can, with caution, be ascribed to the intervention. Patients are generally the main source of data for outcome measurement studies.

A challenge to this approach is that it can be very difficult to find a causal relationship between an aspect of the process of care and the outcome that is being measured. Patients' health is not a simple concept. It encompasses all sorts of areas, such as psychological well-being, pain levels, physical health, emotional status, mobility, ability to work, levels of medication, and activities of daily living. If these outcome measures do not show the expected improvements through treatment, attention then shifts to the actual processes of care and the aspects of practice that may be responsible.

There are many outcome measurement tools that have been developed and tested by researchers which clinicians can use. As development of such measures is time consuming and complex, developing one's own should be approached with a degree of caution.

Defining outcome measures is often difficult, as an assessment of whether the outcome is positive or negative must involve the patient's as well as the clinician's perspective. Many authors suggest that outcome measures must be related to the reasons for developing them and the objectives of the healthcare system (Roberts, 1991).

The purpose of developing outcome measures

Delamothe (1994) suggests the purpose of developing outcomes is to improve the health and the healthcare of the population. However, Calman (1994) states that this must be within the available resources and that clinicians must demonstrate they are delivering a 'value for money' service. Therefore, there is both a clinical and a managerial purpose in pursuing the measurement of outcomes. Since 1992, the Department of Health has been trying to encourage professionals to demonstrate outcomes in clinical care and to use information on outcomes to improve care. Calman (1994) highlighted how the DoH has contributed to this process through the following initiatives:

- **NHS Centre for Coding and Classification** – to aid clinicians in defining a common language for specifying the clinical problem.
- *Effective Healthcare* **bulletins** – so that clinicians know how to treat the clinical issues.
- **National setting of health objectives and targets** – so that clinicians are aware of the objectives of treatment.
- **Health of the Nation Key Handbooks** – to make clinicians aware of the services and standards required.
- **Development of the Audit Information Centre** – so that results are available relating to projects.
- **UK Clearing House for Health Outcomes** – so that information is available to enable clinicians to develop practice.

Anecdotally, colleagues have suggested that outcome measures may be related to the objectives of the healthcare system. This is problematic in its application in the NHS. First, the objectives of the NHS are often not clear – in particular those that relate to the health of the population. Second, outcomes are generally long-term consequences, and many other activities and factors intervene during the timespan, making it difficult to demonstrate a causal link between healthcare and outcome. Very often the outcomes and consequences of ill health cannot be attributable to the healthcare intervention. Thus outcomes occur at an individual and a population level.

Clinicians are interested in determining the intermediate outputs (i.e. what happens before the patient is discharged in the treatment process) and long-term outputs (i.e. what happens when the patients emerge from the treatment process). Long-term outcomes are therefore measured which relate to aspects of healthcare such as:

- life expectancy
- quality of life
- perioperative deaths
- hospital deaths

Short-term outcome measures or intermediate outputs relate to aspects of health such as:

- improving hip replacement surgery (Williams, 1994)
- total knee replacements (Bardsley and Cleary, 1994)

In this way information gained from shared practice and research indicates how to care for patients in a more effective way, to achieve a better outcome during or immediately following the treatment process. Therefore, application of research to patient outcomes is key if clinical practice is to improve and develop.

Using outcome research in practice

Outcome research involves generating, collecting, analysing and applying information about the outcomes of medical and other professional care. The uses of outcome research can include any of the following:

- predicting patient outcomes based on collective experience;
- objective information on patient preferences;
- using the information to influence purchasing decisions;
- identifying best practice in order to develop guidelines for practice;
- improving the quality of care by updating and disseminating knowledge.

Areas in which outcome research is useful are generally those where there is professional uncertainty and little previous clinical research has been undertaken, e.g. benign prostatic hyperplasia. However, even in areas where there is ample research, techniques and practices advance and it is very easy to believe that no further work needs undertaking. Very often developments can be made which have significant impact on the patient's experiences and short-term outcomes. Mulley (1994) suggests that outcome research can identify variations in clinical practice, particularly geographically and in relation to cost and quality of care. Conducting outcomes research involves asking the following questions:

- What is effective treatment?
- Who do they work for and why?
- Which outcomes are valued by patients?

Rigge (1998) suggests that outcomes research would be valuable. However, improved use of existing data would achieve many of the issues related to variations in practice.

The challenge of implementation

There are three specific challenges to implementing outcome research and developing outcome measures in practice. These are technological issues, resource issues and determining patient preference.

- **Technological issues.** Many areas of the NHS do not have sufficient information technology support to provide health professionals with ready access to the kind of information they need to develop more informed knowledge on clinical practice.
- **Resource issues.** This can relate to resources either for undertaking outcome research or for changing treatment as a result of the outcome research. In relation to the former, it must be clear who will interpret the research findings, assume integrity and undertake the research. Each of these has significant resource implications.
- **Determining patient preference.** This is a difficult and as yet underresearched area. Clinicians need to be in a position to offer alternatives depending on the circumstances, and to have full knowledge of the outcomes of the treatment, so that patients can share any decision concerning choice of treatment.

Another challenge is that the use of crude statistics can be inherently misleading. In an article on comparisons of healthcare outcomes, Orchard (1994) notes the following key points:

- Hospital activities are complex and difficult to measure, and their outcomes data need adjusting for casemix.
- Existing casemix systems focus on treatments, but outcomes data need to focus on patients.
- Prognosis itself is inherently uncertain and substantially affected by non-medical risk factors.
- Medical prognoses are multidimensional, qualitative, time specific and disease specific and may be difficult to attribute to specific treatments.
- Using observational data for outcomes measurement means allowing for accuracy, bias, confounding factors and chance.
- Identifying and weighting patient characteristics associated with poor outcomes entails rigorous research.
- Prognostic factors such as severity are difficult to quantify.
- The benefits of casemix-adjusted outcomes data should outweigh the problems and costs of producing them.

Orchard suggests that these problems, though formidable, are not insurmountable.

Once the challenges of outcomes measurement have been identified, consideration also needs to be given to monitoring changes in clinical practice which determine outcomes.

Monitoring outcomes in clinical practice

This is a complex and difficult task which has been identified as part of the NHS Executive's *NHS Information Management and Technology Strategy* (1996). The monitoring strategy at present includes those elements that tend to relate to population level outcome measures, namely:

- asking GPs to collect information on issues such as asthma attacks and related prescriptions, quality of life, etc.;
- using comparative data sets nationally such as Health Service Indicators and Population Health Outcome Indicators;
- Health of the Nation Performance Measures;
- future developments relating to national expert audit which are under development as well as the measures highlighted in the White Paper (Department of Health, 1998).

As Rigge (1998) identifies, using research information currently available (as outlined in Chapter 1) would be an important step in addressing some issues relating to outcome measures and healthcare practice at an individual level. Hence the issue is not just about the research, but about how to disseminate the findings and implement them into practice.

The previous sections have examined how best practice is measured through a series of national initiatives. This next section will examine a number of off-the-shelf audit tools that can be used as indicators for the quality of nursing care.

It is perhaps not surprising that with nurses being by far the largest professional group in terms of sheer numbers, and often cited as providing up to 80% of hands-on care in hospitals, a number of tools have been developed that seek to measure the standards of care provided. We cover only those that we have used in practice. These are presented only as examples from a wide range of similar tools. Other tools have been developed for primary care and the private sector.

NURSING AUDIT TOOLS

Nursing audit tools can be either predetermined standards which are developed, published and used nationally, or standards developed locally in response to a specific problem. However, local audit tools can also be developed by clinical staff to audit practice. These tend to focus on a specific issue that has relevance to that ward or department. Standard-based audit tools can also be developed. In essence, this section aims to show how, having identified best practice (outlined in Chapter 1) and documented this (either through a local guideline or standard, or by using a set of standards that have been developed elsewhere but are viewed as appropriate to the local context), health professionals can measure their own practice measure compliance. Once the measurement is complete, the rest of the audit cycle outlined in Chapter 3 must then be followed, either to improve deficits where identified or to disseminate good practice.

There are three common approaches to developing and using audit tools:

- off-the-shelf audit tools
- audit tools developed from standards based on the Donabedian framework
- criteria-based audit tools

STAFFORDSHIRE
UNIVERSITY
LIBRARY

Off-the-shelf audit tools

Nursing audit tools have been in use for some time. Examples of such tools include *Monitor* (Goldstone, Ball and Collier, 1983), Phaneuf's (1976) and Qualpacs (Wandelt and Ager, 1974). They aim either to measure the quality of care or to indicate quality, retrospectively or concurrently. The next section will describe these tools and outline the advantages and disadvantages of each.

Monitor

Monitor is an audit tool used to indicate the quality of nursing care. It was first published by Goldstone, Ball and Collier, (1983) and is a reformatted version of the Rush Medicus Audit System, which had been used in the USA. Following the widespread use of *Medical/Surgical Monitor*, subsequent versions relating to Paediatric Care (Goldstone and Galvin, 1983), Health Visiting (Goldstone and Whittaker, 1990), District Nursing (Goldstone and Illsley, 1985), Senior (Goldstone and Okai, 1986), Midwifery (Goldstone and Hughes, 1989) and Accident & Emergency (Goldstone, 1991) were developed.

The tool was devised to offer an index to quality (Goldstone and Illsley, 1985), i.e. a pointer, not a measure of quality. However, this principle has been misunderstood by a number of authors (Marsh and Brittle, 1986).

Monitor addresses the 'process' elements of nursing care. It also identifies the impact of laundry supplies, CSSD and domestic services on the ward. *Monitor* has been found to highlight deficiencies in care (Dickson, 1987) and in the care that ethnic minorities receive while in hospital (Corrigan, 1989). Many authors have questioned the validity of this tool (Barnett and Wainwright, 1987), mainly on the basis that an area with a high score may provide poor nursing care and vice versa. This occurs because the majority of questions posed by this tool are based on documentation of care. The assumption is made that whatever is documented is carried out, and to a standard that is acceptable. Also, staff now are often familiar with the content of this audit tool and find it relatively easy to amend their documentation before the study in order to raise their score. Other authors highlight observer bias (Whelan, 1987). This should be eliminated in the training given to assessors, which should also ensure standard interpretation of the criteria. Assessors are also advised not to work in areas where they have close personal friends or have had previous difficulties with colleagues. (However, there have been occasions where assessors, appalled by low standards or pleasantly surprised by high-quality care, have changed their behaviour and attitude accordingly (Corrigan, 1989).) Fortunately, one can identify this during the assessment period on the ward, by frequent communication with the assessors or while analysing and interpreting the results.

The key to a successful audit is a comprehensive implementation plan and training of assessors in order to achieve valid results (Pullan and Chittock, 1986). Some confusion is seen to exist in the underlying philosophy of *Monitor* because it is based on a nursing process framework, yet claims to be applicable to task-orientated nursing. However, staff who organize care using task allocation can still use the nursing process to some degree and, therefore, some of the questions still have relevance.

Steps for implementing a Monitor study

There are a number of steps that are helpful when undertaking a monitor study. These are outlined below.

- Ensure ward staff want to use the tool and that they understand how, when and by whom the study will be carried out.
- Type letters to patients to request informed consent and advising them of the time and date of the study. You may need to approach your local ethics committee for approval.
- Train *Monitor* assessors, discussing issues such as their role, whether to wear uniform and name badges, and the action they should take if they come across an ethical situation they find difficult to handle. An example of this may be finding a blood transfusion running through too quickly and no observations of the patient's pulse and temperature being taken. Assessors are advised to inform a nurse of their observations and record the action of the nurse. If they feel that no action was taken, the facilitator of the study will directly liaise with the nursing management of the ward and the assessor will have no further part in the event. Training usually involves four two-hourly sessions, in which the role of the assessor is fully explained in relation to impartiality and confidentiality. Advice is given relating to being an observer of a clinical practice.
- Inform staff who the assessors are and prepare *Monitor* books.
- Implement the study.
- Analyse the results and prepare a report. The results are fed into a computer, usually with the nurse in charge present. The facilitator and senior nurse identify good practice and areas that need improving. A balanced report is formulated explaining both.
- Feedback the results to ward staff. Feedback is given to staff by explaining both good and poor practice. Specific examples are given, and the staff can question the results or request more information if they require it.
- Prepare an action plan with staff. Once all staff are aware of the results, a meeting should be planned to facilitate the development of an action plan with as many staff as possible.
- Follow up the action plan.
- Re-evaluate progress at agreed intervals.

Monitor's main weakness is that it relies very much on what is documented. Since its development in 1983, some of the criteria could now be perceived as redundant. *Monitor* can be a useful baseline tool and can lead to improvements, depending on action taken subsequent to the audit. Having used this tool numerous times, we have experienced a number of strengths and weaknesses. Two case studies are presented below.

CASE STUDY 4.1   DEMONSTRATING USE OF *MONITOR*

A study was carried out on a 30-bed acute medical ward, which subsequently changed the way the ward was organized and greatly improved the quality of the service offered to patients. Although good practice was highlighted, the main problems following the study were identified as:

- poor assessment of patients on admission
- medically orientated care plans
- poor evaluation of care plans
- lack of written information to patients
- poor clinical practice relating to:
  1 routine observations, e.g. unnecessary taking of temperature;
  2 knowledge relating to a cardiac arrest, e.g. not knowing the procedure;
  3 lifting and handling of patients, e.g. 'drag' lifting up the bed.

With the full support of the manager, the ward staff devised their action plan, which involved:

- a weekly ward meeting to discuss ward issues;
- all staff to undertake further training in record keeping;
- development of a ward information leaflet;
- reviewing the times and frequency of taking observations such as temperature, pulse and respiration;
- review of lifting and handling practice for all staff on the ward.

All the recommendations outlined in the action plan were implemented within six months. This occurred because ward staff were involved from the early stages of planning the project and were not coerced by their manager into implementing change at a pace that was unsuitable for the ward. Furthermore, the manager demonstrated support by attending all ward meetings and assisting wherever possible in facilitating the action plan, without attempting to direct it.

CASE STUDY 4.2 DEMONSTRATING USE OF *MONITOR*

This study was carried out on a surgical unit where staff were told 'you will be monitored next month'. They did not receive preparation regarding the study but had little choice regarding its implementation. The results of the study demonstrated how:

- there were problems with assessment and evaluation of care;
- patients complained of lack of sleep due to nurses talking loudly;
- medications were omitted, and the reasons for this were not recorded;
- clinical practice was poor in relation to:
  1 times of the administration of medication
  2 postoperative observations
  3 wound care, practice and policy

Good practice was highlighted in many areas; however, staff also recognized the problems identified and were willing to act on them with support. Unfortunately they received no such support from their manager, and after a three-month period it was evident that no changes had taken place. The senior ward sister was then formally counselled for failing to act on the findings of the *Monitor*, and was removed from her post to another ward. No further action followed to improve the quality of care on this ward. The result was a demotivated work-force who felt quality assurance was simply a tool to beat staff when they did not comply with the recommendations.

Lessons learned

It can be appreciated that in the above two case studies the importance of the application of the tool was as important as the robustness of the tool itself. Hence a knowledge of effective change management techniques is essential if what we learn from measuring practice is to be useful. These are outlined in the following chapter.

Qualpacs audit

Qualpacs – Quality Patient Care Scales – was devised in the USA by Wandelt and Ager (1974). Qualpacs is classed as a concurrent tool in auditing the quality of care of the patient on the ward.

Like *Monitor* (Goldstone and Galvin, 1983), Qualpacs reviews patients' records and uses patient and staff interviews, observations of patients and observations of staff. It is divided into six categories with a total of 68 criteria:

- Physical   15 criteria
- General   15 criteria

- Communication   8 criteria
- Psychosocial individual   15 criteria
- Psychosocial group   8 criteria
- Professional implications   7 criteria

Following each criterion are instructions that tell the auditor whether the observation is direct (D) or indirect (I). The scoring time for this tool is approximately 4 h, which is similar to the scoring time for tools such as *Senior Monitor* (Goldstone and Okai, 1986). The auditors are advised to intervene if the patient is at risk.

Before carrying out direct observation, the auditor develops a plan of care for the patients based on the information available, and then observes the patient and listens for approximately 2 h. When a nursing action is implemented, the observer scores the item. For example, one of the criteria is 'The "rejecting" or "demanding" patient continues to receive acceptance' and this is rated as either Best Care or Not Applicable or Not Observed. The weighting for each of these ranges from 5 to 1, with 'not applicable' or 'not observed' not scoring at all.

While carrying out this audit, the observer can identify the carer. If a criterion is not observed, the auditor can look in the care plan for evidence of its being carried out.

Once all the items have been scored, the mean for each criterion is determined. These are then totalled and divided by the number of criteria scored.

Qualpacs has the advantage of observing the verbal and non-verbal behaviour of patients, nurses, carers and other members of the multidisciplinary team. Furthermore, it uses more than direct observation to gain information and achieve a full picture of what is happening on the ward. This tool is currently being evaluated in the UK and has been tested extensively in North America; it appears to have overcome the main problems displayed by audit tools such as *Monitor* (Goldstone and Galvin, 1983) and Phaneuf's (1976), i.e. overemphasis on documentation and the nursing process. However, Qualpacs is time consuming and has a complicated scoring system. One could argue that auditors of Qualpacs may be subject to observer bias and that the scoring can be very subjective. Observers may allow their own personal feelings to enter into a situation and score more negatives or more positives depending on the situation.

Users of Qualpacs (Wainwright and Burnip, 1983) have felt that some of the criteria are orientated towards the American style of nursing but also that many others were transferable to the British system of nursing. Qualpacs is a valuable tool, which would need developing to suit British needs. However, it certainly highlights the value of auditing important nursing skills rather than just documentation of care.

We have found it can be useful to ignore the scoring system in any audit tool and to discuss simply the issues identified, not the score.

Phaneuf's audit (1976)

This audit is a retrospective appraisal of the nursing process by reviewing the patient's notes: following discharge of the patient, the nursing kardex and care plan are audited. The tool is therefore based on the assumption that all nursing care is accurately documented. In our experience, this has proved to be a false assumption. Nurses often write a care plan according to the patient's medical diagnosis rather than their individual needs and ability to meet the actions prescribed in a care plan.

The audit was devised around the following topics:

- reporting and recording care
- observations of symptoms and reactions
- supervision of patients
- implementation of nursing procedures
- health promotion via direction and teaching
- the implementation of medical orders
- supervision of those participating in care

It was suggested by the authors of the instrument that approximately five people audit up to ten records monthly postdischarge, and that the maximum time involved would be 15 minutes.

The tool consists of six or seven questions per topic, totalling 50 questions that need to be answered for each patient's record. As in most audit tools the tick boxes are 'yes', 'no' or 'uncertain'. The last is for use by the auditor if they feel the criteria have not been fully met. There is also a 'not applicable' box for the categories relating to nursing procedures and health promotions. The scores are totalled for all the components. Each of the 'yes' boxes has a predetermined weighted score. For example, in relation to the topic of physician/medical orders, if the medical diagnosis is complete and recorded accurately the score is 7. However, in the 'supervision of patient' category, if the nursing care plan has changed in accordance with the assessment of the patient the score is 4.

When all the scores in each section have been totalled, the quality of care is considered 'excellent' if the scores are 161 to 200; 'good' if between 121 and 160; 'incomplete' if between 81 and 120; and 'poor' if between 41 and 80. Less than 40 is considered 'unsafe'.

Phaneuf's audit is a simple tool which is easy to implement and easy to understand. However, there are questions regarding its validity. Although most areas utilize the nursing process to some degree, the tool relies heavily on documentation of care. Not all areas will find the questions applicable, as the nursing process has been interpreted to suit each particular area. Therefore, many areas would 'fail' a question because staff verbally communicate some information, or presume knowledge or actions and would not record all such details in a care plan or kardex. An example of this would be the criteria relating to whether a patient has recreational or diversional activities recorded. This would be considered on a daily basis depending on the needs and wishes of the patient, but would not necessarily be recorded in the care plan.

By carrying out this audit, one measures the quality of nursing documentation rather than the quality of care. This tool was developed in North America and therefore many of the criteria relate to the North American healthcare system.

Advantages of using off-the-shelf tools

These tools require assessors, who may be a staff nurse or the nurse in charge, and individuals can often find this a valuable learning experience. As the tools are easy to implement, the data collected can be collated on software without difficulty. Off-the-shelf tools are easy to use because they have already been developed, tried and tested and are therefore ready for immediate use. The development of an audit tool can be a long process requiring a great deal of time to perfect.

The tools mentioned above give a broad picture of a ward predominantly using criteria-based tools on the nursing process format. They also act as a baseline measure over time and, given that the study could be carried out annually within the same framework, it should act as a reliable indicator of change in care standards. Therefore, these can be replicated in different areas.

Disadvantages of using off-the-shelf tools

Off-the-shelf tools tend to rely on documented care (although Qualpacs does also use the observational skills of the assessor). They tend to have a non-specific focus, in that they cover a wide range of topics and criteria. The use of assessors working in wards and departments often has a halo effect on practice which may result in false observations. Finally, the assumption that what is documented is delivered may not always be true. More importantly the standard and style of care delivery are not addressed if the focus is purely on documentation.

We will now discuss some of the reasons why the use of off-the-shelf audit tools has decreased in favour of alternative methods for auditing quality of care.

The decreasing use of audit tools

It is interesting to note that published literature on the development and application of the tools cited above has dwindled since 1996. The reasons for this could include the following:

- Quality is now more readily perceived in terms of a 'whole systems' approach rather than fixing one piece of the jigsaw.
- The tools attempted to audit a wide range of criteria, some of which were outside the scope of the ward/department when trying to address the issues after the audit. An example of this could be the *Medical Surgical Monitor* (Goldstone, Ball and Collier, 1983), which asks about the numbers of staff and the skill mix. Ward managers may have little influence in changing the skill mix to deliver this standard, and as such would score negatively.
- Using audit tools is time consuming and costly, and there has been a significant reduction in posts that support the quality agenda through the management costs reduction imposed by successive governments. The irony is that with the renewed emphasis in the White Paper on clinical governance, many clinicians who moved into quality posts were made redundant and valuable expertise was lost.
- Clinical audit and medical audit are now reasonably well established and

therefore many of the issues within the audit can be achieved through these programmes.

- Snapshot analysis of quality care has been replaced by an approach using continuous quality improvement.
- Generic audit tools measure only what the author perceives to be important and relevant, which does not necessarily reflect the patient's perspective of quality.

Standard-based audit tools

When we discuss the structure, process or outcome criteria in nursing or the NHS, we tend to place aspects of the organization into one of these categories. Chapter 2 outlined how best practice can be documented using the Donabedian framework, namely:

- **Structure** – which refers to the physical setting, the structure of the organization, financial aspects, objectives, buildings, equipment, attitudes of staff, etc.
- **Process** – which refers to the actions taken by a nurse or member of staff or the care received by a patient.
- **Outcome** – which could be the modification of symptoms of illness, knowledge, satisfaction, skill level, compliance with treatment. 'Outcome criteria consist of assessment of the end results of care usually specified in terms of patient health, welfare and satisfaction' (Donabedian, 1976).

If a standard has been set using the SMARTER criteria outlined in Chapter 2, it is comparatively easy to adapt this into a simple audit tool. The example in Table 4.4 shows a locally agreed standard. This is followed by an audit tool derived from the standard which can then be used to measure compliance with agreed best practice. Staff can then complete the audit cycle by 'closing the audit loop'.

Following the use of structure, process and outcome criteria developed for pressure area care, an audit tool can be developed (see Table 4.5).

Advantages of standard-based audit tools

The advantages of using standard-based tools is that the ward staff 'own' these standards and are therefore more likely to accept them than if they were imposed. The standards and audit tools tend to reflect local priorities for improving practice. Audits of this nature are a natural progression from the formulation of standards and therefore assist staff in developing ideas of what can be suitably measured and what cannot.

It may also be possible to use outcome criteria when looking at clinical indicators for nursing. For example, if one were to assess the rate of pressure sores or hospital-acquired infections, the outcome criteria may indicate that staff have insufficient knowledge to prevent such problems. In this situation, the outcome elements can be improved with limited resource implications.

Table 4.4

Locally agreed standards for pressure area care

Structure

- Registered Nurse or Enrolled Nurse.
- Procedure number 'I' pressure area care.
- Pressure sore prevention protocol and research rationales.
- Aids for pressure prevention, with manufacturer's manual.
- Pressure sore audit forms.

Process

- Each registered nurse (RN) will assess all patients on admission using the Waterlow score.
- All patients with a score of >14 are identified as being at risk and problems, goals and nursing actions are identified.
- The EN evaluates the effectiveness of the care plan.
- The RN uses preventive aids according to protocol.
- The RN attends in-service training on pressure sore prevention within one week of starting on the ward.

Outcome

- The incidence of patients developing pressure sores after admission is reduced to <5%.
- Nurses' knowledge of pressure sore prevention will increase to a score of >90% as indicated by educational score test results following in-service training.
- All patients at risk will have a legible, written plan of care.

Reproduced with the permission of Brighton Health Care NHS Trust.

Disadvantages of standard-based audit tools

There are a few problems associated with this method of auditing. The use of structure criteria can prove problematic because nurses often have little control over many of these variables where deficiencies are identified. There is also a danger in assuming that good care is ensured if all the necessary structure and process criteria are met; for example, instances where wards can be fully staffed yet patients do not receive information regarding their illness and treatment. Thus one cannot attribute a link between structure and process; and furthermore, no evidence exists to suggest links between process and outcome.

Measuring only outcome criteria can be a problem for the following reasons:

- General outcomes should not be used as a single indicator of quality, because patients may have a positive outcome in spite of the care received rather than because of it.
- If staff feel that a patient must achieve a positive outcome within a specified period of time, they may well persuade a patient to achieve a goal at the expense of the holistic needs of the individual.
- It is difficult to discern whether a nurse is solely responsible for a positive patient outcome, because the involvement of the multidisciplinary team and

Table 4.5

Audit tool for pressure area care

	Source	Yes/No	Exemptions
Structure			
• Does an RN administer the patient's pressure area care?	Observe		
• Is the procedure no. 1, pressure area care, available on the ward?	Check records		
• Is the protocol for pressure sore prevention available on the ward?	Check records		
• Are aids for pressure sore prevention in full working order?	Observe Ask nurse		
• Do the nurses use the aids as outlined in manufacturer's manual?	Observe		
• Are pressure sore audit forms available on the ward?	Check records		
Process			
• If the Waterlow score is >14, does the patient have a problem, goal and nursing action documented within 6 h of admission?	Check records		
• Is this problem evaluated on every shift?	Check records		
• Does the nurse administer the care as prescribed?	Observe		
• Is the pressure sore audit form completed and given to the senior nurse following discharge?	Check records		
Outcome			
• Does the nurse attend in-service training sessions on pressure sore prevention within one week of starting on the ward?	Ask nurses		
• Does the nurse achieve >90% in the posteducational test?	Check records		
• Are the plans legible?	Check records		
• Is the annual incidence of pressure sores <5%?	Check records		

Reproduced with the permission of Brighton Health Care NHS Trust.

the patient's own response to treatment can also influence the achievement of outcome measures.
- The lack of research into predicting patient outcomes as a result of direct nursing intervention makes it difficult for the nursing profession confidently to identify achievable outcome measures. Studies into medical practices attempting to link structure and process criteria with an identifiable outcome show either no or limited correlation between the three variables.
- It is possible that close members of the patient's family and friends, or the patient themselves, are also variables influencing recovery.

Some authors suggest reviewing the goals set in comparison with the eventual outcome. In this way, sole use of any outcome can be avoided, giving nurses the opportunity to reflect on other components essential for patient care. However, this approach assumes that nurses have the ability and confidence to set realistic goals and that the nursing process is used effectively by nursing staff. Research into the use of the nursing process by the profession does not support this assumption.

An answer to the above problem depends on support for practitioners from nurse education and nursing research. Research is required to develop standards of care and then predict reliable outcomes for specific patient groups in response to a given nursing intervention. Nurses require further education and knowledge in order to formulate effective goals with patients. A first step to achieving this can be the use of reflective practice. We have found that a useful method is to photocopy care plans for a small group of patients who have been discharged in the last month. The next step is to spend time with the nurses discussing what the outcomes were in relation to the goals set. This may take 1–1.5 hours per month but assists nurses in thinking about the goals they set.

Another useful exercise is for nurses to summarize the progress of a patient with members of the multidisciplinary team for specific groups of patients in an effort to review the overall success of multidisciplinary interventions. In this way, deficiencies in practice, lack of knowledge or needs for further research are identified. For example, the multidisciplinary team may find that during the past year 25% of patients who suffered cerebrovascular accident also developed limb contractions. There is a need to establish whether this is acceptable given the severity of strokes or conditions in which the client was admitted or if massage would have prevented such a problem occurring. What is important is the analysis of why the contractions developed and that standards were set and audited which demonstrate whether the process of care was effective.

The above approach is not without problems. For example, Table 4.6 shows a care plan of a patient with a sacral sore causing pain. Even if the nurse ensures an improved nutritional status, suitable wound care products, pain relief and no pressure applied to the sacral sore, one cannot be certain that the sore will be 1 cm × 1 cm in ten days, or that this patient has the individual capacity for recovery.

Research has not proved conclusively that a combination of the above factors guarantees a predicted rate of wound healing. However, professional experience, gained as a result of caring for wounds, may allow the nurses to predict that the expected recovery rate should be a 1 cm reduction in the wound. Regrettably, nurses often fail to write case studies or reports or to share information of such expertise to allow others to benefit from their experience.

Criteria-based audit tools

Criteria-based audits differ from standard-based audits in that there is not necessarily a standard statement and the issues could be very broad rather than following criteria related to the process. Criteria-based audit tools are relatively simple to devise and use, and their development can stem from a variety of problems and issues.

Table 4.6

Patient care plan: sacral sore

Date	Patient problem	Goal	Nursing action
	Jack feels his sacral sore is causing pain. • Size of sore: 4cm × 4 cm • Colour: yellow/green • Depth: <0.5 cm • Waterlow score: 18	• Reduce pain to <3 on pain scale. • Reduce size to 1cm × 1 cm within 10 days.	• Offer prescribed analgesia 30 minutes before treatment; dose according to severity of pain. • Identify cause of pain. • Obtain wound swab. • Clean area with normal saline; apply a hydrogel to sloughy area according to wound care protocol. Apply non-occlusive dressing. Review treatment every day. • Ask Jack to alter position in bed 2-hourly. • Use Nimbus mattress and pump in accordance with policy. • Assess nutritional state – liaise with dietitian.

Reproduced with the permission of Brighton Health Care NHS Trust.

An example of a predetermined criteria-based audit tool can be found in the Standards of Physiotherapy Practice (1990), which identifies six areas of practice comprising 26 standards relating to practice. Local auditing of these involved composing a criteria-based audit tool.

It can be seen in Table 4.7 that the criteria do relate to a statement and are simple to audit. The standards and criteria apply to all physiotherapists, and local audit tools are similar in design and structure.

Advantages of criteria-based audits
Criteria-based audits are a useful method for:

- tackling a problem that staff feel might exist but whose scale they are unsure about;
- exploring the reasons for the existence of a known problem;
- measuring simple standards that are already predetermined.

Staff at departmental and ward level should be fully included in the whole change process and should therefore feel less threatened by the audit. This involvement also assists in ensuring commitment to implementation of the action plan.

Table 4.7

Documentation standards for physiotherapy practice

Standard: 'Clear, accurate and up-to-date records are maintained' Audit criteria	Yes	No	N/A
Is writing legible?			
Is writing in permanent ink?			
Are all entries recorded within 24hrs of treatment?			
Are all correction to the record initialized?			
Is a clear and logical format used?			
Are judgmental statements of a personal nature made?			
Are all entries dated and initialized?			
Are all attendances dated and initialized?			

Standard: 'Records describe all elements of the care episode' Audit criteria	Yes	No	N/A
Are patient details recorded?			
Is subjective information documented?			
Are findings of objective examinations documented?			
Is a problem list devised?			
Are goals identified?			
Is a treatment plan recorded?			
Are progress notes recorded?			
Is a goal-related discharge summary recorded?			

Standard: 'Records are retained in accordance with existing policies and current legislation' Audit criteria	Yes	No	N/A
Are records retained for a minimum of 8 years after conclusion of treatment?			
Are obstetric records held for 25 years?			
Are records relating to children kept until the patient's 25th birthday, or 8 years after the last entry if longer?			
Are patients' records stored securely?			
Are computerized physiotherapy records registered under the Data Protection Act 1984?			
Are records released with the patient's permission?			

Disadvantages of criteria-based audits

The methods used to formulate a criteria-based audit are based on either predetermined standards or clinical consensus. One could argue that the results obtained
can be specific only for that area. If the audit tool were to be transferable, the
tool would need to be piloted further and tested by a number of assessors to
prove its validity and to identify whether the criteria audited did indeed represent
best practice.

Summary

In our experience, many of the audit tools described above proved useful in beginning the process of changing and improving the quality of care. The main difficulty we experienced was that the whole audit process can quickly accelerate into an unplanned, uncoordinated number of initiatives. In practice, this created three key problems.

First, staff were developing and using audit tools without monitoring and supervision. In some instances, this led to a number of poorly designed tools being used and dubious data being produced. Staff had therefore invested significant time and effort in a project that had limited use. Without proper monitoring of such initiatives, there were also instances of duplication of effort, with several areas developing tools for similar projects, such as auditing nursing documentation and pressure area care management. It also meant that where good practice was identified, there was no mechanism for disseminating this to other areas.

Second, lack of coordination can lead to lack of cooperation from those participating in the audit who may be overloaded with similar requests from different areas. In one instance, this prompted a patient to ask whether it was possible to go to any department in the hospital without feeling obliged to participate in a patient satisfaction survey.

The final difficulty with focusing purely on audit is the lack of systematic approach to resolving deficiencies in care identified through the audit process. Some areas went on to take action to rectify these. Some areas used the results in a punitive way, making staff hostile to future audits. There were also examples where re-auditing several months later identified exactly the same deficiencies in care.

Another approach now gaining popularity seeks to provide an overview of the general indications of quality on a ward. This is called the Quality Pointers Tool (QPT), described below.

QUALITY POINTERS TOOL

The Quality Pointers Tool (QPT) was developed by York University and based on research originally undertaken to examine the effects of grade-mix changes in general medical and surgical wards (Bagust, Oakley and Slack, 1992). The QPT software system allows users to collect and store quality information, to assess the overall quality of care, and to analyse information on the level of care on each ward. The Quality Pointers Tool is basically a questionnaire. Through extensive research involving many clinical-based nurses, a set of simple, yet reliable and valid, questions were formulated to identify the most obvious and visible problems that occur on hospital wards. Each individual question helps to point to the quality of nursing care being achieved, and together they can give a reliable assessment of the overall quality of care that patients are receiving. The researchers who developed the tool identified that as wards got busier, or there were shortages of staff, certain elements of care tended to be omitted. The questionnaire enables these to be identified.

The Quality Pointers Tool is designed as a set of simple Yes/No questions that users can answer quickly and easily. The tool can be used over an extended period to compile a substantial database of quality information. As a result, it is possible to monitor the overall quality of nursing care over time so as to identify patterns and to track changes. It can be used to benchmark an individual ward's performance against itself, as well as against data collected by the York team, which make comparisons with other hospitals used in the study. Responses to the individual pointer questions are especially valuable as a starting point for ward audits, picking out those aspects that show particular strengths or weaknesses. But, crucially, the tool provides evidence on the quality effects of changes at ward level, e.g. staffing patterns, patient throughput, and so on. The tool can be used alone, or in conjunction with workload and dependency measures. Used in conjunction with these sorts of measures, it provides an important method of evaluating the impact of changes in establishment, and helps to identify areas of need in existing establishments. The Quality Pointers Tool provides information in the form of quality indicators, which can prove valuable in further developing measures of outcomes of nursing care. It can provide the following information:

- It identifies elements of care that require improvement, enabling staff to prioritize these.
- It maps trends in the quality of nursing care delivered through assessing:
  - the environment
  - team performance
  - specific aspects of the quality of care.
- It provides a mechanism to compare nurses' subjective professional judgements of the quality of care against objective criteria.
- It is a source of information to complement more subjective quantitative and qualitative information on patient dependency.
- It monitors the quality of care for each individual patient, the time given to each patient, and team levels of care.

In the case study below, we describe how the Quality Pointers Tool was introduced into an acute NHS Trust, and the benefits of the use of the tool to date. Before the introduction of the pilot, there was no systematic way of collecting this information within the Trust. The project was managed using the Projects in Controlled Environments (PRINCE) project management tool advocated by the National Health Service Executive for NHS use.

CASE STUDY 4.3 — IMPLEMENTING THE QUALITY POINTERS TOOL – APPROACH USED

The project team identified the following reasons for adopting this tool:

- to provide a method of objectively evaluating changes in skill mix and levels of activity in ward settings and the subsequent impact on the quality of care delivered;
- to provide a method of identifying areas of concern in relation to the quality of care, enabling further exploration and action planning;
- to provide valuable information to aid in the negotiation of nursing quality standards with purchasing authorities.

QPT project terms of reference
The following steps were taken to set up the project.

- identification of areas to pilot the project;
- installation of computer software and ongoing IT support;
- identification of staff-training programme;
- clarification of effective communication pathways for generating reports and subsequent action plans and evaluations;
- identification of a project roll-out strategy.

Project management
The project board was established, with the responsibilities identified as follows.

Responsibilities of project group members
- **Project board: patient services development group.** This group of senior nurses was responsible for the initiation, direction and review and eventual closure of the project. It held the authority required for committing resources and initiating new work. The Assistant Director of Nursing (who chaired the Project Steering Group) reported directly to the project board.

Project Steering Group: key roles
- **Executive function.** The Director of Nursing held prime responsibility for ensuring the project was capable of achieving the expected benefits and that the project was completed within the costs and timescales agreed by the project board.
- **Senior user.** The senior nurses held prime responsibility to represent the interests of the clinical directorate involved in the project and to monitor project progress against the identified requirements of the clinical directorates for QPT information.
- **Senior technical representative.** The IT department representative held prime responsibility for providing technical expertise for the project.

- **Project manager.** The Assistant Director of Nursing held prime responsibility for ensuring that the project produced the required products, to the required standard of quality, and within the specified constraints of time and cost. The main tasks for the post holder were:
  - overall planning for the whole project;
  - liaison with other related projects, i.e. Nurse Information, Workforce Planning Methodology Group, Clinical Performance Improvement Unit;
  - defining responsibilities for each stage manager;
  - reporting to and taking direction from PSDG as the project board;
  - presenting regular highlight reports bimonthly for the overall project to the project board.
- **Stage manager.** The Nurse Information Coordinator held prime responsibility for day-to-day management of project activities and products. The stage manager worked closely with the project manager to define responsibilities for team members in participating wards and to provide individual ward project plans, guidance and inspiration. The stage manager was responsible for running progress meetings and assisting the project manager in the production of the highlight reports to the senior nurse group.
- **Project assurance team.** Other members of the project steering group.
- **Business assurance coordinator.** The Personal Assistant to the Assistant Director of Nursing held prime responsibility to provide a focal point for administrative control. This individual was not expected to attend planning meetings, but was fed information through the project manager and stage manager.
- **Technical assurance coordinator.** The IT representative held prime responsibility for providing technical advice and support to the project and stage managers and to the team leaders of participating wards.
- **User assurance coordinator.** The Heads of Nursing representatives from each clinical directorate and the ward sister/charge nurse from pilot sites held prime responsibility for providing a link between the pilot project and nurses across the Trust.

In order to map the success of the project and identify the resources in relation to the activities and timescales required to achieve its aims, it was important to be clear about the products the project was expected to deliver. These are shown below.

Deliverables (project products)
- A Quality Pointers Tool programme available in the ward area.
- Trained staff who are able to input data and generate reports.
- A system of using QPT reports to identify action plans and initiate quality improvement in participating areas.
- A system of feeding QPT reports into the existing Nurse Information System.

For each of these products, an action plan with deadlines and resource implications was developed.

Implementation
The IT department installed the software on the ward-based personal computers. A standard set-up was used to assist training. Training was set up to take place after installation and was conducted by the project manager and stage manager. Two of the three wards in the pilots had key staff trained, who then cascaded training to other staff. A third ward requested individual training for all staff. A maximum of 30 minutes was required to train staff to a basic level. Additional training was given to senior staff to show them how to use the reporting system for QPT. Written documentation about the tool and how to use it was given to all staff. Data entry took place at the end of each shift by the nurse in charge. Once they were competent, data entry time was minimal. Each pilot ward was required to draw up objectives for the application of the results.

Figure 4.4 shows one of the many reports it is possible to generate using the QPT. It can be seen from this that staff can identify the number of shifts that scored for an excellent, good, adequate, barely safe or dangerous level of care. Since the introduction of QPT, a trigger mechanism has been put in place which requires remedial action to be taken immediately if dangerous levels of care are reported. The ward managers continually review the data derived from QPT and use them as a basis for identifying quality improvement priorities.

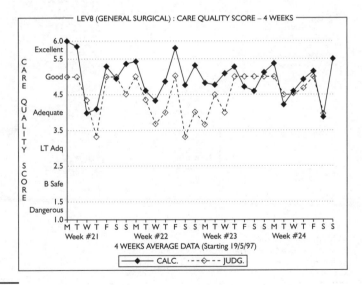

Figure 4.4

Example of a Quality Pointers Tool report (reproduced with the permission of Brighton Health Care NHS Trust)

Achievements following the pilot of QPT

The reports generated have been able to depict accurately the levels of quality of care on the participating wards, and to highlight the impact on quality of issues such as increased patient acuity and nursing skill mix.

Communication has improved at ward level (identified in the QPT evaluation), and between staff levels up to and including general managers. A protocol has been developed depicting the flow of this information throughout the organization (Figure 4.5).

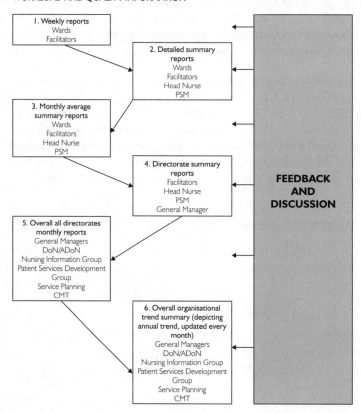

Figure 4.5

Flow of Nursing Information through Brighton Health Care NHS Trust
(reproduced with the permission of Brighton Health Care NHS Trust)

The information produced by QPT complemented other nursing information on workload, quality and skill mix by providing a more specific analysis of team performance, environmental factors, and aspects of care. It has also promoted further development of an information culture, with ward nurses now actively using IT to aid decision making and as a tool to analyse their practice.

As part of the evaluation of the pilot wards, staff were asked how the information from QPT had been useful. They identified that it

- highlighted changes in activity due to changes in patient mix and environmental issues;
- highlighted the effect on quality of the busier periods on the wards;
- prompted discussion relating to standards of nursing care, skill mix, reassessment of priorities, and individual and collective responsibilities;
- encouraged honest and open feedback and support to improve practice.

The pilot wards instituted the following changes as a result of using the QPT:

- Core care plans were designed when QPT identified a delay in writing care plans.
- The staff handover period was redesigned after QPT raised issues about its duration and quality.
- A protocol was developed for admission of patients between A&E and the ward.
- Changes were made in the skill mix and roster to meet increased activity identified in late shifts.
- A shortage of nurses with cannulation skills was highlighted and addressed.
- The fact that staff did not get breaks was highlighted.
- Communication was improved between staff of all grades about quality issues.

Conclusions

There were a few minor problems in the application of the Quality Pointers Tool. Some of the questions in the questionnaire were ambiguous, leading to staff developing their own interpretations. Some questions will not apply to specific wards, e.g. those with no students. The system currently runs in a DOS environment, which undermines the Trust's IT strategy which promotes the use of Windows-based systems only. The QPT was nevertheless found to be a useful and worthwhile investment for reasons outlined above. It was well supported by staff and there are now plans to roll it out throughout the trust.

PATIENT CARE PATHWAYS

Patient care pathways are often termed 'critical care pathways' (Wigfield and Boon, 1996) or 'multidisciplinary care pathways' (Von Degenberg, 1997). Chapter 2 identifies some of the features of care pathways and their use in current practice. This section aims to discuss their application and to show how variance analysis, an integral part of care pathways, can be used to measure clinical practice.

The relevance of care pathways in practice

Care pathways can be useful for:

- **Bridging the acute and primary care interface.** The most effective way to develop a care pathway is to consider the whole episode of care. This should transgress the primary and acute settings rather than observing distinctions based on organizational rather than patient need. Some countries (notably Australia) are also involving social services in the development of pathways.
- **Improving cost effectiveness.** Cost effectiveness can be improved in a variety of ways. Firstly, bed days can be reduced by ensuring that patients who have uncomplicated stays in hospital do not stay longer than required and that this agreement is shared among consultants who perform the same operation.

Cost effectiveness can also be improved by reducing the use of ritualized and often expensive clinical practices. By discussing clinical practice areas such as drugs usage, practice can be reviewed and standardized to prevent wastage and inappropriate use.

Promoting research-based practice and improving quality of care

When designing care pathways, there has to be discussion and agreement on what represents best clinical practice. This is the ideal opportunity to introduce and develop care pathways that are based on evidence rather than 'that's how we've always done it'. Examples have included:

- the routine taking of all observations rather than those that will aid in determining the physiological status of the patient;
- using products that have no benefit and are costly, e.g. antiseptic bath additives and alcohol swabbing;
- starving patients for excessive periods before surgery;
- completing excessive admission details for day surgery patients;
- duplicating personal details by more than one professional group.

Alternatively, clinical practice can be enhanced and developed by discussions that relate to care that patients should (but may not currently) receive, or care that requires development. Examples have included:

- assessment of pain postoperatively
- delivery of timely analgesia postoperatively
- use of anti-embolic stockings
- effective discharge planning

Quality of care can be enhanced by all patients receiving what is prescribed in the care pathway, and audit can assist in addressing why this care was omitted. In a broader sense, issues such as skill mix, staffing levels and poor morale may underpin why care is not delivered, according to the care pathway, especially if variance analysis demonstrates that patients are not receiving certain aspects of care.

Problems can be identified through variance analysis, and this will be discussed in further detail below.

Improving documentation

Care pathways assist in improving documentation for the following reasons:

- Documentation is preprinted in typeface and therefore legible.
- Problems have to be clearly reported in the variance section and causes of variance are recorded.
- The information is available and clearly presented so that patients/clients have access to information that details the care they will receive.

Of course there is no guarantee that staff will deliver the care that is predocumented. However, care pathways do provide information that encourages the professional to sign and record whether care is given or is to be omitted. Care pathway documentation usually takes one of two forms:

- **Outcome-based documentation** – which is used where the physiological status is predetermined for that part of the care pathway. Examples of this include:
  - patient mobile without crutches
  - can carry out hygiene requirements independently
  - wound clean and dry
- **Process-based documentation** – which records a statement thus:
  - Mobilize the patient without use of crutches.
  - Provide assistance with hygiene if required.
  - Check the wound.

The aim of using outcome-based documentation is to promote exception reporting rather than expecting people always to write an evaluation. This of course can be difficult to accept for nurses who have traditionally been used to the nursing process method of assessment, planning, implementation and evaluation. Evaluation is still important when using care pathways, but it is specific and restricted to exceptions rather than being seen as the normal process when documenting care.

One fear is the potential for increased litigation. This fear stems from a conception that if details of care are not recorded in writing, this may be interpreted as the patient having received no care.

This assumption is responsible for the meaningless phrases that abound in many nursing notes and do not really reflect the true physiological or psychological status of the patient. They include:

- 'slept well'
- 'up and about'
- 'NOP' (no obvious problems)

Conversely, some believe that if practice is documented (as in a preplanned care pathway) and then that process is not carried out, the patient/client can undertake legal proceedings for a failure of duty to care.

However, as yet there is no indication that the use of care pathways in the USA or indeed in the United Kingdom has promoted this course of action. This is an untested case. If Trusts and primary care units agree a care pathway via the usual risk management process, then vicarious liability rests with the organization (i.e. one would expect a structure to be in place to endorse such pathways or to challenge them if inappropriate).

Purchaser involvement in the outcomes of care pathways

As yet there are no purchasers who have used care pathways to determine length of stay targets for specific diagnostic groups and thus impose constraints on modes of treatment. However, if care pathways were developed nationally, it is possible that purchasers could work with providers on this issue.

Variance analysis

Variance analysis is a method of measuring care against the pathway. Variations from the plan are recorded; for example, noting reasons for tests not being carried out as per plan. Variance also records activities that were not planned or anticipated as part of that person's care.

Coding variance can be undertaken by using a scale that details what the score of the variance is. Hotchkiss (1997) describes the scale used by the West Glamorgan Hospital, which includes:

1 Patients
2 Family
3 Nurse omission/commission
4 Clinical omission/commission
5 External system
6 Internal system

A code '1' would be given if the patient's condition necessitated other action to be taken which deviated from the care pathway. An example of this might be that a patient refused to eat or drink, or felt unable to.

'Patients' and 'Family' relate to factors concerning the personal or social circumstances of the patient or family where this may affect the progress of the patient. An example might be the family having a problem with broken heating, thus preventing a person being discharged, and therefore a code '2' would be recorded.

'Nurse' or 'Clinical omission/commission' refer to tasks that are either omitted or carried out earlier than expected. Omissions could be because of sickness levels and an imbalance in skill mix, a crisis on the ward, or a professional judgement to omit care for some other reason. A code '3' or '4' would be documented, depending on who was delivering the care.

'External system' refers to factors outside the organization which delay the progress of the patient. Examples might include:

- delays in ambulance transport;
- lost communication between hospitals;
- home support not being available to discharge a patient;
- inability to find urgent accommodation for a previously homeless person who is now unable to care for themselves.

A code '5' would be documented for any of these problems.

'Internal system' refers to all the departments and processes that operate within an organization and result in delays. Examples include the following:

- reduced pharmacy staffing, resulting in delays to take-home medications;
- emergency admissions resulting in the MRI scanner being fully booked and therefore delay in using it for routine investigations.

A code '5' would be recorded on the variance analysis sheet if either of these problems occurred.

The categories above are designed to code the reason and then to document any subsequent action contemporaneously.

Wigfield and Boon (1996) use four categories for classification:

1 Patient variance
2 Clinical, nurse, paramedic
3 System variance
4 Community variance

The variance sheet may look like the one depicted in Table 4.8. Variance analysis can be recorded in the following ways:

- The care pathway can be used to audit what is written and this should become an established part of the pathway.
- The variance sheet can be analysed to find out the source where problems arise for the organization. These can then enter the audit cycle.

Table 4.8

Variance sheet

VARIANCE SHEET			PATIENT LABEL	
Date	Day number	Variance code	Action taken	Effect
25/6/97	2	I (haemorrhage)	Informed medical staff	Return to theatre

The variance analysis should become an integral part of multidisciplinary clinical audit. Changes and developments to practice will then be proactive and the content of the care pathway remain relevant and useful.

Summary

This chapter has described a few of the many approaches used in healthcare to measure clinical practice and clinical and organizational performance. All need to be viewed within the context of the audit cycle outlined in the preceding chapter. It can be appreciated from some of the case studies that the ability of any measurement tool to effect change in clinical practice lies as much in its application as in the tool itself. Hence an understanding of effective change management techniques is fundamental to the application of the audit cycle. The next chapter will outline some of the theories of change management.

References

Bagust, A., Oakley, T. and Slack, R. (1992) *Ward Nursing, Quality and Grade Mix*, North Western Regional Health Authority, Manchester, p. 42.

Bardsley, M. and Cleary, R. (1994) Auditing the outcome of total knee replacement, in *Outcomes into Clinical Practice* (ed. T. Delamothe), BMJ Publishing Group, London, pp.70–80.

Barnett, D. and Wainwright, P. (1987) Between two tools. *Senior Nurse*, 614, 40–2.

Blythe, Lord (1995) Charter Mark Awards 1997 – Guide for Applicants, Charter Unit, London.

Bullivant, J. (1996) Benchmarking in the UK NHS. *International Journal of Health Care Quality Assurance*, 9(2), 9–14.

Calman, K. (1994) Introduction, in *Outcomes into Clinical Practice* (ed. T. Delamothe), BMJ Publishing Group, London, pp.1–13.

Corrigan, P. (1989) *Evaluation of Monitor Project*, Seacroft and Killingbeck Hospitals, Leeds.

Delamothe, T. (1994) *Outcomes into Clinical Practice*, BMJ Publishing Group, London.

Department of Health (1991) *Patients' Charter*, Department of Health, London.

Dickson, N. (1987) Do you measure up? *Nursing Times*, 83(44), 25.

Donabedian, A. (1976) *Some Issues in Evaluating the Quality of Health Care in Issues of Evaluation Research*, American Nurses Association, Kansas City, MO.

General Medical Council (1998) *Maintaining Good Medical Practice*, GMC, London.

Goldstone, L. (1991) *Accident and Emergency Monitor*, Newcastle upon Tyne Polytechnic Products, Newcastle upon Tyne.

Goldstone, L. and Galvin, J. (1983) *Paediatric Monitor*, Newcastle upon Tyne Polytechnic Products, Newcastle upon Tyne.

Goldstone, L. and Hughes, D. (1989) *Midwifery Monitor*, Newcastle upon Tyne Polytechnic Products, Newcastle upon Tyne.

Goldstone, L. and Illsley, V.A. (1985) *District Nursing Monitor*, Newcastle upon Tyne Polytechnic Products, Newcastle upon Tyne.

Goldstone, L. and Okai, M. (1986) *Senior Monitor*, Newcastle upon Tyne Polytechnic Products, Newcastle upon Tyne.

Goldstone, L. and Whittaker, C. (1990) *Health Visiting Monitor*, Gale Centre Publications, Loughton.

Goldstone, L. Ball, J. and Collier, M. (1983) *Monitor: An Index of the Quality of Nursing Services on Acute Medical and Surgical Wards*, Newcastle upon Tyne Polytechnic Products, Newcastle upon Tyne.

Health and Safety Executive (1997) *Successful Health and Safety Management*, Health and Safety Executive, London.

Hotchkiss, R. (1997) Integrated care pathways. *Nursing Times Research*, 2(1), 30–7.

JCAHO (1988) *Accreditation Manual for Hospitals*, JCAH, Chicago, Ill.

Marsh, J. and Brittle, J. (1986) Monitor – definition of measurement. *Nursing Times*, 82, 36–7.

Maxwell, M. (1983) *Accreditation: The Way Forward in the NHS*, Keele University, Keele.

Maxwell, M., Kennedy, T. and Spours, A. (1996) Clinical benchmarking – results into practice. *Journal of Health Care Quality Assurance*, 9(14), 20–3.

Mulley, A. (1994) Outcomes research implications for policy and practice, in *Outcomes into Clinical Practice* (ed. T. Delamothe), BMJ Publishing Group, London, pp.13–28.

NHS Benchmarking Reference Centre (1994) *Introduction to Process Mapping*, NHS Benchmarking Reference Centre, Wrexham.

NHS Executive (1994) EL(94)16: Report of the independent enquiry relating to deaths and injuries on the children's ward at Grantham and Kesteven General Hospital during the period February to April 1991 ('the Allitt Inquiry'). Letter by Sir Duncan Nichol, Chief Executive NHS Management Executive, Department of Health, London.

NHS Executive (1996) *NHS Information Management and Technology Strategy*, NHS Executive, London.

NHS Executive (1997) *The New NHS: Modern, Dependable*, Department of Health, London.

NHS Executive (1998) *A First Class Service: Quality in the New NHS*, Department of Health, London.

NHS Executive (1998) The New NHS: Modern, Dependable — A National Framework for Assessing Performance Consultation Document.

Orchard, C. (1994) Comparing healthcare outcomes. *British Medical Journal*, 308, 1493–6.

Phaneuf, M. (1976) *The Nursing Audit*, Appleton Century Croft, New York.

Price, J. (1997) Accredited nursing, *Nursing Standard*, 11(24), 26–7.

Pullan, B. and Chittock, J. (1986) Quantifying quality. *Nursing Times*, 82(1), 38–39.

Rigge, M. (1997) Keeping the customer satisfied. *Health Service Journal*, 107(5577), 24–7.

Royal College of Physicians (1996) *The Consulting Physician: Responding to Change*, Royal College of Physicians, London.

Scally, G. and Donaldson, L. (1998) Clinical governance and the drive for quality improvement in the new NHS in England. *British Medical Journal*, 317, 61–5.

Scrivens, E. (1995) *Protecting the Professional or the Consumer*, Open University Press, Buckingham.

Shaugnessy, P. (1998) *What Exactly Are Outcomes?*, Internet, Olsten Health Services http//www.okqchomehealth.com/whatsnews/.

Standards of Physiotherapy Practice (1990) Chartered Society of Physiotherapists, London.

Tannahill, A. (1985) Reclassifying prevention. *Public Health*, 99(6), pp.364–6.

United Kingdom Central Council for Nursing, Midwifery and Health Visiting (1996) *Guidance for Professional Practice*, UKCC, London.

Vincent, C. (1995) *Clinical Risk Management*, BMJ Publications, London.

Vincent, C. (1997) *Risk, Safety and the Darker Side of Quality*, British Medical Journal, 314, 1775–6.

Von Degenberg, K. (1997) Integrated care pathways. *NT Research*, 2(1), 37.

Wainwright, P. and Burnip, S. (1983) QualPacs at Burford. *Nursing Times*, 2 February, 36–8.

Wandelt, M.A. and Ager, J. (1974) *Quality Patient Care Scales*, Appleton Century Crofts, New York.

Whelan. J. (1987) Using monitor-observer bias, *Senior Nurse*, 7(6)

Wigfield, A. and Boon, E. (1996) Critical care pathway development: the way forward. *British Journal of Nursing*, 5(12), 732–5.

Williams, M. (1994) Using outcome information to improve acute care: total hip replacement surgery, in *Outcomes into Clinical Practice* (ed. T. Delamothe), BMJ Publishing Group, London, pp.56–70.

5 STRATEGIC PLANNING AS A MECHANISM FOR IMPROVING PROFESSIONAL PRACTICE

INTRODUCTION

Chapter 1 outlined the significant impact practitioners have on influencing the quality and cost of healthcare through the way in which they practise. Healthcare professionals clearly do not practise within a vacuum, and the quality of the service they are able to offer patients is influenced by the environment in which they are practising. The impact of the physical environment – the equipment, drugs, support services, etc. – is obvious. Less tangible, but equally important, is the organizational culture. Is it an open and questioning organization in which innovations are encouraged and welcomed? Or is it one that stifles creativity and conspires to silence those who question the status quo? Creating a climate that encourages quality improvement is a challenge for many organizations, and approaches for attempting to do this are covered in this chapter. These look at the organization as a whole, but it can also be argued that, to understand the whole, we must appreciate its component parts, understand how they work and identify mechanisms to keep them functioning and healthy.

The NHS has a rich cultural history, as do the professional groups that function within it. The way in which these professional groups are organized and managed (if we accept many of the rational change management theories), or self-organize and function (if following complex adaptive models of change management), will affect both the performance and behaviour of the professional. We believe that the development of professional practice can be enhanced through creating a strategic plan to develop the profession (and professionals) to meet the needs of the public it serves.

This chapter therefore outlines some of the principles of strategic planning and change management, and uses a case study based on our own experience of developing, implementing and evaluating a strategy for nursing and midwifery in an NHS Trust. Although this is a nursing case study, we contend that these principles are relevant to any professional group seeking identity and leadership within the increasingly complex healthcare systems of today. The underpinning theory and lessons learned from our attempts to provide a strategic framework for the development of professional nursing can, we believe, be applied equally to the medical profession and may also offer some advantages to pharmacists, physiotherapists, dietitians, occupational therapists and other professions allied to medicine. The challenge for the latter groups is securing a mechanism for influence at board level. We believe that strong alliances between these groups and the nursing and medical director can be mutually advantageous.

Why have a strategy for nursing?

In 1989 the Chief Nursing Officer for England launched *The Strategy for Nursing* (Department of Health, 1989). This document outlined the strategic direction for nurses in England and identified a number of targets to be achieved locally. This was followed by *A Vision for the Future* (Department of Health, 1993). For many hospitals and NHS Trusts, these DoH documents provided the framework for the development of local strategies to meet the targets set. Hence in many NHS Trusts the rationale for the development of local strategies for nursing was driven by a wider national directive.

The development of strategies for nursing is a relatively new phenomenon. An extensive literature search of both commercial and library databases (including those in the Royal College of Nursing) yielded comparatively few articles, with none cited before 1988. This mirrors the growing number of articles in recent years expressing concerns about the leadership and direction of the nursing profession. It could be argued that the two issues are interconnected. The title of the second Department of Health (1993) document, with its reference to a 'vision', implies a promise of better and brighter things for the future. Making the vision a reality is the challenge for the nurse leaders of the future. As Nelson Mandela wrote,

> *Vision without action is merely dreaming, action without vision is just passing the time of day; but combine action with vision and you can change the world. (Mandela, in Brown, 1996)*

The next section seeks to identify the skills required by nurse leaders if they are to realize this vision. Relevant literature is then reviewed in an attempt to identify a framework to effect the necessary changes.

Nursing leadership in the UK

> *The concept of nursing leadership in the UK would appear to have reached a crossroads. The NHS reforms, coupled with changes within the nursing profession, have emphasised the distinction between the 'nursing management' of the past and the qualitatively different 'nursing leadership' model of the future'. (Stamp, 1992)*

This observation is significant in all nursing leadership positions, from the chief nurse right down through the nursing structure. The role of senior nurses in purchasing has been subject to speculation and would appear inadequately represented in spite of the acknowledgement that they have a significant role to play (NHS Executive, 1993). The new White Paper (NHS Executive, 1997) seeks to address nurse involvement at board level by incorporating nurses on primary care group boards.

There are also changes in NHS Trusts, with many executive nurses responsible not for the operational management of nurses (now devolved to clinical directorates), but for providing professional advice to the board as well as leadership and direction to nursing staff. The distinction is thus made between managing nurses and leading nursing. This distinction is more than academic, since, devoid of the hierarchical power of the past, the executive nurse director requires a new armoury of skills very different from the old-style, operationally focused Director of Nursing (DoN). A recent survey exploring the roles and perceptions of nursing in NHS Trusts established a number of findings that are relevant when considering the role and function of nurse executives (NHS Executive, 1995). The report sought to clarify perceptions with regard to the value that DoNs bring to the board. The perceptions of nurse directors and chief executives (CEs) are shown in rank order in Table 5.1.

Table 5.1	Director of Nursing	Chief executive
Where DoNs bring value to the board: DoN and CE perceptions compared	• Strategic development	• Quality assurance
	• Clinical practice development	• Clinical practice development
	• Quality assurance	• Strategic development
	• Education contracting	• Clinical audit
	• Operational management	• Operational management
	• Service reconfiguration	• Education contracting
	• Clinical audit	• Complaint handling

Source: NHS Executive (1995).

It can be seen that nurse directors place strategic development first, whereas the chief executives place this as the third most valuable contribution. This has implications for Directors of Nursing; first, in that the chief executives rank only third what the DoNs view as their most valuable asset, indicating they need to raise the profile of this work. Second, there is clearly an expectation from the CE that the DoN take a lead in quality assurance and clinical practice development at board level. It would, therefore, seem prudent for nurse executives to examine their work profile and ensure that these expectations are being met. This offers real opportunities with respect to the clinical governance agenda.

These findings need to be considered alongside others in the NHS Executive report (1995) which indicate that nurse managers spend most of their time on, and bring added value to, day-to-day issues such as staff management and development and operational management. The report showed a disparity between the high value attached to clinical practice development and the lower amount of time spent on this activity. The report suggests that clinical managers are more reactive than proactive (p. 20). Hence in spite of the *value* placed on strategic development and the development of clinical practice through strategic planning, the *reality* is that clinical managers clearly do not have the time to develop this. Recognition therefore must be given to the key role of the DoN in driving the strategic vision for nursing. As the report notes (p. 15), 'If clinical managers are not spending enough time on clinical practice development, the delivery of the nurse director's operational and strategic agenda may well be compromised.'

Skills and competencies for nurse leaders

Another study (Prospect Centre, 1992) identified the skills and competencies necessary for nursing directors. These are shown in Table 5.2. This table has been amended and regrouped to take account of the top three priorities listed in Table 5.1 with the relevant skills grouped below each heading. Issues pertaining to leadership are also listed.

In reviewing the competencies in Table 5.2, it is interesting to note the similar themes that arise when compared with two authors' definition of strategic planning:

Table 5.2

A competency framework for Trust Directors of Nursing

Strategic development (including management of change)

- Sees the organization as a total system: takes a 'helicopter' view of the Trust as a whole, within a bigger healthcare system.
- Challenges the status quo: thinks innovatively and creatively about new ways of doing things to improve organizational practice.
- Influences planning and management of change: understands the importance of clarity about what is to be achieved; establishes goals for its achievement and monitors progress; understands the value of projects in promoting involvement in change and develops ownership of the change process.
- Champions the human consequences of change: understands the need for people to have time to acclimatize to change; anticipates the impact of change on the organization and takes appropriate steps to address it; recognizes the importance of people to the development of the organization.
- Uses basic concepts of business management: understands the fundamental elements and processes of running a successful independent business enterprise.
- Understands the evolving role of the nursing director: identifies the development needs of self and others; assesses and judges people's potential for career advancement.

Clinical practice development

- Effectively delegates decision making to others: understands the importance of supporting others' development; involves them directly in activities for which they will assume authority; is tolerant of their mistakes as part of the learning process and progressively releases control.

Quality assurance*

- Articulates what constitutes effective patient care: demonstrates a commitment to health care and the importance of the patient as a customer deserving of the highest quality of care.

Leadership

- Motivates nurses to bring about change: displays strong leadership skills; employs effective communication skills; recognizes the importance of encouraging feedback from the workforce.
- Employs personal networks to promote change: gains the respect and credibility of others.
- Builds constructive relationships with non-nurse management: builds teams; is diplomatic and receptive to others' points of view; possesses clarity about own and others' roles.

---

* Encompasses the broader concept of quality improvement rather than narrower definitions of quality assurance.
Adapted from Prospect Centre, 1992, p.40.

The term 'strategic' expresses deliberate and conscious articulation of direction. An explicit strategy allows for co-ordination of activity; it provides direction for people, rather than merely reacting; people can begin to plan, change and establish priorities. (Peters and Waterman, 1988)

Now we have made the observation that there is a fundamental difference between managing nurses and leading nursing, and have described the competencies necessary for the latter, the attraction of strategic planning as a tool for helping the new nurse leaders in their much altered roles can be appreciated. There would appear to be an overlap between the *competencies* of future nurse leaders, and the theories of strategic planning. Hence the two are interlinked. Nurse leaders need a mechanism to turn the *Vision for the Future* (Department of Health, 1993) into a reality, and strategic planning and implementation is the *process* that enables them to do this. Effective strategy development and implementation are dependent on leaders with the vision and competencies to promote that vision through the strategic planning process. This therefore answers the question posed at the beginning of this section: 'Why have a strategy for nursing?' Leaders with vision need a clear strategy to achieve that vision, or, in Mandela's words, 'combine action with vision and you can change the world' (in Brown, 1996).

Given that strategic planning is relatively new to nursing – and given the links and interrelationships between strategy, quality assurance and change management – the next section reviews the literature to explain the theories and rationale for the approach used in the Brighton Health Care Strategy for Nursing and Midwifery (Appendix 1). This is followed by a case study outlining the practical application of these theories and assessing their usefulness. In the words of one author, 'If you don't know where you are going, you will probably end up somewhere else' (Bera, in Stransen 1988).

WHAT IS A STRATEGY OR STRATEGIC PLANNING?

The *Collins Dictionary* defines 'strategy' as 'a particular long term plan for success, especially in politics, business etc'. This emphasizes the long-term rather than reactionary approach, the notion of developing some kind of plan, and the concept of working towards 'success' or agreed aims.

From reviewing the literature on strategic planning in nursing, some other definitions are offered. Hoffman (1990) stresses the importance of widespread consultation to ensure multiple viewpoints are heard, and recommends a participatory approach.[1]

Hastings' (1990) model for a professional practice environment is shown in Table 5.3.

It can be seen from the above definitions that there are similarities between the strategic planning process and the competencies for nurse leaders in

---

[1] Nursing is used to include Nursing, Midwifery and Health Visiting

Table 5.3	1	Establish the mission, leadership, vision and sense of direction for that organization.
A model for the development of a professional practice environment	2	Identify and communicate organizational priorities and strategic direction.
	3	Operationalize the professional practice model through:
	•	standards of care
	•	allocation of resources and design for delivery system
	•	systems to support professional practice:
		– education
		– governance
		– research and evaluation

Source: Hastings (1990).

Table 5.2. This 'rational' approach is one that is favoured by a number of authors. Boisot (1995), for example, defines strategic planning as 'essentially a rational approach where the availability of the right kind of data and a judicious application of the appropriate analytical tools means the strategic environment can be adequately grasped'.

Strategic planning, therefore, is used to give a sense of direction to corporate endeavours. The use of such rational planning models makes a number of assumptions:

- that there is adequate data/analysis available for planning;
- that the instruments used to collect data are accurate, valid and reliable;
- that the environment into which the strategy is introduced does not experience any unpredicted changes to the status quo.

The latter point is particularly problematic in the NHS, which can be affected by numerous unpredictable factors that can confound even the best-planned strategy; for example, changes in epidemiology, the development of the HIV virus and multiresistant bacteria, changes in government policy, introducing the internal market into the NHS, developments in technology (e.g. the introduction of keyhole surgery) and many other factors.

In such circumstances, the application of a rational planning approach is more difficult in the absence of comprehensive information. In a more turbulent (rather than predictable) organization, the development of 'strategic intent' may be a more appropriate approach.

Heavy turbulance

Intended strategy ⟶ Realised strategy

Figure 5.1

Strategic intent (reproduced with the permission of McGraw Hill, Developing Strategic Thought: Rediscovering the Art of Direction Giving, M. Boisot (1995))

'Strategic intent' describes the process of coping with turbulence through direct, intuitive understanding emanating from the top of an organization and guiding its efforts (Boisot, 1995, p. 36). It therefore relies on developing a vision to give it unity and coherence. It succeeds by remaining simple and intelligible and by avoiding a level of detail that might quickly be rendered obsolete by unpredicted events. This is illustrated in Figure 5.1.

For example, an NHS Trust may set a standard to reduce the incidence of pressure sores by 5% within one year (the 'intent'). The methods used to *achieve* this standard can vary widely, depending on the client group, new research, development of new pressure-relieving aids, and unpredictable events (such as an outbreak of *Clostridium difficile* in a care-of-the-elderly ward leading to an increased risk). The actions to be taken towards realizing the intent are therefore identified using local expertise.

Rational planning and strategic intent approaches have their supporters and critics, largely dependent on the strategic environment into which these various strategic approaches are introduced. It has been our experience that the most important factor would seem to be suiting strategic planning to the type of organization into which it is to be used. In the literature on strategic theory, as well as overlap with some of the conceptual components of leadership, strategic theory also seemed to have links with other approaches to healthcare management and practice. It would appear that strategies aspire to a vision of the future, and as part of that vision goals, targets or objectives (nomenclature depending on the author) are set in order to communicate that vision to others. All would appear to stress the importance of participation of other individuals in this process. Cited authors also mention the importance of leadership in aspiring to these goals and inspiring others to do the same. Many see the process of development and implementation of strategy as a mechanism for moving along a continuum, from *what used to be* to *what will be in the future*, using a variety of approaches. This is important, since it can be appreciated that what many of these authors are talking about is instigating a change of some kind. Moreover, they would argue that the point of change (i.e. their 'vision') is justified, because it will bring about some form of quality improvement (QI). Hence the theories of change management and quality improvement all need to be considered as part of the strategic planning process.

Concepts from each of these three disciplines were used to underpin the development of the Strategy for Nursing in Brighton Health Care (BHC). The challenge was therefore to identify, from the wide range of literature on leadership, change management and quality improvement, a robust framework for developing, implementing and evaluating a strategy that

- incorporated contemporary professional nursing issues;
- was aligned to the strategic direction of the organization;
- took account of the strategic direction of the NHS;
- was sensitive to local professional issues and built on the existing wealth of good practice;

- was owned by nurses and midwives within the Trust and enabled them to actively participate.

The literature from each discipline was reviewed in an attempt to inform this work (Parsley, 1996).

The change management theories reviewed fell into five categories. Some identified a cyclical approach to managing change (Fretwell, 1985). Others identified them as a movement along a continuum, through a series of discrete steps or phases (Plant, 1987; Cuba and Clark, 1978; Rogers, in Welch, 1979). These had some conceptual overlap with the rational planning theorists through setting clear goals and using a systematic process that moves through a series of discrete phases or steps in a predictable and rational way (Tables 4.2 and 4.3 in Chapter 4). The quality assurance literature also has examples of such rational models; for example Lang's QA cycle (1976), and the audit cycle or spiral (Figure 3.1 and 3.2 in Chapter 3). The assumptions underpinning such models are based on a view of the world which links *cause* with *effect*. The difficulties inherent in isolating a variable to prove that doing x will cause y are well rehearsed in Chapter 1, where this difficult issue is explored as it relates to evidence-based practice. Proving such links in social science is just as complex and fraught with difficulty because of the numerous variables involved.

A third group of theorists describe models that take account of the fact that change does not always occur in such a planned and rational fashion; opponents of change can push the change agenda backwards as readily as its proponents can propel it forwards (Lewin, 1953). The emphasis in these approaches is therefore to understand and analyse the context into which change is to be introduced, and to make efforts to strengthen the driving forces and reduce the restraining forces. The above theories are outlined in more detail below.

CHANGING PRACTICE

This section provides an overview of the different change management theories in respect of organizations, teams, individuals and the role of the change agent. Some of the tools that may be useful when planning and undertaking change will be examined. The reasons why change efforts may fail will also be explored.

Change: a definition

The phenomenon of change has been explored using a variety of theoretical models, including the sociological, psychological and organizational or systems perspective. Sociologists define three basic stages of change:

- initiation, which involves the launching of new ideas;
- legitimization, which involves the arguments for change being communicated;
- congruence, the process of reconciling the value systems of those proposing the change with those who are the targets of the change.

The above stages can be applied to both individuals and organizations. The next section describes some of the change management theories that can be applied to understand and manage both organizational and individual approaches to change management.

Change and the organization

Organizational change is a developing area of research and application and many theories have been developed.

Imershein (1997), drawing upon the work of Kuhn, conceptualized the process of change in scientific and technological areas in terms of a paradigm shift. Innovation occurs in a revolutionary form when the existing paradigm cannot provide the answers to significant problems. Imershein acknowledges an in-built resistance to change, suggesting that slight modification of the existing paradigm often occurs as an intermediate measure to solve recalcitrant problems. Should this fail, there will be a search for a new paradigm to accommodate both the already manageable and the now unmanageable problems. This leads to a revolutionary shift to the new paradigm. Within this context, major innovations therefore tend to occur against a background of crisis, at a time when tensions are often high.

Imershein's observations about change can be applied to quality improvement in healthcare. Imershein makes the distinction between small, incremental improvements versus a massive paradigm shift that occurs when new knowledge is required to address recalcitrant problems. Healthcare has seen numerous examples of such paradigm shifts: the discovery of anaesthetics, antibiotics and antiseptics, to name but a few.

A number of theorists believe that such changes cannot be studied in isolation. The impact they have on a wider social system is profound and far reaching. The next section outlines this approach to change management, namely that of systems theory.

SYSTEMS THEORY

A system is an entity that maintains its existence and functions as a whole through the sum of its parts. Chaos theory is defined as the study of complex and non-linear dynamic systems (Glass, 1996). Chaos theory is not about disorder but dictates that minor changes can often cause huge fluctuations. One of the central tenets of chaos theory is that, although it is impossible to predict the state of a system, it is possible to model the overall behaviour of the system. Comprehension of a system cannot be achieved without a constant study of the forces that impinge upon it (Katz and Kahn, 1966). Ramstrom (1974) advocates systems thinking as a means of gaining a full appreciation of the increased interdependencies between the system and its environment, and between various parts of the system. Classical and non-classical theories have been found wanting because of their emphasis on organizations as fragmented and closed social systems acting independently of external forces (Baker, 1973).

STAFFORDSHIRE UNIVERSITY LIBRARY

Flower (1995, p. 10) uses the terms 'control' or 'para-control' to describe his view that rather than 'driving' systems, we 'shepherd' them. He explains this process by referring to the natural world, using the example of sheep in a field 'doing their own thing, eating the grass, finding their own water, producing the wool'. Sheep dogs will keep them in a group; the shepherd keeps them in the general location and then harvests the results. Flower believes that this is the sort of system, the kind of management, that we will see in future.

In today's complex organizations, computer software evolves rapidly, adapting to its environment, communicating with software throughout the world, finding out and learning about other systems. He believes many of our systems are now approaching a level of complexity where they are beyond our control, meaning that surprises are inevitable and we may not always understand exactly what is happening. As the things we create become more and more complex, they acquire almost a biological nature of their own.

Systems theory challenges many of the traditional approaches to strategic planning, which have been based on rational planning models. Such models were useful in a stable environment, and writers on the subject typically describe a number of stages for strategic planning:

- Assess the environment for strengths, weaknesses, opportunities and threats.
- Develop the strategy for change.
- Implement the strategy.
- Evaluate progress against objectives.

The chaos theorists challenge the usefulness of this four-stage approach in a turbulent environment. In new industries such as computing, the concept of a ten-year plan is absurd because there may be rapid paradigm shifts within one or two years. Similarly, in healthcare, application of rational planning models can prove problematic because:

- Healthcare organizations are becoming increasingly complex and health needs increasingly unpredictable.
- Owing to the rapid and complex nature of constant change, healthcare managers and clinicians find it difficult to formulate detailed long-term strategies. By the time strategies are developed, the environment and context into which they were to be applied has changed, often radically. Hence detailed 5–10 year strategic plans may need to be significantly modified over time.
- Healthcare organizations are becoming larger and not developing along the simple lines previously developed, e.g. combined Trusts, partnerships with private care facilities, multisite development, etc.

Some aspects of healthcare are more easily predicted: the growing elderly population, and the shrinking pool of teenagers available to enter nursing. Rejecting long-term planning would be foolish. If we acknowledge that the rapid rate of change is a fact of life in today's healthcare institutions, then it follows that we need to identify mechanisms for coping with this phenomenon.

Kelly (1995a,b) argues that a centralized, top-down approach to deal with change does not work. He believes effective decision making needs to be spread throughout the organization, and that changing things from the top down works only when things are stable. Managing change should therefore involve the bottom of the organization and the fringes, where new approaches can establish their usefulness without being stifled by the inertia of the orthodox system. However, Senge (1994) identifies that 'it is not about having a top-down or bottom-up approach, but participation at all levels'.

Interdependency of systems

Other theories that relate to organizational change include those offered by Senge (1994), who identified that understanding the interdependency of systems is crucial. This included:

- **Strategy** – involvement in setting the direction of change.
- **Structure** – of the organization.
- **Skills** – including those of staff.
- **Style** – the way in which management acts.

These elements should, therefore, feed into any plan relating to undertaking change on an organizational basis.

Key messages relating to change management in more complex organizations include the following:

- Set short term goals.
- Communicate at all levels throughout the organization to ensure the participation of anyone who is likely to be affected by the change.
- Be prepared for the unpredictable and to alter plans to meet new pressures.

Another phenomenon described by the complex adaptive systems theorists is that of *emergence*, i.e. unpredicted and unexpected effects that may generate a complete paradigm shift. The recommendation from writers such as Kelly (1995a,b) is to embrace new ideas that emerge, rather than (as is typical in a more traditional organization) to restrict the changes in an effort to maintain the status quo. Examples of the latter include the Swiss watch industry, which once held a stranglehold on the world market. Sceptical of the marketability of the new quartz watch, the Swiss did not pursue this new development. The patent was bought by the Japanese, who then took over from the Swiss as the world leader. Healthcare too is littered with new ideas, rejected by many in their time, which are now accepted: the theories of evolution and germ theory, to name but a couple. More recently, patient pathways – a form of standard care plan, once rejected – are now in ascendancy, as is the role of 'nurse consultant' as opposed to the old historical view of doctor's handmaiden.

STAFFORDSHIRE UNIVERSITY LIBRARY

Individual/team responses and change

The component parts of any organization, i.e. the teams and the individuals who work within them, inevitably influence the potential for that organization to adapt and evolve.

As Plant (1987) observed, 'Unless behaviour changes, nothing changes.' The individual members of an organization clearly affect the change process within it. Dyer (1984) reflected that 'the organisation is . . . an abstraction. Organisations do not change their behaviour, although change in organisational structure or process can impact upon behaviour. What actually occurs is that a collection of people who share common orientations consciously or unconsciously decide . . . to change.'

Basset (1971) offered insight into the way change takes place within an individual. At this individual level, three elements are identified as prerequisites in order for change to occur:

- **The rational element** – the recognition that change must occur.
- **The affective element** – the acceptance at an emotional level of the need for change.
- **The achievement element** – the belief that effective change is possible and the individual can contribute to it.

Other authors have made similar observations. Dalton (1970) stated that, for the change agent to take action, the individual has to perceive 'a felt need' strong enough to motivate him or her. This notion underpins most of the popular theories on models of management behaviour, which all have a disparity condition built into them. They are based on the assumption that the change strategy will involve the individual seeing the difference between what they are doing and what they should, or could, be doing. Management development programmes often involve an examination of the minimum/maximum positions of that particular theory with the aim of pushing the individual to the upper end of the continuum (Table 5.4).

Table 5.4	Minimum position	Maximum position
Maximum and minimum positions in Douglas McGregor's management theory	Theory X	Theory Y
	Assumption that managers had about people – they dislike work, want security, need direction and want direction.	Assumption of managers – the worker likes work, is self-motivated and accepts responsibility.

Adapted from Dyer (1984).

Rogers (in Welch, 1979) expands these stages and identifies five phases through which the individual has to move (Figure 5.2). Rogers' theory is underpinned by two factors. First, the individual needs to be interested in the innovation; and second, they need to be committed to making the change occur.

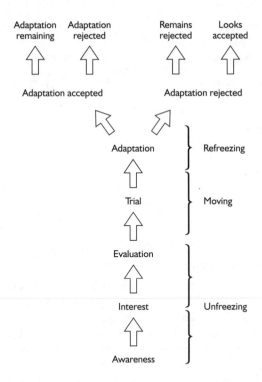

Figure 5.2

Rogers' theory of change (from Welch (1979))

Pratt (in Greaves, 1982), defines five categories into which individuals may fall, based on their response to the change process within the organization. These are:

- **Enthusiasts** – the initiators of the change. These may hold subordinate positions within the organization.
- **Supporters** – who are often respected and powerful members of the organization. Their views may be less radical than those of the former group, but they are easily persuaded by arguments for the need to change.
- **Acquiescers** – who tend to follow the line of least resistance and adopt the change, even if only superficially, in response to pressure from the supporters.
- **Laggards** – who tend to be introspective and are unable to take a global view of the need for change. They tend to be sceptical and reject change until it is widely accepted by their peers.
- **Antagonists** – who actively or passively resist all change attempts as they are introduced.

The challenge is to devise change management strategies that take account of all five groups.

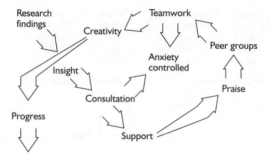

Figure 5.3

Fretwell's demographic model of change (Source: Fretwell (1985))

Demographic model of change

In our experience of managing teams, we are aware of the limitations of devising a strategy based purely on individual responses. Other variables also need to be considered. The first such variable was the influence the team has on the attitudes and behaviour of the individual. Hawthorne (cited by Dyer, 1984) demonstrated that individuals can be, and often are, influenced in their judgements, decisions and actions by the way group members behave towards them. It may not be possible to predict the changes to specific individuals, but an overall effect can be seen.

Fretwell's (1985) demographic model of change (Figure 5.3) illustrates factors that can move teams through the change process. Key factors from this model that we identified as crucial are:

- consultation
- support
- praise
- peer groups
- teamwork
- anxiety control

Stocking (1984), in her studies of innovation within the NHS, reiterated some of the themes of earlier theories, but introduced some other factors for consideration. She identified that, to make an innovation diffuse, some or all of the following would have to be evident:

- **Identifiable enthusiasts** – individuals who invented or discovered the idea, who are keen to disseminate it, and who put in considerable time and energy promoting it.
- **Lack of conflict** – with current national policies or established climates of opinion among professionals and other groupings.

- **Local appeal** – the innovation should appeal to those who have the power to promote change.
- **Relevance** – the innovation should meet the perceived needs of patients and staff. It should not require major role or attitude changes and should be simple to organize.
- **Adaptability** – the innovation should suit local circumstances.
- **Low cost** – little finance or other resources should be required, unless such requirements can be hidden or increased resources made available.

This model can be used in conjunction with Lewin's forcefield analysis, outlined later (Lewin, 1953). Essentially, all of the above components represent driving forces. Noting their presence and/or absence can be a useful exercise when predicting the likelihood of successful change. Lewin identified three stages of the change process, which are relevant to individuals and teams:

- unfreezing
- moving to a new level
- refreezing

The first, 'unfreezing', involves the process of becoming aware of the problem and the need for change. There is also a need to believe that there is potential for improvement before the change process can progress.

'Moving to a new level' involves clarifying the problem and planning action, which involves 'identification' and 'scanning'. Identification involves subjects being influenced by someone who has power or for whom they have respect. Scanning involves seeking information about potential options from a variety of sources (Marriner-Tomey, 1988). A variety of strategies provide staff with information at this opinion-forming stage. 'Refreezing' is the integration of the change into one's personality and stabilization of that change.

Covey's circle of influence

Another model that can be helpful when planning change is Covey's circle of influence/circle of concern. Covey's model was derived from his studies of what makes people effective (Covey, 1992; see Figure 5.4).

Covey highlighted that to be truly effective we need to focus within our circle of influence and make changes in things that are within our control. Less effective individuals spend much of their energy working on their circle of concern, i.e. worrying about things that they have no power to influence. In this model it has been shown that if we work on the inner circle, as we make changes and impact, so our circle of influence grows as those outside see our successes and wish to work with us.

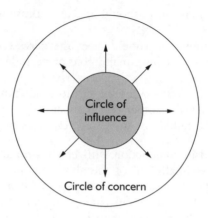

Figure 5.4

Covey's model of the circle of influence versus circle of concern (Source: Covey (1992))

CHANGE MANAGEMENT

The change agent

Chinn (in Bennis, Benne and Chinn 1988) identified three key strategies that can be used as approaches by the change agent when managing change. These are: empirical rational; normative re-educative; and power coercive.

- **Empirical rational strategy** – based on the assumption that people are rational and behave according to rational self-interest. Using this model, it is expected that individuals will be willing to adopt change if they accept that it is justified and see that they will benefit from it.
- **Normative re-educative strategy** – based on the assumption that people act according to their commitment to sociocultural norms. The rationality and intelligence of individuals are not entirely excluded, but attitudes and values are also taken into consideration when planning change.
- **Power coercive strategy** – involves compliance of the less powerful with the leadership of the more powerful. Conflict is a common feature of this strategy. The conflict theory of social change contends that at the basis of most organizational change is some form of conflict, i.e. dissatisfaction, alienation and frustration experienced by members of the organization. These members, in order to resolve or eliminate these conflicts, attempt to change the circumstances within the organization. These efforts of change usually lead to conflict with other groups who do not perceive any difficulties with the existing system.

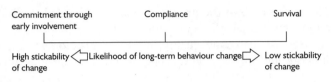

Figure 5.5

The change continuum (reproduced with the permission of HarperCollins Publishers Ltd from *Managing Change and Making It Stick*, Plant (1987))

Another strategy advocated by many authors is the notion of 'ownership' of the change by the individuals it will affect. This strategy stems from early studies by Coch and French (1948), who identified the importance of involving everyone affected by change in the plan. In this industrial-based research, methods that used little or no worker participation led to worker resistance, turnover and production loss; the trial group showed the fastest rate of relearning and surpassed previous output by 14% in 30 days. There were no resignations, no absenteeism and no grievances in the trial group. Plant (1987) emphasizes the importance of worker involvement as crucial to the likelihood of long-term behaviour change by showing it at points along a continuum (Figure 5.5). Gillies (1989) extends this further by incorporating a feedback loop into the process.

A change strategy that incorporates this philosophy of 'ownership' is the change agent model, which focuses on the use of communication skills and the development of a good working relationship between the leader (or change agent) and the person or people of the target system. Based on a normative, re-educative strategy, five steps are described (Tappen, 1989):

- **Step 1 – Build a relationship.** This assumes the need to build trust and respect. Actions recommended to achieve this include good communication techniques; openness and honesty; providing information about your skills and credentials; and demonstration of ability.
- **Step 2 – Diagnose the problem.** This is the identification of the 'felt need' to change. Methods used include meetings, conferences, informal discussions, surveys and questionnaires. Consensus building is also stressed. ·
- **Step 3 – Assess resources.** This includes motivation and commitment to change; knowledge and skills needed to implement the actual change behaviour; sources of power; and influences that support the change. It also includes economic resources and elements such as time and energy.
- **Step 4 – Set goals and select strategies.**
- **Step 5 – Stabilize, consolidate and reinforce change.**

Another group of change management theories looks at the role and function of hierarchy and power when change is being implemented (Harrison, 1994). Proponents of these theories identify that the success or failure of rational plans can largely be attributed to ensuring that those who hold power within an organization are supportive of the proposed changes. These observations are also found in the QA literature, with many authors citing the importance of ensuring that any structures for managing quality in an organization place responsibility for this within the line management structure. Hence managing quality carries equal responsibility with managing contracts or finance. There is much evidence to suggest that treating quality as extra or special, and divorcing it from the main stream of the business, severely undermines its status and effectiveness within an organization.

We were heavily influenced by Harrison's views on how to create an effective organizational structure, and his descriptions of the 'black hole' mirrored some of our previous casualties in implanting change, casualties we were not keen to suffer again. Harrison's structure for a successful change management initiative is shown in Figure 5.6.

In Harrison's model, the 'targets' are those who will be affected by this change. As the author points out, one often does feel like a target if change is poorly executed. This model emphasizes the importance of the most senior individuals in the organization legitimizing or authorizing the change. The authorizing sponsor (CEO) works with the first target group, who then become the reinforcing sponsors for the next layer in the organization. This process is repeated through the organization.

This model emphasizes the importance of a cascade process and securing the involvement of all stakeholders (those affected by the change). Harrison's second structure (Figure 5.7) shows an example of poorly managed change, in which

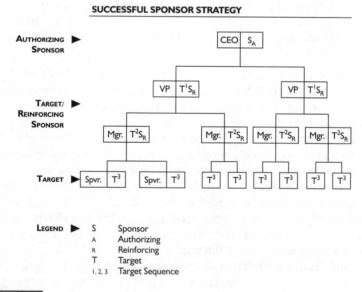

Figure 5.6

Harrison's model for a successful organizational structure to manage change (copyright © IMA 1996, see Harrison (1994))

the 'black hole' is representative of lack of ownership of the change initiative by middle management and the blockage of effective two-way communication.

Harrison (1994, p. 6) also depicts change management as a 'wave' with a series of different stages which can typically occur through the change management process (Figure 5.8). One can reduce the amplitude of the wave by careful management of change, but it will never disappear altogether. Hence the predictability of these various stages can be effectively anticipated so as to minimize the impact of resistance to change.

Why change fails

Change is often viewed as a destination, i.e. a one-off single event rather than a journey. This perception prevents the process of managing change being viewed as a learning experience with the potential for failure which can itself be the catalyst for constructive change. Traditionally, and currently, change is often seen as a top-down event structured around committees or groups who are selected to implement the change.

From the literature on the subject of change and change management, we have identified core reasons why change fails:

- lack of vision;
- lack of planning and preparation;
- long-term goals which are outdated before implementation;
- poor communication leading to people not understanding the need to change;
- a legacy of previous poorly managed change;
- finally, the cries of 'we've always done it this way' which are sometimes heard in organizations; this often denotes underlying resistance and fear of failure in the staff who may be most affected by the changes.

These problems can be minimized by using the techniques of forcefield analysis and/or stakeholder analysis.

Tools that aid change management

Each of the tools presented here can be used alone or in combination. They are intended to help guide change agents through the change management process and reduce the likelihood of mistakes.

Forcefield analysis

Forcefield analysis was devised by Lewin (1935) and is defined as 'the diagnosis and evaluation of enabling and restraining forces that have an impact on the change process'. The tool enables the change agent to identify enabling and constraining forces within the change process.

First, the change objective must be clearly defined and linked to the strategic vision of the organization. If it is a major project, the change objective must be linked to the operational goals. From here, the enabling and constraining forces can be identified.

UNSUCCESSFUL SPONSOR STRATEGY

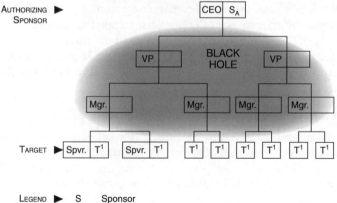

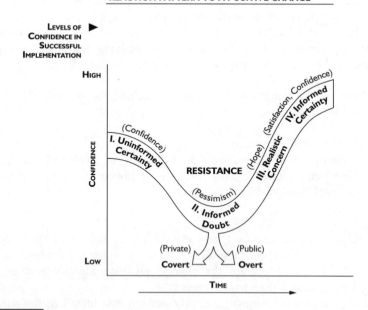

Figure 5.7

Harrison's 'black hole' (copyright © IMA 1996, see Harrison (1994) adapted from the work of D. Conner)

Figure 5.8

The positive change curve (copyright © IMA 1996, see Harrison (1994) adapted from the theories of D. Kelley and D. Conner)

The next step is to decide how powerful the respective enabling and constraining forces are. This encourages dialogue and reveals individual perceptions of identified problems. Measuring these forces can be carried out using either of the following methods:

- scoring each force as having high, medium or low impact;
- scoring each force numerically on a scale of 1 to 5.

So that shared understanding can be reached, participants need to rationalize why they have categorized each force as an enabler or constrainer. Forcefield analysis can be applied to macro or micro level change and also at various stages of the change process.

Stakeholder analysis
Stakeholder analysis is another method for identifying issues that may influence a project or organization, and how these influences will affect the change process.

First, we need to identify who the key stakeholders are at any phase of the change process. As with the forcefield analysis, these need to be weighted as having high, medium or low influence.

Secondly, the change agent must evaluate whether these stakeholders are currently supportive of the change, against it or indifferent. Once this is complete, the following questions need to be asked:

- How can the balance be shifted in terms of the stakeholders' views, and/or can new stakeholders be brought in to shift the balance?
- Is there a way of boosting or reducing stakeholder influence?
- Can the change objective be redefined to reduce resistance?

Using the above questions can enable a project group to decide how difficult the change process is going to be and the value of attempting the change if there are no supporters. Other methods to gain support may need to be sought before the project goes ahead.

Preliminary summary

This section outlined some of the theories on strategy development, nurse leadership and understanding and managing the change process from organizational, team and individual perspectives. Change theories were included here because it is apparent that when seeking to improve clinical practice the need for change at one or more of these levels is fundamental. The preceding chapters have dealt with identifying, documenting, measuring best practice and strategic planning. These have predominantly focused on the practice of the individual clinician. This section has introduced the notion that for changes to be made, it is not just the individual who is required to make changes for the better, but the organization within which they work. Strategic planning and leadership can (we believe) be used alongside change management theories to develop an organizational approach to assist clinicians in developing their own professional practice.

This next section presents a case study on the development and implementation of a strategy for nursing and midwifery in an NHS Trust. The study describes the approach taken and some of the findings of a research study to evaluate the work. In developing the strategy, the author drew on an eclectic mix of the theories outlined in the previous section. These were influential in underpinning plans to develop and implement a Trust-wide strategy for nursing and midwifery. The final section of this chapter reflects on which of these theories were most useful in practice. In describing the case study, Donabedian's structure–process–outcome framework is used to try to explain the approach taken.

The *structure* incorporates the hierarchical structure necessary to cascade this process and adaptation of Harrison's (1994) model. The *process* explains what was actually done with the structural groups and describes what happened as a result (or some of the outcomes). The *outcomes* (interestingly) fell into two categories: those that were broadly anticipated and planned for (as shown in the example of the strategy document in Appendix 1) and those that emerged as a result of the new structural groups that were created and the alliances that arose from them. The next section therefore describes an approach to establishing the structures, the process used for implementation and some of the outcomes for the Brighton Health Care (BHC) Strategy for Nursing and Midwifery.

CASE STUDY 5.1 DEVELOPMENT AND IMPLEMENTATION OF THE BRIGHTON HEALTH CARE STRATEGY FOR NURSING AND MIDWIFERY

Background to case study

This case study took place in Brighton Health Care NHS Trust (BHC). BHC comprises four hospitals that together provide the hospital services on the Sussex coast. BHC's immediate catchment population is approximately 300,000. The Trust is a pilot site for developing a patient-focused care philosophy, called 'integrated patient care' or IPC (Garside, 1993). This initiative is an attempt to focus all services around the needs and locality of the patient.

The Trust's organizational chart, showing where the nursing directorate fits, is shown in Figure 5.9.

BHC became an NHS Trust in 1993. As shown in Figure 5.9, the Trust adopted a clinical directorate structure based around five clinical directorates, each with its own general manager, clinical director (all doctors) and business manager. There were five central directorates, each with a director. Like many NHS Trusts, with the establishment of this structure the nursing workforce no longer reported through to the Director of Nursing, but through the clinical directorate

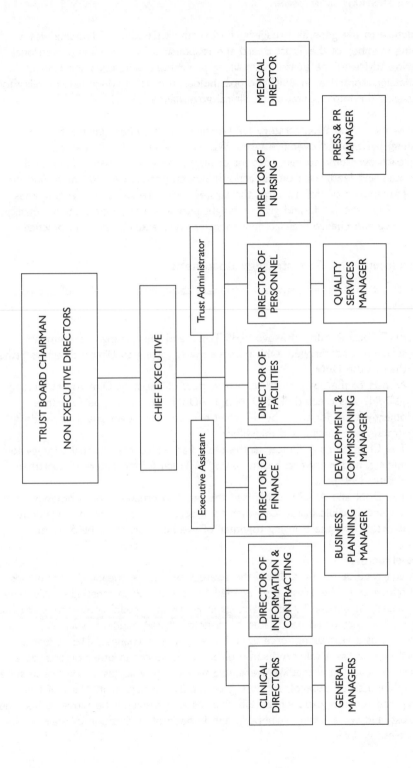

Figure 5.9

Brighton Health Care NHS Trust – Management structure (reproduced with the permission of Brighton Health Care NHS Trust)

structure to the general manager. The Executive Director of Nursing was a voting member of the Trust Board and responsible for providing professional nursing advice to the board, maintaining professional standards and leading professional practice. In BHC the post holder also has a wider responsibility for managing the implementation of clinical governance.

The work on the BHC Strategy for Nursing and Midwifery (at the time of writing) has evolved over five years. We have developed and adapted the approach over time to take account of new professional and organizational priorities and feedback from an action research project carried out to find out the perceptions of staff towards the strategy, capture some of the outcomes arising from the work, and give us insight into which strategic planning, quality assurance and change management theories were actually useful in practice.

Developing the first strategy document

The thrust to develop a strategy document came from a number of quarters, namely:

- BHC became a fourth-wave NHS Trust, and the nursing management structure had changed, with nurses now reporting to clinical directors rather than to the DoN.
- As part of the new structure, a new post of Assistant Director of Nursing (ADoN) was created. The DoN and ADoN had specific performance objectives set for them by the chief executive to develop a Trust-wide strategy for nursing and midwifery
- The Chief Nursing Officer at the DoH had issued the national strategy for nursing, midwifery and health visiting, A Vision for the Future (Department of Health, 1993).
- The DoN and ADoN recognized the need to create a new framework for developing clinical practice which took account of the new management structure and the bringing together of five hospitals in an NHS Trust.

The structure

It was agreed at the time that if the strategy was to be meaningful for nurses and midwives in the Trust, they needed to be involved in creating it. We were also heavily influenced by the warnings in Harrison's model about the 'black hole' (Figure 5.7) that could be created by disenfranchized middle management and could act as a restraining force against any proposed changes. This struck a chord with us, as it mirrored some of our experiences in other organizations, where we had found that we were able to instigate changes in practice in spite of, rather than because of, support from middle management. Many of this group had recently experienced job changes as a result of the move to become a Trust, and were feeling vulnerable and in need of clarification of their new job roles.

It was agreed that the Director of Nursing would chair a nursing policy committee consisting of the patient services managers. The committee would be responsible for setting broad policy and direction, and members took the decision that the responsibility for developing and implementing the strategy for nursing should rest with the 20 heads of nursing.

The process: what we actually did
A one-day workshop was held with all the heads of nursing, facilitated by the Assistant Director of Nursing. The objectives for the day were:

- to explore with the participants the role and function of the newly created heads of nursing posts and begin to build the team;
- to review current policy documents and contemporary nursing and midwifery issues;
- for the ADoN to present differing approaches to strategic planning to inform a discussion on how to begin to develop a strategy for nursing and midwifery in BHC;
- to develop a first draft of the BHC Strategy for Nursing and Midwifery.

The day focused on getting a first draft of the strategy completed. Although the objectives were ambitious, these were met. Following the review of contemporary nursing issues, the group brainstormed over 200 items that they felt needed addressing within the Trust. A second workshop enabled these to be grouped into key themes as a way of breaking this huge agenda into bite-sized chunks.

At the end of the day we had identified the following eight key issues that were to form the framework for the development of nursing practice across the trust. These were:

- clinical leadership
- staff development and education
- communication
- quality
- accountability
- purchasing, commissioning and marketing
- research
- equal opportunities

For each of the eight issues, we drafted a purpose statement identifying what we were seeking to achieve in addressing each issue. The 200+ list of issues and concerns was collated by the ADoN following the first workshop and was used to form the basis of draft objectives grouped under each of the eight key issues.

This draft document was circulated to the Nursing Policy Group and the heads of nursing for comment, and amended and approved at a subsequent meeting.

However, as we acknowledged at the time, writing the document was only the start. The challenge was to ensure that it did not go the way of countless other strategic planning documents and end up on the shelf gathering dust. For this reason the decision was taken not to circulate the document at this point; it was recognized that further work needed to be done to make it into a working document that was useful and meaningful to practising nurses and midwives.

Creating a structure to develop the strategy

Following the approval of the strategy document in principle by the key nursing groups, it was agreed that ultimately the power to decide whether or not these objectives were met would depend on the ward sister or charge nurse. In exploring with the heads of nursing how we could engage sisters and charge nurses in working towards these objectives, they observed that the new clinical directorate structure had done much to fragment the corporate nursing focus. Nurses seldom got the opportunity to meet colleagues from other clinical directorates, and even in the preliminary stages of developing the strategy we had encountered numerous examples of duplication of work: for example, five different groups who had been working independently with each directorate setting standards on discharge. We were therefore cautious about presenting the document to the sister/charge nurse group and giving them sole responsibility for implementing the objectives in their clinical areas. There were two reasons for caution. Firstly, the devolution of budgets and other responsibilities following the disappearance of many clinical nurse manager posts had significantly increased the workload of sisters and charge nurses. Secondly, we did not want to duplicate work through issuing a list of objectives to be introduced by the sisters and charge nurses. For example, an objective under the staff development and education brief was to ensure all nurses and midwives had an annual appraisal and review. It became apparent that there was no corporate approach for nurses to do this. We wanted to avoid each area having to develop their own appraisal documentation and training.

Other examples where a corporate approach was felt to be advantageous included:

- the need for nurses to undertake clinical audit and set standards for practice (the need for an educational programme to facilitate this process was also identified);
- a review of the principle of the 'named nurse' and sharing models of good practice;
- preparing nurses for PREP (Standards for Post-Registration Education for Practice);
- clarifying job descriptions, with particular reference to succession-planning criteria;
- a corporate review of patient literature and the need to develop standards for its production and publication;

- increasing nurse understanding of the UKCC code of conduct and scope of professional practice (United Kingdom Central Council for Nursing, Midwifery and Health Visiting, 1992);
- the need for a multidisciplinary Trust-wide group to give 'approval in principle' to professionals expanding their scope of practice; assuring competence to do so and developing policies to support these practitioners;
- preparing preceptors for their preceptorship role;
- learning how apply research findings to practice;
- reviewing access to all sites for disabled patients and staff.

The list is not exhaustive, but provides a flavour of some of the issues the heads of nursing felt could be tackled collaboratively rather than expecting each sister and charge nurse to tackle them independently. The list may also seem dated, given that it is taken from work completed in 1993. The priorities and objectives have obviously moved on since then. The 1998 Strategy for Nursing and Midwifery objectives are reproduced in Appendix 1. These were based on the latest issues believed to be important for the strategic development of nursing practice.

We were also mindful of the fact that presenting sisters and charge nurses with a new programme of work might lead to concerns about their own workload and ability to deliver this agenda. We were keen to engage a wider group of nurses and midwives in the whole project, not least as a way of doing a quick reality check on developing our ideas on how to take the project forward. It was agreed that we would establish eight nursing focus groups (NFGs), whose job would be to put the meat on the bones of our strategy. Their task was to ensure that when we presented this work to a wider audience, it was not merely to say 'This is what we want you to do', but 'Here are some ways in which we can help you to do it.'

The focus groups were set up, supported and coordinated by the ADoN. Members were recruited from volunteers responding to an introductory letter sent to staff in all clinical areas explaining the role and purpose of the focus group, the purpose statement (to give staff the opportunity to contribute to topics that were of particular interest to them), and the dates of the first meeting that it was mandatory they attend.

The response to the introductory letter was encouraging, securing a broad cross-section of staff nurses, sisters/charge nurses, some enrolled nurses and a few nurse practitioners, with representation across all clinical directorates and across all sites. We had identified that focus groups should ideally have between six and ten members to keep them to a manageable size, encourage everyone to participate and keep focused on the task in hand. All the focus groups were chaired by the ADoN, which ensured that at least one individual had an overview of what all the groups were doing and could ensure that there was no duplication of effort.

Managing the focus groups

There were a number of underlying principles that were adopted when managing the groups. These were important in ensuring their effectiveness and in achieving the initial task set for all the groups, namely to produce all the supporting materials in preparation for the launch of the BHC Strategy for Nursing and Midwifery. All groups had an eight-week deadline. A consensus conference was arranged for ten weeks after the commencement of the work, where all the focus groups would present their completed work to date and outline future plans. This was a challenging target, which was met through adopting the following techniques:

- Time in meetings was kept to a maximum of one hour to ensure time out from the clinical areas was kept to a minimum.
- The meetings all had timed agendas, with the emphasis being on reaching decisions on actions to be taken.
- The actions were then assigned to group members and a deadline was agreed. The majority of the work was therefore carried out and completed outside the meeting.
- Subsequent meetings were arranged only as necessary, and timed to fit in with the completion of all of the current actions so that these could be reviewed.
- All groups developed a tight project plan with clear responsibilities, tasks and deadlines.
- Handwritten minutes were kept in the meeting, noting only key decisions and agreed actions and deadlines. These were photocopied and distributed at the end of the meeting. Administration was therefore kept to a minimum.

All group members were committed to the work and worked enormously hard to deliver against agreed objectives. At the end of the eight weeks, all the groups had completed the preliminary work as agreed. This was pulled together in a supporting set of appendices to go alongside the BHC Strategy for Nursing and Midwifery. So, for example, the focus group responsible for staff development and education had produced:

- guidelines on preceptorship and dates for a series of seminars they had devised on becoming a preceptor to support the objective stating that all newly qualified staff will be supported by a preceptor;
- guidelines on preparing a PREP portfolio for the UKCC along with dates for seminars they had developed, to support the objective that all nurses and midwives in BHC will have developed a PREP[2] portfolio in preparation for re-registration;

---

[2] The Nurses, Midwives and Health Visitors (Periodic Registration) Amendment Rules Approval Order 1995, Statutory Instrument 1995 No. 967

- documentation to support the appraisal process using proformas, a set of guidelines on how to conduct appraisal and agreed dates when the personnel department would run training for appraisers and appraisees, to support the objective that all nurses and midwives in BHC will have an annual appraisal and regular review.

All the focus groups also produced resource packs for their link workers, a role that is explained later in this chapter.

Pulling the preliminary work together

A consensus conference was arranged for the 70 focus group members (including the 20 heads of nursing who had been spread evenly across all the focus groups, which they had selected on the basis of a specific interest, an area of expertise, or both). The purpose of the conference was to share the work of each group, present a set of proposals on how to take the work forward, and identify a strategic plan to actively engage the 1200 'whole-time equivalent' (WTE) nurses and midwives across BHC in transforming the words on paper into a dynamic process that both improved patient care and developed nurses and nursing across the Trust.

The groups had prepared the presentations themselves, and all the focus group members contributed. For many it was the first time they had spoken in public to such a large group, and they were offered coaching and support if needed. Those who could not face the challenge of public speaking contributed by preparing handouts or the overheads. The mood of the conference was positive and buoyant, with a sense of pride at what had been achieved in such a short space of time. One of the comments on the evaluation forms for the day captured the overall theme of the feedback:

> *It is very exciting; if this is what 70 of us can do in 8 weeks, who knows what 1200 of us can achieve over the next year!*

The final part of the conference was devoted to developing a strategic framework to implement the proposals.

The vision was now complete, and we felt we had a good strategy to take to the staff. We needed to find a way of winning their interest and commitment and to get their help in taking the objectives forward in all clinical areas.

Implementation framework

According to Harrison's model (Figure 5.6), we had secured the ownership of the heads of nursing group at an early stage. The eight themes had then been developed by a cross-section of nurses from all grades and across all sites. We felt that this had ensured a wide cross-section of as representative a sample of nurses as we could practically achieve. The more junior staff had challenged and amended the original objectives drafted by the heads of nursing group, and there was agreement at the consensus conference that all of the objectives in the strategy were priority issues for nursing, realistic (but challenging) and achievable.

The next tier we wanted to target, therefore, were the sisters and charge nurses. We already had some champions at this grade, as 20 sisters and charge nurses had been involved in the focus groups. We had taken advice from them as to how best to proceed. The overriding concern from this group was the huge amount of work involved to implement the strategy objectives in their ward area, and concern that they may be expected to undertake a significant amount of extra work without help. We also appreciated that in order to make a real difference at the bedside, we needed to find a way to involve all nurses at ward level, not just the sister or charge nurse. The idea of 'link workers' was proposed as a solution to both of these problems. The role of the sister or charge nurse was therefore to plan and coordinate the implementation of the strategy objectives at a local level, not necessarily to do the detailed work. This would be done by the staff nurses and enrolled nurses. The role of the link worker is outlined below.

Role and function of the link worker

It was agreed that each clinical area (typically a ward or department) would identify a named link worker for each of the eight focus group themes. It was left to the sister or charge nurse to identify how to recruit link workers, although it was advised that they should be 'interested volunteers'. Some smaller units doubled up and had a link worker covering two areas, whereas the bigger units encouraged staff to pair up and have two link workers per focus group. All the link workers' names were entered into a database and the focus groups communicated with them directly. The focus group members had responsibility for dividing the link workers between them so that each member had a cohort of around eight to ten link workers. This was normally done on a geographical basis; for example, the focus group member for quality working at the children's hospital would liaise with all the quality link workers at other sites. The focus group member was to be responsible for communicating with their cohort of link workers and informing them of link worker meetings and study days, ensuring they were issued with the resource pack prepared by all the focus group members. This pack gave information on how to achieve the objectives, indicated where to go for help and assistance, and set the objectives for link workers for the forthcoming year.

So (for example) when the Staff Development and Education focus group were working on the aim 'all nurses in BHC should have a PREP portfolio', the link workers were contacted by the focus group and advised of the dates of forth-coming workshops. At the workshop they were given an overview by focus group members on what PREP was all about, and shown a PREP portfolio, specifically developed for all BHC staff, which included written guidelines on how to complete the portfolios. An interactive component enabled them to ask questions and begin to develop their profile. Link workers were then advised on how to help their colleagues develop these for themselves. Their objectives were to ensure that all their ward colleagues were informed of what they had learned; to act as a resource for staff who were unsure what to do about PREP; and to actively encourage all staff to develop their portfolios. Link workers were also responsible for feeding back to the focus group so that the group could audit the impact of their work. The sisters and charge nurses felt that the use of link workers was a helpful way of achieving the nursing strategy objectives at ward level, and this cascade structure for the strategy was therefore the final approach that was approved. The structure is shown in Figure 5.10. It can be appreciated that this has similarities with the model presented by Harrison (1994).

We also took the sisters' and charge nurses' advice on how to disseminate the strategy and communicate its contents. There was overwhelming advice that the launch needed to be done face to face rather than the document be sent round with a covering letter, particularly since all the supporting material meant the document was by now large, at over 100 pages including appendices. Although logistically quite difficult to organize, it was agreed to take a roadshow round all the sites and target all 110 sisters and charge nurses. This was done over a four-week period. The roadshow comprised an initial presentation by the DoN/ADoN explaining the work to date, outlining proposals for the future and stressing the important role of the sisters and charge nurses in taking nursing forward. After a question-and-answer session, the participants then viewed poster presentations prepared by all eight focus groups and were able to talk informally with focus group members (all their peers or colleagues) about the specific focus group objectives, what was required of them and their link workers, and what help would be forthcoming for the link workers.

Overall the evaluation from these sessions was extremely positive, although there was cynicism from some. Others, although positive about the work, were concerned about the additional workload. Some took a more pragmatic view, summed up on the evaluation form by one participant:

> *It looks a lot of work, but actually, you can't argue that any of the eight issues or objectives are not relevant to nursing. In fact, the majority of them are core components of the Sr/CN job description. If this works out it will be a big plus for us, as rather than trying to tackle this huge agenda on our own, we have the focus groups and link workers to help us. If we don't do this, we're not really doing our jobs.*

Action planning workshops
Following the roadshow, sisters and charge nurse were asked to review the document, talk about it with their teams and sign up for a follow-up session four

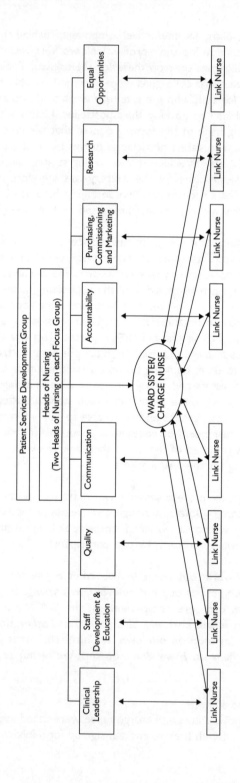

Figure 5.10

Structure for implementing the Strategy for Nursing (reproduced with the permission of Brighton Health Care NHS Trust)

weeks later. The purpose of the follow-up session was to allow more considered discussion on the strategy and then to give sisters and charge nurses some time and assistance in thinking about how to take work forward in this area. The session included an introduction to project planning, and then participants split into smaller groups facilitated by the heads of nursing. They worked systematically through each of the objectives for each of the eight issues, and identified specific objectives and target dates for their clinical areas loosely based around these. So (for example) under 'staff development and education' many lists included:

- Identify link worker.
- Send link worker to workshop on PREP portfolio.
- Meet link workers and agree objectives for the year.
- Review progress against objectives with link workers every three months.
- Schedule time at ward meeting and training session for link workers to inform and teach PREP.

A project plan was drafted in the workshops, taken back to the clinical area and reviewed and amended in consultation with the link workers; sisters and charge nurses were encouraged to display the plan for the year and return the master copy to the ADoN/HoN for a central record to be kept. An example of such a plan is shown in Figure 5.11.

Throughout the first year, the focus groups continued to meet, compare their work against their original objectives and offer support to the link workers and sisters/charge nurses. The ADoN remained the central coordinator of all the work, and monitored the progress made in conjunction with the heads of nursing.

One year in: the next phase

At the end of the first year, a workshop was arranged by the ADoN to review the progress to date with the heads of nursing. Before this date, the heads of nursing held sister/charge nurse away days within their individual directorates to review progress against the original action plans. Overall, the progress was viewed as positive; a summary of the dissemination framework and key achievements of each of the focus groups is shown in Figure 5.12.

It was agreed by the heads of nursing to pursue this approach and review, update and relaunch the strategy objectives. They also commissioned a major research study to capture feedback about the impact of this work during the second year of the Strategy for Nursing and Midwifery. 'Strategy II' was therefore launched at a conference for mainly sisters/charge nurses and focus group members, 15 months after the first strategy document. Following the conference and launch of the revised objectives, the cycle followed in the first year (summarized in Figure 5.13) was repeated.

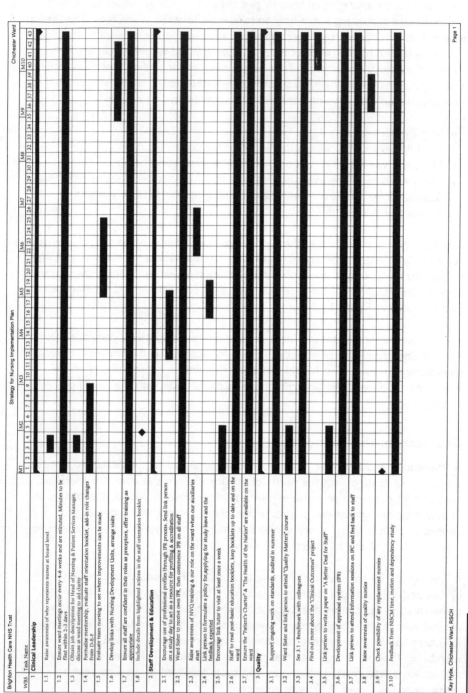

Figure 5.11a

Example of a project plan (reproduced with the permission of Brighton Health Care NHS Trust)

WBS	Task Name
4	**Communication**
4.1	Update organisation chart in staff motivation booklet
4.2	Encourage staff to read Bulletin, Newsflash & memos
4.3	Member of staff to attend crash team briefing / written feedback
4.4	Evaluate admission packs on the ward
4.5	Evaluate Named Nurse project – ask patients who their's is
4.6	Add information on patient's advocate to admissions booklet
4.7	Add information on complaints procedure
4.8	Introduce audit of ward meetings using App. 4.7 audit tool
4.9	Show App. 4.8a, raise awareness of documentation issues
4.10	Annual Audit with School of Nursing
4.11	Staff to see Melinda Stone re: documentation
5	**Accountability**
5.1	Ensure staff read documents on the ward and understand the relevance to their work. Link person attends workshops / feedback
5.2	Obtain a copy of the local document. Explore issues such as cannulation, venepuncture and what they mean to our workload
5.3	Find more information on "Scope of Practice"
6	**Purchasing, Commissioning and Marketing**
6.1	Discuss involvement in contracting with Head of Nursing
6.2	Link person to attend marketing module
6.3	Sister to attend Business Management modules run by the Training Department
6.4	Meet with accountant monthly to discuss budget statement
6.5	Make people aware of the Business Plan
7	**Research**
7.1	Raise awareness of research in out area
7.2	Encourage staff to think about issues of research that could be done on the ward
7.3	Link person to join a research interest group
7.4	Link person to develop a folder of research issues and articles for the ward
7.5	Brainstorm ideas
8	**Equal Opportunities & Awareness**
8.1	Raise awareness of "Opportunity 2000" and the new Opportunities Officer
8.2	Raise awareness of the EC directives on manual handling

Column headings: M1 (1, 2, 3, 4), M2 (5, 6, 7, 8), M3 (9, 10, 11, 12, 13), M4 (14, 15, 16, 17), M5 (18, 19, 20, 21), M6 (22, 23, 24, 25), M7 (26, 27, 28, 29, 30), M8 (31, 32, 33, 34), M9 (35, 36, 37, 38), M10 (39, 40, 41, 42, 43)

Figure 5.11b

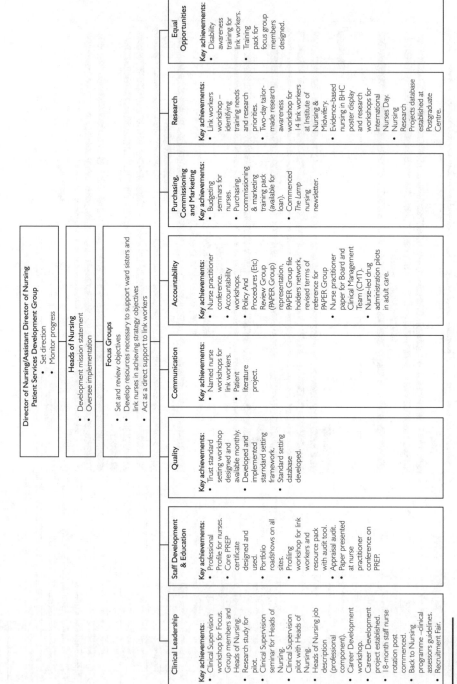

Figure 5.12

Summary of the dissemination framework and key achievements of each of the Focus Groups (December 1996) (reproduced with the permission of Brighton Health Care NHS Trust)

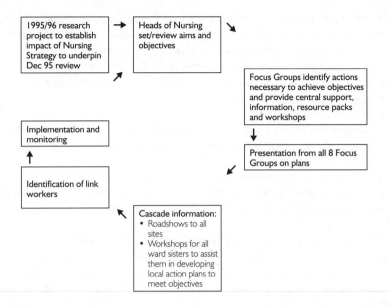

Figure 5.13

Cycle for launch and review of Strategy for Nursing and Midwifery (reproduced with the permission of Brighton Health Care NHS Trust)

Research project

It was agreed when Strategy II was published that it would be helpful to conduct a more rigorous evaluation of the impact the strategy had achieved, with regard to both developing clinical practice and how it was received by nurses working within Brighton Health Care. The Director of Nursing carried out a research study between May 1995 and February 1996 as part of the dissertation for her master's degree (Parsley, 1996). The purpose of this study was to inform and develop the third cycle of the strategy objectives and identify any changes that needed to be made, either in the structure or with the implementation process to make it more effective.

Aims and objectives of research

Aims
The aims of the study were:

1 to evaluate methods used for developing and implementing the BHC Strategy for Nursing and Midwifery;
2 to develop and enhance this strategy.

Objectives
The objectives of the study were:

1 to review the literature on leadership, strategic planning, change management and quality assurance theories which could be used to implement and evaluate the BHC Strategy for Nursing and Midwifery;
2 to find out from nurses and midwives in BHC their perceptions of:
   ● the hierarchical structures put in place to drive the initiative
   ● the process of implementation
   ● the resulting outcomes;
3 to analyse the findings and explore whether the theories of leadership, strategic development and change management were helpful in underpinning the approach used;
4 to critique the original implementation framework and use this as the basis of recommendations for adapting the approach to BHC and any other organizations that may wish to adopt this approach.

Description and rationale for research method selected
This study of the BHC Strategy for Nursing and Midwifery used a non-experimental design, since the area under investigation did not lend itself to the strict laboratory-type control of an experimental method. It used a combination of qualitative and quantitative methods in an attempt to fulfil the research aims. Qualitative data were generated from semi-structured focus group interviews to find out from key stakeholders their views on the methods used to implement the Strategy for Nursing and Midwifery. This enabled the interviewer to explore in more depth with the focus groups their perceptions and views. The focus group interview transcripts formed the basis of a questionnaire which allowed a much larger sample to be surveyed and to generate quantitative data for analysis. Techniques from 'action research' were utilized which enabled the researcher to feed back research findings throughout the research and adapt the change process according to participant feedback. Steps were taken to ensure the validity and reliability both of the interview data and the integrity of the questionnaire. In total 294 questionnaires were distributed and 204 were returned, giving a highly satisfactory response rate of 69%. This response means that the representation error is less than 2%. The types of respondents are shown in Figure 5.14.

The changes recommended to the BHC Strategy for Nursing and Midwifery (outlined later in this chapter) are based on the findings of the research and have been developed in conjunction with the key groups shown in Figure 5.9. Findings that may be of specific interest to those developing strategies for professional development are outlined below.

Selection of some of the key findings

The Strategy for Nursing and Midwifery document
Ninety-three per cent of respondents agreed there was a need for a document that gave a clear direction on how the profession is to develop. It is encouraging to note that 67% of respondents believed that the Strategy for Nursing and

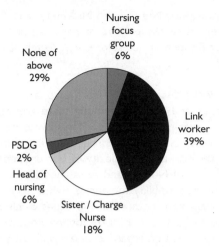

Figure 5.14

Pie chart showing hierarchal position of all respondents (n=204) (reproduced with the permission of Brighton Health Care NHS Trust)

Midwifery should continue. In terms of the theories of change management, this was a positive finding: Rogers (in Welch, 1979, Figure 5.2) identified that for change to be accepted, individuals need to be interested in the innovation and committed to making it occur. This result therefore indicates that well over half the nurses in BHC meet Rogers' criteria.

Comments endorsing the *Strategy for Nursing and Midwifery* document itself (Brighton Health Care, 1994) included the following:

> *I think it is a really good document ... the whole core of it is what nursing needs.* **(Head of nursing)**

> *I think its strength lies in the fact that it has made explicit and tangible for a lot of nurses and midwives a lot of issues that were not clearly understood or given the necessary priority before the document's existence.* **(Patient services manager)**

Cascading the work of the strategy

One of the key findings of the research was that there is a high degree of ownership and involvement from the Patient Services Development Group, heads of nursing, focus group members, and ward sisters and charge nurses. Of the other groups surveyed, the link workers and the 'none of the above' group (i.e. those who had not directly been involved in the early stages of the strategy) showed a significantly higher response rate, scoring 'neither agree nor disagree' to the responses in the questionnaire. Such respondents may have a lower awareness of the Strategy for Nursing and Midwifery, and therefore do not have any strongly held opinions (either positive or negative) on the topics concerned. A major challenge for Strategy III, therefore, was to target these nurses and involve them more.

Although initially we were disappointed with the apparent lesser awareness about the Strategy for Nursing and Midwifery among these groups of nurses, a slightly different interpretation was placed on this when viewed from the perspective of change management theories identified through the literature review. This indicated that, given the size and complexity of our organization, coupled with the fact that the Director of Nursing and Assistant Director of Nursing do not have line management responsibility for nurses (which some authors cite as a barrier to change management because of the issues of hierarchical power), the fact that large numbers of senior nurses responded positively to the Strategy for Nursing and Midwifery has to be regarded as a significant achievement. Other implementation frameworks that could have been used (for example, targeting more junior nurses directly) could prove problematic if those who manage them (e.g. patient services managers, heads of nursing, sisters and charge nurses) are not supportive of the initiative. This could act as a significant barrier to change, and on reflection we felt we had taken the right approach. In terms of Stocking's (1984) model outlined earlier, this finding indicates that another of her critical success criteria for implementing change – that the innovation should appeal to those who have the power to promote change – was met.

Commitment to the strategy by senior Trust managers
Forty-three per cent of respondents agreed that the Trust Board is committed to the implementation of the Strategy for Nursing and Midwifery, and 38% agreed that the general managers are committed to the implementation of the strategy.

Outcomes of the BHC Strategy for Nursing and Midwifery
The questionnaire sought to ascertain nurses' perception of some of the outcomes that had occurred as a result of the introduction of the strategy. A series of statements in the questionnaire asked the respondents to score responses on a Likert scale. A summary of these findings are outlined in Table 5.5.

It is encouraging to note the positive responses to these statements and the perception by nurses that the strategy led to a number of significant achievements within two years. It also shows that another of Stocking's (1984) initial success criteria for implementing change – that the innovation is viewed as relevant for key stakeholders – was met. The simplicity of the statements in Table 5.5 belies the amount of work that has gone into some of the developments. For example, there was an urgent need to update the clinical procedures, protocols and guidelines underpinning nursing practice. The UKCC document *Scope of Professional Practice* (United Kingdom Central Council for Nursing,

Table 5.5

Outcomes from BHC Strategy for Nursing and Midwifery

Outcome	% of respondents who agree
Awareness of nurses' accountability and scope of professional practice increased	76.1
Clinical procedures, protocols, guidelines being updated	75.9
An increase in the number of nurses expanding the scope of professional practice	74.6
An increase in the number of new activities undertaken by nurses expanding the scope of practice	73.5
Nurses in BHC more aware of current professional issues	71.5
Nursing projects by staff which have led to improvements in their clinical areas	70.5
More nurses now managing budgets	69.1
Setting of nursing standards has developed and increased	62.1
Nursing audit and nurses involved in multidisciplinary audit have increased	60.8
The number of nurse practitioners has increased	58.6
The quality and quantity of patient information literature has increased	58.6
The Strategy for Nursing and Midwifery has contributed to the professional development of nurses involved	57.4
Objectives set which have brought about changes in clinical practice	53.1
Nurses had greater understanding of how nursing in Brighton is to be developed	52.5
The quality and quantity of appraisals for nurses has increased	51.5
Senior nurses have developed longer-term objectives for developing nursing rather than focusing on day-to-day crisis management	49.0

Reproduced with the permission of Brighton Health Care NHS Trust.

Midwifery and Health Visiting, 1992) led to nurses expanding their scope of practice by undertaking activities traditionally done by other professional groups. Robust policies and procedures were needed to underpin this role expansion to ensure the safe delivery of effective care. Producing these documents was extremely time consuming, and significant progress had been made through the establishment of a Policies and Procedures (etc.) Review ('PAPER') Group. This multidisciplinary group oversaw the development of evidence-based policy and procedure documents and ensured they were disseminated throughout the Trust.

Barriers to implementation
The research findings indicated that the commitment and enthusiasm nurses expressed towards the BHC Strategy for Nursing and Midwifery, coupled with the value nurses placed on this work, were strong driving forces in maintaining its development and success. Part of the research also sought to identify potential barriers to implementation. The three key barriers are outlined below.

Conflict with other Trust/national priorities
A significant barrier was the large number of other change initiatives/priorities currently being developed within BHC and the NHS. Sixty-seven per cent of

respondents agreed there were many other change initiatives/priorities competing with the Strategy for Nursing and Midwifery. This was constantly referred to by interviewees, for example:

> I think you have to acknowledge we are trying to introduce something in a situation where everybody is really overstretched. I don't mean managers, I mean the actual troops ... They have just got so much to do, so much to think about. (Patient services manager)''

> We are not just here to do seven hours' patient care, some of that seven hours must be taken up with development and at the moment it [development work] isn't seen as that. (Focus group review)

The conflicting priorities include *Patients' Charter* (Department of Health, 1992) initiatives and other associated quality initiatives. Hence the importance of one of the components of Stocking's (1994) model, namely the lack of contact with current priorities, was borne out in practice.

Increasing ward workload
There is also a perception from nurses that they are experiencing difficulty delivering direct clinical care and as a consequence they are not able to devote time to important practice development work. Seventy-seven percent of respondents *did not* feel there were sufficient nurses to deliver clinical care as well as develop practice. This was worrying for two reasons. First, it can be seen that many of the strategy objectives (Appendix 1, pp. 5–7) are fundamental to the quality of patient care. It is crucial for the development of nursing that nurses have the opportunity to reflect on and develop their own nursing practice in order to remain responsive to changing health needs. Development activities cross a broad spectrum and include nurses preparing themselves and others to expand their role (for example, taking on new activities as a result of changing practice, reduction in junior doctors' hours, or new technology). Second, the responses to questions on staffing levels raise issues about the current establishment and skill mix and the need to resource development work adequately. In the words of one nurse,

> I think it needs to be stated very clearly if BHC is going to support taking nursing forward to the next century they have got to be prepared to put some resources in. This is what it has cost to set up in nursing time and actually put a business plan for the nursing strategy forward – do it the same way as any other directorate which has to put in a plan. (Focus group review, 1984)

Of all the theories of change explored, only Stocking's (1994) stresses the importance of cost, i.e. that little finance or other resource should be required unless such requirements can be hidden or increased resources made available.

Since Stocking's work was based on the NHS (others are more generic models), this is an important factor to note. Resource allocation (lack of appropriate resources) was the biggest restraining force identified.

Time

One of the most significant barriers identified both through the questionnaire and the focus group interviews was the lack of time to develop nursing practice and enhance patient care. Eighty per cent of respondents felt that insufficient time was allocated to do the work; 89% agreed that much of the work done to date was done in nurses' own time; 88% agreed releasing staff to attend meetings was a problem and 81% believed that meetings were important to progress the implementation of the Strategy for Nursing and Midwifery. Finally, 91% of nurses surveyed believed that the Strategy for Nursing and Midwifery could be better implemented with more time. As some nurses noted,

> ... *when you go to meetings in work time you feel guilty because you've left colleagues rushing around doing what you've left them ...* (**Focus group review**)

> ... *this needs doing but the agenda's too full, other things have priority, just getting through the work of the day has priority.* (**Patient Services Development Group**)

> *I am sure there's quite a few of us here today and I'm sure I shouldn't really be here today. I'm putting extra pressure on my colleagues, but I know it's important.* (**Focus group review**)

A highly significant finding from this research is the importance respondents placed on the resources necessary to achieve the objectives in the Strategy for Nursing and Midwifery (see Appendix 1, pp. 5–7). Numerous references were made about the importance of having sufficient nurses on the wards and dedicated time for nurses to carry out professional development work. References were made in the tape transcripts to the importance of having allocated sums of money to progress this initiative. This has to be balanced with a natural resistance to change, and one could argue that the comments that there are insufficient resources were excuses, because the threat of change and the challenge to the status quo make nurses feel uncomfortable. However, if this *were* the case it does not explain another significant finding in the research, namely that nurses have undertaken significant amounts of this work in their own time, off duty. Following presentation of the research findings to the board, £10,000 was set aside for the third cycle of the strategy to allow for replacement costs for focus group members undertaking strategy-related work. Interestingly, few nurses actually chose to use the funding. It appeared that the principle of management being seen to make resources available (i.e. demonstrating commitment) was more important than the need for actual funding.

The role of the sister/charge nurse

It was also clear from the tape transcripts and questionnaire (1996) that the sisters and charge nurses group perceive they were spending significant amounts of time giving direct clinical care. This raised questions about where the leadership of more junior nurses is coming from if sisters and charge nurses are not given sufficient time out from clinical work to carry out staff appraisal and supervision; to develop and audit professional standards, policies and procedures; to put research findings into practice; to teach more junior nurses new skills and assess their competence; and to develop education programmes for and with patients. These were all key themes in the Strategy for Nursing and Midwifery, and are the components of the sister/charge nurse job description which distinguish them from more junior posts. Hence when ward activity increases, the more senior staff take a caseload of patients and focus on care delivery rather than managing and developing the ward. This is not problematic when it happens occasionally, since there will inevitably be fluctuations in workload. However, there is evidence to suggest that in some areas sisters and charge nurses doing direct care, rather than leading the ward, was the norm rather than the exception. In reviewing this finding with sisters and charge nurses, it was agreed that achieving the strategy objectives was inherent to the practice of good nursing and high quality patient care. As Harper (1986) notes,

> *The quality of care can only be as high as the competence of the person providing that care.*

And Pembrey's research (1978) reminds us,

> *The Sr/CN role as a leader in ensuring competence of all nurses is one of the most significant factors affecting the quality of nursing care.*

Greater emphasis was therefore placed on developing local leadership in the role of the sister/charge nurse in Strategy III. Similarly, it was identified that further work needed to be done to give sisters and charge nurses dedicated time to fulfil their leadership role.

The role of the Director of Nursing

Another theme running through the research was respondents' perceptions of the Director of Nursing role. Importance was placed on the value of a unified strategic approach to the development of nursing practice which is coordinated centrally and at a senior level. Interestingly, over half of the nurses surveyed agreed that working in clinical directorates had made it more difficult for nurses in BHC to share good practice. In the words of one nurse,

> *I think with division [within a Trust] into directorates, we don't meet each other as much as we used to. I don't know what's happening*

next door. . . . having something that unifies the nursing teams is of great value. **(Link worker)**

The importance of a professional figurehead to lead and develop nursing practice is further endorsed through some of the tape transcripts. As some participants noted,

I think we need a nurse because . . . there are so many managers who are non-nurses . . . you need . . . a nurse who is committed to it and . . . you know can help us just to say . . . I support you. **(Link worker)**

I think the Director of Nursing is there as the figurehead: captain of the ship, if you like, and fighting her corner. You are there as the representation of nursing in Brighton Health Care and you reflect the issues and the values . . . **(Focus group review)**

The importance of leadership in ensuring effective change is noted by many of the references cited in the section at the beginning of this chapter (Figure 5.1). It was therefore encouraging to note that nurses felt positive about the contribution made by the Director of Nursing.

Changes made in the BHC Strategy for Nursing and Midwifery following analysis of research findings

Structure
It was clear from the research findings that the more senior groups of nursing staff had a heavy commitment to, and high amounts of involvement with, developing and implementing the strategy. It was felt important that they should be encouraged to continue with their contribution. The challenge was to identify changes in the structure which ensured that more junior nurses became more aware of, and more closely involved in, the work of the strategy. A number of steps were taken to ensure this occurs in the third cycle.

Nursing focus groups
The value of having nursing focus groups was strongly endorsed by the research findings. Eighty per cent of respondents agreed or agreed strongly with the principle of establishing focus groups to coordinate the implementation and the monitoring of the Strategy for Nursing and Midwifery; 86% responded positively to the need for focus groups to do extra work to support the sister or charge nurse and link workers. Importantly, 83% of nurses who were focus group members agreed that being on a nursing focus group served as a valuable source of personal development.

Numerous examples exist of focus groups tackling objectives where a corporate approach is more desirable than individual directorates or wards attempting to

STAFFORDSHIRE
UNIVERSITY
LIBRARY

tackle significantly sized pieces of work in isolation. It has also ensured that such work is overseen by the Director and Assistant Director of Nursing to provide the necessary support and professional advice.

It was agreed that focus groups needed to continue and that more junior representation on these groups would be sought. It was also recognized that some focus group members had been contributing for nearly three years and it was probably time to seek replacements. A campaign to recruit new members to the focus groups, which secured both new members and a greater proportion of more junior staff, was successful.

Link workers
It was clear from the research that where the link worker network was working well the impact of the Strategy for Nursing and Midwifery was significantly greater. Similarly the awareness and understanding of all nurses in areas where this system was working well appeared to be greater. A key objective for the third cycle was, therefore, to strengthen the link worker network, providing the link workers with the necessary education to contribute meaningfully to the achievement of their strategy objectives and the resources necessary to disseminate the strategy achievements to their colleagues. Link workers contributing in this way were able to use this work as evidence for their PREP portfolio, and help was given to them in preparing the evidence for their personal profile. This was important, since there was a commonly held misperception by nurses that the mandatory five study days every three years were classroom based. We ensured that development work undertaken by link workers was used towards the mandatory study hours. This approach had the benefit of contributing to organizational as well as personal development.

Reviewing focus group effectiveness
The research also explored respondents' perceptions of the effectiveness of the eight focus groups and their contributions. The findings were reproduced in a league table, shown in Table 5.6.

There was clearly a statistical difference in respondents' perception of the relative effectiveness of each focus group. The question posed by the researcher was whether this was a reflection on the efficiency of *the group itself* or simply indicative of the respective values and priorities placed by clinical nurses on each of the *eight issues*. Hence, for a staff nurse working in the ward, issues around quality of nursing care, nursing accountability, etc. may be given much higher priority than issues surrounding purchasing, commissioning and marketing. This led to a number of changes being made to the Strategy III document to reflect these concerns. At the conference to review the research, it was agreed that some of the focus group names needed changing to make more explicit what it was they were trying to achieve. The amended focus group titles reflect input from more junior nurses who feel more comfortable with the names used.

Table 5.6

League table of focus groups, indicating respondents' views on the effectiveness of each focus group

Focus group	Likert scale (%)					Aggregate score (%) 4+5
	1 disagree strongly	2 tend to disagree	3 neither agree nor disagree	4 tend to agree	5 agree strongly	
Quality	1.8	19.0	36.3	35.1	7.7	42.8
Accountability	1.8	17.4	38.3	32.9	9.6	42.5
Staff Development & education	2.4	19.2	36.5	34.7	7.23	41.9
Communication	1.8	20.2	35.1	33.9	6	39.9
Clinical leadership	3.6	18.7	40.4	32.5	4.8	37.3
Research	1.8	19.8	43.1	30.5	4.8	35.3
Equal opportunities	2.4	22.9	42.8	28.3	3.6	31.9
Purchasing, marketing & commissioning	3.0	24.8	44.8	24.2	3.0	27.3

Reproduced with the permission of Brighton Health Care NHS Trust.

Two more fundamental changes were made. Firstly, a workforce planning group was created in response to a growing problem with recruitment, combined with work beginning on a capital redevelopment programme which would eventually consolidate the currently disparate services onto one site. Significant work therefore needed to be done to address both short-term and long-term issues of workforce planning. Secondly, the communication focus group was disbanded since many of its objectives had become what we referred to as 'maintenance objectives'. This term was used for objectives that had been running for at least two years and were relatively well established within the clinical areas. It was agreed that these should therefore form a regular part of the way in which wards were run rather than remaining as a specific objective in the strategy. The only objective that had not been met was more effective communication of work originating from the Strategy for Nursing and Midwifery. It was agreed that this objective could usefully be adopted by the marketing focus group. The problem with having a 'communication' group was the danger that it might abrogate focus group responsibility for communicating their work from the other groups. Responsibility for communication and dissemination is now vested firmly with each focus group.

Key lessons learned

Through the findings of the research, a consensus conference and numerous other regular forums, we have had the opportunity to reflect at length upon what we did, where it was successful and how, if we were to start again knowing what we know now, we would do things differently. This exercise was important in ensuring that we did not fall into the trap outlined by Freud, that 'those who do not learn from their past are forced to re-live it'.

Some of the lessons we learned are presented here, so that those developing a similar approach elsewhere might avoid having to relive our experiences.

Communication

The importance of good communication cannot be overemphasized (Fretwell, 1985; Figure 5.3). Although the establishment of the focus groups and the workshops for the sisters and charge nurses proved time consuming, they were essential so that individuals had the opportunity to contribute to, and own, the subsequent work. The research confirmed this approach. However, we had made the assumption that if we could be effective down to this level, the sisters/charge nurses and focus groups would ensure the rest of the staff were afforded similar opportunities. This happened in some areas but not consistently. To rectify the limited dissemination of the Strategy for Nursing and Midwifery below sister/charge nurse level, we instigated a number of different initiatives, including:

- making much more explicit the role of the sisters and charge nurses in leading this work through the appraisal process; giving them time in regular seminars to review their progress, share good practice and work though any difficulties;
- reviewing and updating the link worker database and formalizing the relationship between focus groups and link workers to stress the responsibility of the focus group members in ensuring all link workers are supported through written updates, meetings and workshops;
- developing a 'ward portfolio', adopting the principles of a PREP portfolio but focusing on the Strategy for Nursing and Midwifery (This document contains an introductory section on the BHC Strategy for Nursing and Midwifery and the objectives for all the focus groups for the forthcoming year. The portfolio is completed by the sisters/charge nurses and link workers, who develop an action plan to achieve the strategy objectives. Link workers have responsibility for building evidence of their achievements and progress, and incorporating this work into the portfolio to share with colleagues. For example, quality link workers can include information on the in-house courses they have attended on quality and standard-setting, and a summary of what they learned. The required project work (a compulsory part of both courses), such as standards set or audits completed, will also be included in the portfolio. This then provides a dynamic resource for staff to review and update. (It also provides information on all focus group members and how to contact them.);
- a bimonthly Trust-wide nursing newsletter, *The Lamp*, with regular updates on the work and activities planned;
- two internal conferences targeted specifically at more junior staff.

Education

The importance of education as a strategy for effecting change has been identified (Bennis, Benne and Chinn, 1988). We therefore appreciated that education was vital if staff were to meaningfully participate in achieving the strategy objectives. For example, before the strategy, staff were critical of requests to 'do' audit or 'do' quality assurance without having been given them the necessary knowledge and skills. Like many Trusts in the late 1980s, nurses in BHC had become involved in setting numerous standards. A review of the 80 standards found in the central file revealed that only a tiny proportion of these had been audited; while a review indicated that 70% of standards contained unmeasurable statements and criteria. This was a powerful lesson learned in view of the concerns highlighted in our research about the conflicting demands on nurses' time. Although significant amounts of time and effort had gone into setting these standards, it was difficult to provide objective evidence that it had actually led to any beneficial changes in practice, except in a very few areas. However, as a result of our educational programme, standards and audit are now developed properly and audited on a regular basis.

The other area we had underestimated was the hesitancy on the part of more junior staff to contribute to the focus group meetings. Some felt intimidated by the process, and there was a danger that we were just paying lip service to 'shared governance'. Further work is being done to rectify this, buddying up more experienced members with more junior ones, offering coaching for things like chairing meetings and speaking in public. With hindsight, we should have put on a short workshop for all new focus group members to prepare them to contribute as an active member of the group. Hence the theoretical models that show change as a cyclical process (such as, for example, Fretwell, 1985; Figure 5.3) were borne out in practice.

Evaluation

The research project proved invaluable in identifying how we were doing and what we needed to change. Again, with hindsight, we could have begun this after the first cycle. We also needed to find more effective ways of illustrating the impact that the strategy had on direct patient care. Evaluation is now being addressed at a local level through the construction of the ward-based profiles outlined above. For example, link workers for quality have been involved in the implementation of a pressure damage prevention strategy and have contributed to a Trust-wide audit showing a drop in pressure sore prevalence from 17% in May 1994 to 1.34% in 1998.

However, finding objective evidence of the benefits of some of the softer issues, for example the improvement in both quality and quantity of patient literature, has proved more difficult.

SUMMARY AND CONCLUSIONS

At the beginning of this chapter we set out some of the theories reviewed from the disciplines of quality assurance, leadership and change management which we considered to help us in our search for a model to develop and implement our strategy. Some of these have been alluded to in the case study, where we felt the theories helped us to understand some of the findings of the research evaluation. Some theories we set out to incorporate explicitly into our approach – for example, Harrison's structural approach (1994) and Covey's circle of influence (1992). The rational planning models (such as those in Boisot, 1995; Tappen, 1989) were also influential in the approach we developed. As can be seen in Figure 5.13, we worked systematically through a series of steps to effect the desired changes, setting aims and objectives. Having completed these steps, the importance of developing the strategy further, evolving and maturing the approach in order to sustain momentum gained, became apparent. Change models such as Fretwell's (1985), which stressed the cyclical nature of continuously improving and changing, seemed to fit with our own experience of putting the strategy into practice.

As with the need to ensure that clinical practice is underpinned by evidence, we observed that management practice needs a similar foundation. Our experience in undertaking a change management project of this size seemed merely to endorse the key principles outlined in the literature. Where things did not go so well, it was inevitably because we had overlooked (or chosen to ignore) some of the theories. For example, midwives were underrepresented on the focus groups, and were the most alienated group as far as ownership of the strategy was concerned. Hence more attention to Fretwell's (1985) model with respect to consultation with the midwives could have avoided this problem. Similarly, use of Plant's (1987) change continuum could have predicted low compliance and low stickability of the strategy objectives (Figure 5.5). This is being addressed by working with the heads of midwifery to amend the strategy so that it falls in line with their own priorities and expectations. Similarly, some of the other professional groups viewed the strategy as exclusive and elitist. This has been addressed partly through better communication with these groups (specifically on the benefits arising as a result), and partly through extending the membership of the focus groups to include them where relevant, having recognized the importance of ownership and effective communication as outlined in the literature.

We found specific examples where the theory helped us to understand why things were not working so well in practice. We found examples of 'black holes' (Figure 5.7) in our organization through the consistent message from some areas that more junior staff were not getting information. We went though the 'change wave' (Figure 5.8), which helped us to understand why things seemed to run out of steam after the first year, and come up with an annual plan to put the momentum back into the strategy work. We found that where things were not going to plan there were clear 'restraining forces' that we had overlooked (Lewin, 1953). Where things were going well, the driving forces were easily identified in terms of clear leadership, ownership by staff and following a clearly agreed plan.

What was intriguing was the way theories provided us with different perspectives on a complex strategic change project, which the adoption of a single model would not have provided. The rational planning approach helped us to set some clear objectives we needed to achieve. Setting aims and objectives was important in helping staff understand exactly what was expected of them and enabling us to develop clear programmes of work. It also provided us with a way of articulating to non-nurses why the strategy was so important. Communicating the importance of the strategy was essential, since there was evidence from the research (Parsley, 1996) that some stakeholders did not value the strategic importance of this work. We challenged this view, reminded sceptics that nurses represent 43% of the workforce and consume £23 million of the payroll budget. Maintaining the integrity of professional nursing practice through the Brighton Health Care Strategy for Nursing and Midwifery is an essential component underpinning all of the Trust's strategic objectives. Setting clear objectives for improving practice (and therefore, by proxy, patient care) we stressed as being as fundamentally important as achieving the Trust's financial and activity targets. We ensured the work focused on issues that were given high priority either at a national level (e.g. named nurse) or by nurses and patients themselves. Hence the rational planning model provided objectives grounded in the real world, a plan for achieving these and a mechanism for communicating the vision of nursing's future direction, both to nurses in BHC and to a wider audience. It was, therefore, a useful prospective approach.

Conversely, the complex adaptive systems theory proved a useful framework for retrospective analysis. We certainly saw numerous examples where unexpected or unpredictable things occurred as a result of new relationships or alliances created by bringing together staff who in the normal course of their work would never meet. For example, the clinical leadership focus group started off with an objective to provide succession planning for nurses in the Trust. When the objective was originally set, it was initially envisioned by the heads of nursing that this would involve the identification of succession planning criteria for each of the nursing grades. What emerged was something startlingly different, with more junior staff challenging the hierarchy; setting themselves up as a project steering board and creating a whole career development programme based around cross-hierarchical action learning sets. They went on to train as facilitators themselves and are currently running a programme for 18 staff, which is now being developed still further. Emergence of new and unexpected ideas as a result of creating new teams created a whole that, as systems theorists note, is more than a sum of the parts.

Complex adaptive systems theory also helped us to come to terms with the fact that some things *are* messy and unpredictable, and wilfully do not go according to plan. It gave us a framework to understand what was happening and a useful balance to the rational planning theories, where, in spite of following all the right rational steps, things did not go as anticipated. However, as a prospective model, it is probably less culturally acceptable in the NHS. It would be a brave (or possibly foolish) Director of Nursing who made a presentation to the board on the strategic direction for the profession based around forming a few new alliances and waiting to see what exciting consequences emerged. It is also a high-risk strategy: there is a balance between tapping into the creativity of staff and keeping a focus on delivering against national and corporate priorities.

The advantage of our eclectic approach was that it enabled a mixture of both. The rational part, with its objectives that provided an overall intention, rather than being overly prescriptive, ensured that staff had a clear vision of what needed to be achieved, but enabled those involved in the process to address these in dynamic and creative ways.

The other theory that proved useful was Covey's (1992) circle of influence, described earlier in this chapter (Figure 5.4). In explaining the habits of highly effective people, Covey notes that ineffectual people tend to spend a lot of time focused on the outer circle of his model, that is, paying attention to things that are of concern to them but over which they have no influence. This was something we observed with some nurses who focused on barriers such as lack of money, insufficient staff, lack of time, poor working environment, poor equipment or lack of cooperation from medical staff. These barriers were used to rationalize why things could not change. Our strategy focused specifically on our own areas of nursing practice over which we had direct influence. Covey's model advocates changing and improving things over which we have influence, so the circle expands as others note the impact and wish to collaborate.

Thus it was with our Strategy for Nursing and Midwifery. We started small, with things that we felt mattered to patients and staff, and were in line with corporate and national policy. There were some cynics, but we focused on specific achievable goals and used our influence to make a difference. As we were able to demonstrate improvements, the interest of others in the strategy grew. More people got involved; new nurses joined the focus groups and became link workers. Other professions expressed an interest in making a contribution and dietitians, pharmacists, chaplains and clinical audit, personnel and medical staff have all got involved in project work started by the focus groups. We also have representation from our local university from nurse educationalists and researchers. Successful projects, such as

- nurse-led drug administration
- a medication error review policy
- pain guidelines
- development of a multidisciplinary education programme on quality improvement
- a career development programme
- reducing hospital-acquired pressure damage

– (and many others) have demonstrated significant improvements which have helped to strengthen interest in and commitment to the strategy.

In conclusion, strategic planning, underpinned by change management and leadership theories, were helpful in developing, implementing and evaluating the strategy presented in the case study. The strategy proved to be an effective organizational tool for enabling clinicians to work together in an organized way to make significant improvements in their clinical and professional practice.

The next chapter explores an approach from industry which seeks to involve all its employees in working together to improve quality; this is known as total quality management.

REFERENCES

Baker, F. (1973) *Organisational Systems: General Systems Approaches to Complex Organisations*, Irwin, Homewood, IL.

Basset, G.W. (1971) Change in Australian education. *Australian Journal of Education*, 15(1).

Bennis, W., Benne, K.D. and Chinn, R. (eds) (1988) *The Planning of Change*, Holt, Reinhart & Wilson, New York.

Boisot, M. (1995) *Preparing for turbulence: the changing relationship between strategy and management development in the learning organisation*, in Developing Strategic Thought: Rediscovering the Art of Direction Giving (ed. B. Garratt), McGraw Hill, Homewood, IL, pp. 29–46.

Brighton Health Care (1994) *Strategy for Nursing and Midwifery*, internal publication, Brighton Health Care NHS Trust, Brighton.

Coch, L. and French, J.R.P. (1948) Overcoming resistance to change. Human Relations 1, in Covey, S.R. (1992) *The Seven Habits of Highly Effective People*, Simon & Schuster.

Cuba, D. and Clark, D.L. (1978) Planned organisational change in education, in *Curriculum Innovation* (eds A. Harris *et al.*), Croom Helm, London.

Dalton, G. (1970) Influence and organisational change, in *Organisational Change and Development* (ed. L.P. Griener), Irwin Dorsey, IL.

Department of Health (1989). *A Strategy for Nursing: A Report on the Steering Committee*, Department of Health Nursing Division, London.

Department of Health (1992) *Patients' Charter*, HMSO, London.

Department of Health (1993) *A Vision for the Future: The Nursing, Midwifery and Health Visitor Contribution to Health and Health Care*, National Health Service Management Executive, Leeds.

Donabedian, A. (1966) Evaluating the quality of medical care. *Millbank Memorial Fund Quarterly*, 44(2), 166–206.

Dyer, W.G. (ed.) (1984) *Strategies for Managing Change*, Addison Wesley, Reading.

Flower, J. (1995) The structure of organised change. *Healthcare Forum Journal*, 38(1), 1–11.

Fretwell, J.E. (1985) *Freedom to Change: The Creation of a Ward Learning Environment*, Royal College of Nursing, London.

Garside, P. (1993) *Patient Focused Care: A Review of Seven Sites*, National Health Service Management Executive, Leeds.

Gillies, D.A. (1989) *Nursing Management: A Systems Approach*, 2nd edn, W.B. Saunders/Harcourt Brace Jovanovich, New York.

Glass, N. (1996) Chaos, non-linear systems and day to day management. *European Management Journal*, 14(1), 98–106.

Greaves, F. (1982) Innovation, change, decision making and the key variables in nursing curriculum implementation. *International Journal of Nursing Studies*, 19(1).

Harper, L. (1986) Skill mix: All mixed up. *Nursing Times*, 82(48), 27–31.

Harrison, D. (1994) *Accelerating Change: A Practical Guide to Implementation*, Workshop for Institute of Management Studies, London. Implementation Management Associates Inc., Denver.

Hastings, C. (1990) Career development and advancement in a hospital setting. Paper presented at the annual conference of the American Nurses Association Council on Continuing Education and Staff Development, Baltimore, 12–14 October.

Hoffman, S.E. (1990) Building a power base through strategic planning. Paper presented at the annual conference of American Nurses Association Council on Continuing Education and Staff Development, Baltimore, 12–14 October.

Imershein, A. (1997) Organisational change as a paradigm shift. *Sociological Quarterly*, 18(1), 33–43.

Katz, D. and Kahn, R.L. (1966) *The Social Psychology of Organisations*, John Wiley, New York.

Kelly, K. (1995a) *Out of Control: The New Biology of Machines*, Fourth Estate, London.

Kelly, K. (1995b) The structure of organised change. *Healthcare Forum Journal*, 38(1), 602–607.

Lewin, K. (1935) *A Dynamic Theory of Personality*, McGraw, New York.

Lewin, K. (1953) *Studies in Group Decisions in Group Dynamics: Research and Theory* (eds D. Cartwright and A. Zander), Row Person, Evanston, IL.

Mandela, N., cited in Brown, S. (1996) *The Strategy for Nursing*, presentation to Brighton Health Care Trust Board, Brighton.

Marriner-Tomey, A. (1988) *Guide to Nursing Management*, 3rd edn, Mosby Mission, St Louis, LA

NHS Executive (1993) *Building a Stronger Team: The Nursing Contribution to Purchasing. A Report on the Impact of Nursing Skills and Experience on the Purchasing Process*, Department of Health, UK.

NHS Executive (1995) *Sharpening the Focus: The Roles and Perception of Nursing in NHS Trusts*, Newchurch & Company, London.

NHS Executive (1997) *The New NHS: Modern, Dependable*, Department of Health, London.

Parsley, K. (1996) An evaluation of the Brighton Health Care Strategy for Nursing: an application of the theories of quality assurance, change management, leadership and strategic planning. Master's degree thesis, Nuffield Institute for Health, University of Leeds, Leeds.

Pembrey, S. (1978) The role of the ward sister in the management of nursing: a study on the organisation of nursing on an individualised patient basis. PhD thesis, University of Edinburgh, Edinburgh.

Peters, T. and Waterman, R. (1988) *In Search of Excellence*, Harper & Row, London.

Plant, R. (1987) *Managing Change and Making It Stick*, Fontana, London.

Prospect Centre (1992) *A Competency Framework for Trust Nursing Directors*, South West Thames Regional Health Authority, Kingston-upon-Thames. In Hennessy, D.A. and Gilligan, J.H. (1994) Identifying and developing tomorrow's Trust Nursing Directors. *Journal of Nursing Management*, 2, 37–45.

Ramstrom, D.O. (1974) Toward the information-saturated society, in H. Leavitt.

Rogers, cited in Welch, L.B. (1979) Planned change in nursing. *Nursing Clinics of North America*, 14(2), 311.

Senge, P. (1994) *The Fifth Discipline Fieldbook*, Nicholas Brealey Publishing, London.

Stamp, G. (1992) *One Year On: The Nurse Executive*, National Health Service Management Executive, Leeds.

Stocking, B. (1984) *Initiative or Inertia*, Burgess & Son, Oxfordshire.

Stransen, L. (1988) Strategic planning: an effective management tool for nursing. *Nursing Management*, **19**(5), 80.

Tappen (1989) *Nursing Leadership and Management: Concepts and Practices*, 2nd edn, Davis, Philadelphia.

United Kingdom Central Council for Nursing, Midwifery and Health Visiting (1992) *The Scope of Professional Practice*, UKCC, London.

Welch, L.B. (1979) Planned change in nursing. *Nursing Clinics of North America*, **14**(2), 311.

6 TOTAL QUALITY MANAGEMENT

Earlier chapters explored different frameworks and quality assurance tools commonly used in healthcare aimed at improving clinical practice. As outlined in the last chapter on strategic planning, the success or failure of such initiatives by healthcare professionals are likely to be strongly influenced by the organizational culture and the attitude of management towards such initiatives. Many professionals (see, for example, Hayward, 1996) point out that the quest for ensuring all clinical practice is based on robust evidence does not appear to be mirrored by health service managers and policy makers when it comes to making management and policy decisions.

The problem experienced by many clinicians adopting some of the aforementioned quality improvement frameworks was that these often occurred within an organizational vacuum, with no overarching corporate approach or strategic vision of how to improve quality systematically throughout the whole organization. In the mid-1980s, as medical audit and nursing standard-setting were evolving, there was comparatively little in the health service literature about organizational frameworks for improving quality. This was soon to change, with a number of different approaches being developed or adopted to fill this vacuum. These next chapters set out two such approaches; first, total quality management (TQM), an approach adapted from industry, along with a case study of applying this to an NHS Trust and second, in Chapter 7, patient focused care, a framework initially developed in the USA, followed by a case study of applying this in an NHS Trust.

DEFINING TQM

A review of the literature on the application of TQM in the management of healthcare in the UK shows little published before 1988. TQM was a new phenomenon within this arena, and began to attract interest from managers and professionals in the National Health Service (NHS), as well as the private sector, at about this time. Finding a clear-cut definition of TQM from publications pertaining to the health service, and from the more prolific texts on applying this approach in industry (where it has been established for significantly longer), proved difficult, as many authors use differing terminology to explain TQM.

Although the terminology used by authors varies, there are similarities that run through all the various approaches. These are as follows.

Total

TQM involves everyone and everything that happens within the organization, from the part-time cleaners to the chief executive; from the specifications for a multimillion-pound hospital to the process of emptying the rubbish bins. There is an understanding that, without this total involvement, the other components of this approach will fail, or have only limited success.

This totality of approach expands across professional and departmental boundaries, as it is widely accepted that a high proportion of quality problems occur at these interfaces. For example, the ward may have an effective system to ensure patients are prepared for theatre, and the theatre an effective system for dealing with the patient on arrival. Yet the system often breaks down when portering staff are unable to transfer patients from the ward to theatre on time. Closer inspection of the problem often reveals a lack of communication between these three areas, and a lack of understanding about the whole process. Each area concentrates on a discrete part, without central coordination. 'Total' also refers to the timeframe required in adopting this approach, i.e. it is a continuous process or journey, not a short-term project or programme.

Quality

The second theme running through the texts on TQM is that of 'quality' – specifically, what this term means and how it can be consistently achieved. Definitions include:

Fitness for purpose or use

(Juran and Gryna, 1980)

The totality of features and characteristics of a product or service that bear on its ability to satisfy stated or implied needs

(BS 4778, 1987)

The total composite product and service characteristics of marketing, engineering, manufacture and maintenance through which the product and service in use will meet the expectation by the customer

(Feigenbaum, 1983)

Conformance to requirements

(Crosby, 1979)

Inherent in all of these definitions (made explicit when placing them in context of the whole approach outlined by these authors) is the connection between the customer and supplier in the quality chain. Hence for all products or services there will be a supplier/customer relationship. Part of this chain will, therefore, involve determining what it is the customers want, and the suppliers meeting these needs.

'Customer' is a term used in its broadest sense. It also incorporates the next person in line to receive the product or service, as well as the ultimate customer.

For example, the porter collecting a patient for theatre from the ward is a 'customer' of this process. He or she has certain needs, such as the patient being ready for transfer, the appropriate paperwork being complete and the porter being informed in sufficient time to collect the patient. He or she then becomes a 'supplier' to the theatre, which requires the porter to deliver the patient safely, with appropriate paperwork and at the right time.

Defining 'quality' is an important part of the TQM approach, as it is a word that means different things to different people. This can make the management of quality in large organizations difficult, as for some it means 'excellence' or some kind of unattainable standard of perfection, whereas others may work from a set of minimum standards, or within an acceptable level of error. For example, a 'quality standard' that 70% of outpatients are seen within 30 minutes may be set. Some may view meeting this goal as a quality service, while others may focus on the service the other 30% receive as inadequate.

The definition of quality, and the recognition of the customer/supplier relationship are important to the TQM approach, as it is from these concepts that the third common theme is derived. Understanding the needs of the customer and recognizing the customer/supplier relationship creates the potential to have some sort of control over the quality of products or services being produced. This concept is expanded by many experienced in the TQM field, who believe that if enough is understood about the work process it is possible to control, reduce and (some believe) eliminate completely the number of errors that occur within that process.

This leads to another common observation about quality: that it does not just happen of its own accord, it has to be managed.

Management

TQM is concerned with achieving a culture change within the organization. Many authors acknowledge the limitations of the management styles of the 1950s, and the resultant impact on the organizational culture. These were based on macho management – treating employees as an easily replaceable commodity, a poor attitude towards the customer, accepting waste and error as inevitable (but continually cutting costs), discouraging change, buying from suppliers who offered the cheapest option and competing on price. Such an approach could be successful only if (Mortiboys, 1990):

- employees remained subservient;
- demand exceeded supply;
- customers' expectations increased very slowly;
- the worldwide situation remained static.

In fact, this was not the case. Britain's share of world trade in manufactured goods fell from 13% in 1960 to 7% in 1980. By 1986 it had fallen still further to 5.5% (Mortiboys, 1990). During this time, there was an increase in the number of competitors, an increase in customer and employee expectations and unpredictable financial systems, all occurring against a backdrop of rapid change. This pattern was mirrored in the health service, with the introduction of self-governing Trusts competing for their share of the healthcare market. These pressures caused some managers in the health service to investigate claims that TQM offers an effective solution to these problems, with the Department of Health sponsoring a number of pilot sites in the UK. Latterly, the White Paper *The New NHS: Modern, Dependable* (NHS Executive, 1997) seeks to integrate continuous improvement in healthcare with the introduction of clinical governance.

Much of the literature stresses the importance of 'management style' and 'organizational culture'. 'Culture' can be difficult to define in this context, but a simplified yet powerful assessment can be made by observing what happens in an organization immediately a problem has been identified. In some organizations, staff will not report the problem. This is usually a result of previous experience, where identifying problems led to an immediate hunt for the 'culprit' or perceived initiator of the problem, followed by punishment. In others, staff will not bother to identify problems, as previous experience has shown they are met with apathy and lack of action. An organization practising TQM will acknowledge the problem and those involved in the work process will be given the time and resources necessary to effect an acceptable solution.

The culture change is achieved through a structured framework of implementing quality improvement which incorporates a fundamental change in management style. Common themes running through various approaches include:

- recognizing the need for effective leadership and management to enable employees to contribute to improving the quality of their work ('management through people');
- recognizing the role that all employees can play in improving the quality (or lack of it) of the work process they are involved in;
- developing a strategy to effect the culture change;
- developing work-based teams to monitor and improve quality;
- adopting concepts, tools and techniques that facilitate a greater understanding of the work process (such as statistical process control);
- improving the customer/supplier relationship;
- reducing (and for some eliminating completely) errors or mistakes.

These themes crop up continually in the writings of some of the widely acknowledged authorities in this field (Crosby, 1986, 1988, 1991; Deming 1986; Juran and Gryna, 1980; Juran, 1988). Hence it is difficult to attribute some ideas to one specific author, as many writers appear to adapt and develop the ideas of others. Another difficulty in criticizing some of these approaches is that most of these experts have founded their own consultancy firms, with much of the educational material they supply to clients subsequently being subject to strict copyright agreements, and not available for general use. This means that the books written are only a part of the material available, with the most recent developments being kept in commercial confidence for the use of clients only.

However, of the better-known authorities in the TQM field, a number have defined certain elements that they believe essential in adopting TQM. These are outlined briefly below. All these authors stress the need to place the key elements of their approach within the context of the totality of their work, as criticizing certain components of the approach in isolation precludes an understanding of the vital interactions of the various concepts, tools and techniques.

This chapter ends with a case study that explores the implementation of one such approach to examine the application of these concepts within a hospital setting (as opposed to the more common industrial case studies outlined by many of the authors referred to below).

INTRODUCTION TO THE NOTABLE AUTHORITIES ON TQM

W. Edwards Deming

W. Edwards Deming is an American statistician who went to Japan in the late 1940s. He is widely acknowledged as the initiator of the use of statistical quality control measures, which were utilized extensively and successfully by Japanese industry. At the time, Deming preached a message founded on statistics, based on his extensive experience of sampling techniques gained whilst working for the American Bureau of the Census.

Drawing on the work of Shewhart (1931), Deming advocated the need to focus on problems of variability in the manufacturing process, and the need to identify their causes. He divides these into 'special causes', which are those effects assignable to individual equipment, machinery or operators, and 'common causes', such as faulty raw materials, which are shared by several operations and are therefore the responsibility of management. He criticizes the approach used in many companies of attempting to look for the cause of chance variation, which typically occurs in the absence of statistical methods. He recommends the use of statistical methods to measure performance in all areas, not just conformance to product specifications. He believes it is not enough to meet specifications, it is necessary to continuously reduce the amount of variation as well. His underlying philosophy is that productivity improves as variability decreases and, as all things vary, statistical methods of quality control are needed.

Deming promotes the need to ensure worker participation in decision making. He blames management for poor quality, stating that they are responsible for 94% of quality problems, and points out that it is management's task to help people work 'smarter, not harder'.

Deming is a severe critic of motivational programmes because he believes that 'doing one's best' is insufficient – one needs to know what to do and have the correct resources to do it. Consumer research is also cited as important, as the needs and requirements of the customer are always changing.

Like many other writers in this field, Deming is sceptical of the application of inspection as a method of quality control when used in isolation, as he believes this neither improves quality nor guarantees it. He is also critical of 'acceptable quality levels' (e.g. meeting the required standard 80% of the time). He also notes that simply checking the specifications of incoming materials is insufficient if the material encounters problems in production; it is important that the supplier understands what the material is to be used for.

There were some initial difficulties with Deming's approach, particularly in relation to employee resistance and management uncertainty as to their role in quality improvement, and one criticism was that too much emphasis was placed on the statistical aspects. These problems were addressed by those later Americans who followed Deming to Japan – Juran and Feigenbaum. Deming's later work (1982) also expands beyond statistical methods, including a systematic approach to problem solving – the Deming 'plan, do, check, action' (PDCA) cycle (Figure 6.1). Deming also emphasized the need for senior managers to become actively involved in the organization's quality improvement programmes.

Deming is well known for his 14 key points, which he cites as essential for the transformation of American industry. These points can apply to any size of organization, as well as to divisions within it, and are:

1 Create constancy of purpose to improve product or service.
2 Adopt the new philosophy.
3 Cease dependence on inspection to achieve quality.
4 End the practice of awarding business on the basis of price tag alone. Instead minimize total cost by working with a single supplier.
5 Improve constantly and forever every process for planning, production and service.
6 Institute training on the job.
7 Adopt and institute leadership.
8 Drive out fear.

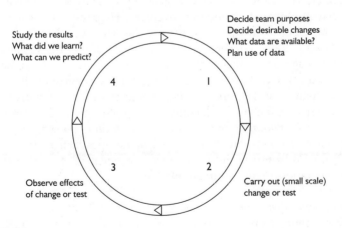

Figure 6.1

Deming's action cycle (Source: Deming (1982))

9 Break down barriers between staff areas.
10 Eliminate slogans, exhortations and targets for the workforce.
11 Eliminate numerical quotas for the workforce and numerical goals for management.
12 Remove barriers that rob people of pride of workmanship. Eliminate the annual or merit system.
13 Institute vigorous education and self-improvement for everyone.
14 Put everyone in the company to work to accomplish the transformation.

These underpinned Deming's quality improvement programmes. Another American was similarly influential in transforming the thinking behind Japanese manufacturing – Joseph Juran.

Joseph M. Juran

Juran's background lay in engineering. His other wide-ranging accomplishments, however, include that of university professor. Along with Deming he is credited with influencing the success of Japanese industry in the post-war years. He was invited to Japan in the early 1950s, where he lectured on management and quality. He is noted for dealing with the broad management aspects of quality; identifying the important role of communications, coordination of functions and the human element; and stating that an understanding of the human situations associated with the job will go a long way to solving the technical problems and that such an understanding may be prerequisite for a solution.

Juran emphasizes the vital role of management, with the strong message that quality does not happen by accident, it must be planned. In his opinion, 80% of quality problems are caused by management, and he advocates the training all managers in quality to enable them to oversee and participate in quality improvement projects. He views the project-by-project approach by problem-solving teams as the way to secure overall quality improvement. He stresses the need to include top-level management in this process, because he perceives that the major problems in organizations are interdepartmental. He questions the instinctive belief of many top managers that they already know what needs to be done and that training is for others. He also warns of the dangers of departmental goals undermining the company's overall mission. He promotes the use of statistical process control, although warning of this leading to a 'tool-orientated' approach.

His book, *Juran on Planning for Quality* (1988), outlines his structured approach to company-wide planning. He defines a tripartite approach to this: (1) quality planning; (2) quality control; and (3) quality improvement. Key elements as part of the implementation of the strategic planning are:

- identifying customers and their needs;
- establishing optimal quality goals;
- creating measurements of quality;
- planning processes capable of meeting quality goals under operating conditions;

- producing continuing results in improved market share, premium prices and a reduction in error rates in office and factory.

Juran stresses the importance of securing consistency from one's suppliers in achieving a quality product or service and, thus, emphasizes the role of the purchaser. This should include training in methods for rating vendors, with the customer making the investment of time, effort and special skills to help poor vendors improve.

Along with others, he differentiates between the end customer, who receives the final product or service, and other internal and external customers. This incorporates his concept of quality, since 'fitness of use' will need to be ensured at every customer/supplier interface.

He is critical of quality drives based on slogans and exhortations because he does not believe they elicit the required behaviour change. This was usually because such initiatives gave no specific tasks or projects to be tackled; did not allocate individual responsibility for doing the necessary tasks; provided no structured process for implementation; and did not revise systems used for judging manager performance. He states that 'The recipe for action should consist of 90% substance and 10% exhortation, not the reverse' (Juran, 1988). His views are often voiced by clinicians who are cynical about importing concepts such as mission statements and 'visioning' to the NHS.

Juran lists ten steps to quality improvement:

1 Build awareness of the need and opportunity for development.
2 Set goals for improvement.
3 Organize to reach the goals (establish a quality council, identify problems, select projects, appoint teams, designate facilitators).
4 Provide training.
5 Carry out projects to solve problems.
6 Report progress.
7 Give recognition.
8 Communicate results.
9 Keep score.
10 Maintain momentum by making annual improvement part of the regular systems and processes of the company.

These underpinned the implementation of his TQM programmes.

Philip B. Crosby

Philip Crosby is an American with a background in quality control. A quality manager on the first Pershing missile programme, he later became Corporate Vice President and Quality Director of ITT in the USA. His bestselling book, *Quality is Free*, was first published in 1979, and he has written a number of books that expand his original ideas (Crosby, 1967, 1972, 1984, 1986, 1988, 1990). He has established his own consultancy company, Philip Crosby Associates.

The Crosby approach to TQM is outlined later in this chapter, in the case study applying TQM in an NHS setting.

J.S. Oakland

Author of *Total Quality Management* (1989), this British authority on the subject is Professor of TQM at the European Centre for Total Quality Management at the University of Bradford Management Centre. As with many other authors, he stresses the importance of the customer/supplier interface, which he illustrates by the use of a 'quality chain', with the customer and supplier forming the vital links. The chain can therefore be broken at any point if an individual or other essential piece of equipment does not meet requirements. Oakland examines the management of quality through two central concepts: (1) quality of design; and (2) conformance to design.

- **Quality of design.** This is defined as 'A measure of how well the product or service is designed to meet its purpose'. This involves establishing what the product or service will be used for. The most important feature of the design is the specification. Specifications also need to be established at each point in the customer/supplier interface.
- **Conformance to design:** This is the extent to which the product or service actually achieves the quality of design. Oakland stresses the need to build statistical process control into the production process, and details this further in his book *Statistical Process Control* (1986). He also emphasizes the need to build prevention into the work process.[1]

Central to achieving the above two factors is the notion of 'work' being a series of interdependent processes, with clear inputs and outputs. Oakland recognizes the need for a coordinated, corporate-wide framework to integrate these concepts into practice, and utilizes a 13 step implementation plan, as illustrated in Figure 6.2.

OTHER LEADING AUTHORITIES ON QUALITY

There are a number of other notable figures whose thoughts and writings have influenced the development of total quality management in the industrial sector. To date, little has been written about the application of these specific approaches in service industries, perhaps owing to the technical nature of some of the approaches used, which were designed for use specifically in industry. These are briefly mentioned below, including some of the pioneering approaches within the NHS.

---

1 Author's note: These concepts are interesting in considering the implication of the principles with Chapters 1 and 2. Hence 'quality of design' has some transferability to ensuring that clinical guidelines, pathways, protocols etc. are based on sound evidence and fit for purpose. The second variable in terms of patient outcome is 'conformance to design', i.e. the extent to which professionals comply with the specifications in the guidelines. Both elements need to be present to secure a good outcome.

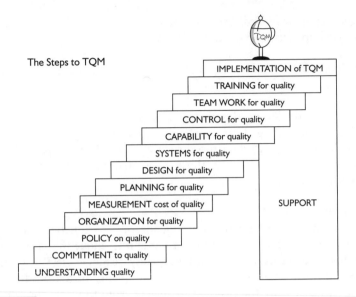

The Steps to TQM

IMPLEMENTATION of TQM
TRAINING for quality
TEAM WORK for quality
CONTROL for quality
CAPABILITY for quality
SYSTEMS for quality
DESIGN for quality
PLANNING for quality
MEASUREMENT cost of quality
ORGANIZATION for quality
POLICY on quality
COMMITMENT to quality
UNDERSTANDING quality

SUPPORT

Figure 6.2

Oakland's steps to quality management (reproduced with the permission of Butterworth-Heinemann, *Statistical Process Control*, Oakland (1986))

Armand V. Feigenbaum

Author of *Total Quality Control* (1983), Feigenbaum defines quality control as 'an effective system for coordinating the quality maintenance and quality improvement efforts of the various groups in an organization so as to enable production at the most economical levels which allow for full customer satisfaction'. Like other authors in this field, he does not use the term 'quality' as synonymous with 'the best' or 'excellence'. He defines it as 'best for the customer use and selling price'.

His approach expands beyond the mechanics of quality control to include the human relations aspects of quality management. To this end, he stresses the need for a channel for communication for product–quality information, and a means of participation for all staff in the overall plant quality programme.

He defines this total quality system as:

> *The agreed companywide and plantwide operating work structure, documented in effective, integrated technical and managerial procedures, for guiding the co-ordinated actions of the people, the machines, and the information of the company and plant in the best and most practical ways to assure customer quality satisfaction and economical costs of quality.*

The management tool used to achieve this is a four-step approach that involves:

- setting quality standards;
- appraising conformance to these standards;

- acting when these standards are exceeded;
- planning for improvements in the standards.

Another key focus of this approach is the notion of 'quality costs', which are divided into:

- prevention costs (including those of quality planning);
- appraisal costs (including those of routine inspection);
- internal failure costs (including those such as rework or scrap);
- external failure costs (including those generated through warranty and dealing with complaints).

Genichi Taguchi

Taguchi's approach is well known for its 'quadratic loss function', a statistical approach that illustrates that a reduction of variability about the target leads to a decrease in loss and subsequent increase in quality (Taguchi, 1979). In contrast to many other authors, Taguchi (1981) defines the quality of the product as 'the (minimum) loss imparted by the product to society from the time the product is shipped'. This therefore incorporates not only the loss to industry in terms of scrap or rework, maintenance costs, machine downtime and warranty costs, but also the costs to the customer as a result of the product's unreliability, which leads ultimately to further knock-on costs to the manufacturer, as a subsequent fall in market share will inevitably occur.

The focus for this approach is therefore very firmly at the design stage, when rigorous testing minimizes product variability and ensures that quality targets are consistently met. This 'off-line' approach to quality control is managed in three stages: (1) system design; (2) parameter design; and (3) tolerance design.

This final stage offers a mechanism to further reduce variation within the production process. This is achieved by tightening factors that are shown to cause variation. It is at this stage that the 'loss function' is utilized, with more money being spent on better material or equipment, incorporating the Japanese philosophy of 'invest last' rather than 'invest first' (Taguchi, 1979).

Kaoru Ishikawa

Ishikawa is best known for pioneering the quality circle approach in Japan during the 1960s (Ishikawa, 1976, 1985). Use of this tool by the Japanese incorporated the education of workers into statistical quality control, an approach slightly different from the use of this tool in the West. The 'seven tools of quality' taught to all employees were:

- Pareto charts
- cause and effect diagrams
- stratification
- check sheets
- histograms

- scatter diagrams
- Shewhart's control charts and graphs

Shigeo Shingo

Shingo is most famous for his 'poka yoke', 'Defect = 0', or the concept of mistake proofing that appears in many of the other approaches outlined above (Shingo, 1986). The need for statistical sampling is eliminated because whenever a defect occurs the whole production process ceases, the cause is defined and action is taken to correct it. As part of this approach, inspection is used to identify errors before they become defects. This is usually achieved by instrumenting machines with immediate feedback.

Hugh Koch

Hugh Koch is one of the few authors who has started to produce work detailing the practicalities of implementing total quality management in a healthcare setting (Koch and Chapman, 1991; Koch, 1991a, b).

He identified a number of difficulties in the application of the concepts to TQM in healthcare settings, namely:

- lack of top management commitment and vision
- 'flavour of the month/year' attitudes
- hospital community service culture and management style
- poor appreciation of TQM concepts, principles and practices
- lack of structure for TQM activities
- ineffective leadership

In Koch's model (Figure 6.3), the following key components are identified. First, the services must be:

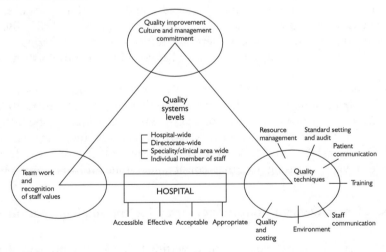

Figure 6.3

Koch's TQM model (reproduced with the permission of H.C.H. Koch, *International Journal of Healthcare Quality Assurance* (1991b))

- accessible
- effective
- acceptable
- appropriate (to patients, purchasers and the Department of Health)

Second, the services have to be organized with the appropriate quality input for:

- clear management commitment, leadership and capabilities;
- optimum teamwork and recognition of staff value;
- implementation of quality techniques (clinical audit, standard-setting, information/monitoring, communications);
- monitoring and identification of performance against contract specification and reduction of 'non-conformance'.

This model identifies the need to consider service quality at four levels:

- directorate
- speciality/clinical area
- individual member of staff

TQM IN THE HEALTH SERVICE

The texts of the above authors expand on the concepts of their particular approach, and some offer practical advice for its implementation. However, the application of TQM in the health service in the UK is relatively new and (with the notable exception cited above) the majority of texts have not yet diversified to include this area. Other countries, notably Canada and the United States, have experimented with TQM in the healthcare setting (Wilson, 1987; Berwick, Glanton and Roessner, 1990) but there are difficulties in transferring some of the lessons learnt because of the differences between British and North American healthcare.

These differences cause problems for those wishing to adopt this approach within the NHS. Some may opt to try it for themselves and others to utilize services from the growing number of management consultants who offer this facility. Many management consultants have recognized the lucrative market offered by the NHS and are keen to get a foothold. There are advantages and disadvantages in using external consultants, some of which are outlined below.

The use of management consultancy firms for the implementation of TQM

It can be useful to have people with expertise helping to apply complex and different approaches to a hospital or healthcare setting, particularly in the early stages. In our experience, these people commonly fall into the following two categories:

- those with significant experience within the health service, particularly in quality assurance, technology development or financial support, but with limited experience of TQM;
- those with extensive experience in implementation of TQM in industry, but with limited knowledge of the health service.

There are advantages with the former group, in that they are familiar with the health service and, as such, may be more acceptable to staff, who tend to resist 'non-health professionals'. The difficulty arises when the learning curve of the consultant, with regard to applying TQM in the NHS, is matched by that of their clients. Absence of such experience should be viewed with caution. A good indicator is whether or not the company has in place the structural components associated with their approach to TQM. For example, if they mention company-wide training, then have all their employees undertaken this? If they advocate the use of problem-solving teams, then how many do they have and what kinds of problems have they solved? If they refer to statistical control methods, then when and how did their company last use this tool?

There are advantages in using the second group of consultants if they have a proven track record of implementing TQM in an industrial setting. This gives an assurance that the approach has been validated elsewhere, and can work. The difficulty arises in deciding whether or not the approach is 'culturally acceptable' to the NHS, and whether it can be adapted to this setting. We use the term 'culturally acceptable' guardedly, as one of the aims of TQM is to change the organizational culture, and one needs to differentiate between what is a threat to the traditional style of management and what could be a genuine difficulty in transferring a particular tool or concept to a healthcare environment.

Consultants also offer a variety of educational packages, for all levels of the organization, and their experience in teaching TQM courses. This can be an advantage when one considers the time, effort and money that would need to go into producing such packages from inception. However, these materials must be suitable for the target groups at the outset.

There are major advantages to developing a successful in-house TQM packages in those cases where there is sufficient in-house expertise. The course can be geared to local needs; it is taught by those who have developed it, giving a strong commitment to making it work; it can prove cost effective, and hospital staff who develop such a package have the option of competing on the consultancy market themselves and generating income.

An obstacle to creating such a package is in avoiding infringement of copyright when utilizing work previously published by specialists in this field. Consultancy companies are protective of their materials and there are already cases in the industrial sector of substantial payments awarded for use of such material without permission.

A good consultancy firm will aim to promote self-sufficiency for the client developing TQM. This should involve developing local staff to enable them to teach these courses. It can be advantageous in the early stages for the training

STAFFORDSHIRE
UNIVERSITY
LIBRARY

273

at executive board level to be done by someone from outside the organization who is well versed in the principles of TQM. First, it is essential to gain the commitment and good understanding of senior executives if TQM is to be adopted throughout the organization (and few in-house course facilitators would relish the thought of running their first course with the top management in the hospital if they have limited practical experience in the TQM field). Second, the consultant can work with the executive board to create a local framework for managing quality. Third, if the executive board has selected consultants in whom they have confidence and respect, then they are likely to be receptive to their suggestions, working in partnership to adapt the approach to local needs.

From our experience, we would recommend that the consultant and client need to work together in drawing up the specifications for the TQM approach. Difficulties may arise if a particular approach is too rigid to incorporate the local culture. Similarly, there is a danger of the client drawing up a list of specifications for a TQM approach from a very scant knowledge of what is required, rather than encouraging input from the expertise of the consultant at the specification stage. The traditional approach of selecting a number of consultants to present a short synopsis to a panel, members of which then choose a consultancy at the end of a day's interviewing, is beset with problems. It is crucial that time and effort are dedicated to select the right approach to fit with the hospital culture, not least because of the significant resources this enterprise will entail.

A major disadvantage in employing external consultants is the cost. TQM is not a short-term project, it is a long-term process. Similarly, developing a home-grown version can incur significant costs, even though these may be hidden in terms of staff time devoted to the project. Funding therefore needs to be considered on an ongoing basis. Considerable financial benefits may be gained from this in-house approach, but an initial investment of cash is required to start the process of implementation, of which the staff training consumes a high proportion of the budget.

Once the particular approach (or combination of approaches) to TQM has been determined, the process of implementation begins. In our experience, the difficulties of this challenge were exacerbated by the lack of practical advice available on where to begin, what to do and how to sustain the momentum of such an extensive process.

The textbooks talk about concepts such as 'commitment', 'involvement', 'education', 'error costs' and 'measurement', all of which we could appreciate and comprehend. What we needed to know was how, in an average NHS hospital, these concepts can be realized in practice. For example, how does one gain commitment? How can it be sustained? How can we involve everybody and coordinate their involvement in a systematic way? What are the logistics of educating everybody? What are we going to teach them? How much are all the errors in our processes costing us? How do we reduce these costs? How and what should we measure? What do we do with the measurement data? These were just some of the questions that faced us at the time. They are also typical of the questions often posed by others considering TQM.

In an attempt to provide an insight into what can be involved in the implementation of TQM in a health service setting, we finish this chapter with a case study based on our personal experiences. The purpose of outlining how we did it is to give others considering adopting TQM an appreciation of what this can entail, some of the pitfalls we identified and some general ideas that may be considered useful. As noted in the introduction to this chapter, common themes run through all approaches to TQM. These include addressing the practicalities of developing a structure to manage quality, embarking on organization-wide education, introducing measurement, securing and demonstrating management commitment, solving problems and giving recognition to staff and raising awareness. All total quality managers will have to face these issues, albeit under a different handle. The Crosby approach to TQM is cited in this case study because it was the consultancy company appointed at the time. It is not the intention to recommend this approach over any other. Without direct experience of implementing any other approach, we cannot offer comparative critiques of other approaches. The intention is simply to offer practical suggestions for the implementation of TQM rather than an 'armchair critique' of the different theories.

AN INTRODUCTION TO THE CROSBY APPROACH FOR TQM

The philosophical foundation of Crosby's approach is based upon five central concepts, of which 'All work is a process' (explained in detail in Chapter 2) is key, and what he referred to as 'the four absolutes' of quality management. Crosby does not use the term 'total quality management' but refers to his approach as the quality improvement process (QIP). This is subtly different from the common definitions of TQM and is explained more fully later in this chapter.

The four absolutes are the answers to four questions concerning quality that Crosby believes it is absolutely essential to answer. These are:

- What is the definition of quality?
- How is it achieved?
- What is the performance standard?
- How can it be measured?

The answers to these questions and their application within a health service context are explored below.

6.5.1 What is the definition of quality?

A typical list of common responses when posing this question to NHS staff are:

- 'Excellence'
- 'Expensive'
- 'Durability'
- 'Luxury'

- 'Reliability'
- 'Marks & Spencer' – whose marketing approach has clearly succeeded in making them synonymous with quality in the public's perception!

It can be appreciated from this list that there are two major problems when attempting to use such definitions in the NHS. First, people's perceptions of 'quality' vary widely. This can make it difficult to address quality issues because differing interpretations of quality can prove a barrier to communication. Second, such definitions are subjective and unquantifiable, making it difficult to measure quality. It is difficult to assess whether a service is more 'excellent' or more 'luxurious' this year than last year.

To generate further discussion, staff were asked to consider a standard-issue hospital chair (the plastic stacking type) and debate whether it was an example of a 'quality' chair. This added a further dimension to the debate. It was agreed that the chair was no antique, but this raised the issue of whether or not a 3-foot wide, leather, £500 chair was a desirable substitute. It was decided not, on the grounds it was not easy to clean, was too expensive and required too much storage space. An important factor in judging the quality of the chair was therefore its intended use. A list of requirements was drawn up for a chair that was only intended to be sat on for periods of no more than two hours (such as visiting times or meetings) and which needed to be stored between use owing to limited space in the ward.

The revised verdict on the chair, based on these new criteria, was that it was a quality product. It was relatively easy to list quality requirements for a product such as a chair, but there were concerns this would not be as easy for a service-oriented organization such as the NHS.

Referring back to the original list of definitions, we underlined the use of 'Marks & Spencer' as being synonymous with quality. Staff brainstormed a list of criteria that they believed were important in judging a service organization (such as shops, banks or restaurants) to be one that offered good quality. These included:

- pleasant, helpful staff;
- staff with good knowledge about the service who could give informed advice (for example, if things were delayed, how long the customer would have to wait; specific expertise on the service offered);
- environment (for example, tasteful decor, furnishing and carpets in good repair, cleanliness);
- good car-parking facilities;
- prompt service (staff felt they should not have to wait more than five minutes in a bank or shop queue);
- a wide choice of goods or services;
- clear signposting;
- customer complaints dealt with courteously and efficiently, with easy access to senior management;

- value for money;
- open at convenient hours;
- privacy (many disliked the communal changing rooms in some clothes stores).

Hence it was possible to establish criteria for services as well as products. Using this list of criteria, we scored our own hospital's performance using a score of one to ten, and noted that there was scope for improvement. It was identified that part of the process for establishing criteria would entail determining the expectations of the customer, which could be done via market research.

There were some difficulties when transferring this approach to the NHS. For example, when going out for a meal, the customer has clear expectations of the restaurant and the food, based on a set of known requirements. When coming into hospital, the majority of patients are unaware of what many of their requirements are. Some are easy to establish, for example being treated courteously, short waiting times, environmental and comfort factors (the 'desired' requirements). However, patients are unable to define other requirements of the service they receive, such as the technical and professional aspects of their care. Most would not be able to identify the requirements of a 'quality' appendectomy, or judge the 'quality' of the equipment used to treat them. In this instance, the professionals involved in treating the patient need to define these 'needed' requirements for them. This is possible if one refers back to the concept that 'all work is a process'. What actually happens to a patient on admission to hospital is a series of many different processes (for example, admission, diagnosis, treatments and discharge). The requirements of each of the processes (both from the perspective of the patient and the professional) can be identified using the process model worksheet (Chapter 2, Figure 2.1). Crosby acknowledges this by differentiating between 'desired', 'needed' and 'mandatory', i.e. (government and professionally mandated) requirements for each process.

In view of the lack of knowledge the majority of the public have about the processes in hospital, there are difficulties in applying definitions of quality such as 'satisfying the customer' or 'exceeding customer expectations'. We identified that many patients have differing expectations of the service, and they are able to judge the care only by comparison with treatment received in other hospitals. A patient who waits four hours in casualty in one hospital, and two hours in another, might therefore consider the second hospital as having a reasonable waiting time, as they expected to wait four hours. This presents problems when trying to determine patient satisfaction levels using survey techniques.

Staff also identified that, often, patient satisfaction did not always concur with what staff perceived as 'quality' care. Examples were given of a patient whose surgical treatment was a technical success, and saved his life. He wrote a letter of complaint about the poor quality of service in the hospital because the food was not to his liking, staff kept waking him up at night to take his blood pressure, and a pair of his pyjamas had gone missing. At the other end of the scale was a patient whose treatment and resultant problems resembled a report to the health service ombudsman. Yet she thought her care was excellent because 'everyone has been so kind'.

Crosby's first absolute of quality management

The definition of quality is conformance to requirements.

If managers want people to 'do it right the first time', then employees need to know what 'it' is, and have the resources to achieve 'it'. 'It' is the requirements that are essential to the process, as identified through the process model work-sheet (see Chapter 2, Figure 2.1). The agreement of these requirements between all of those involved in the process is an essential part in maintaining a quality service. Once the requirements are established clearly, the process of auditing them to see if they are being met becomes possible.

What is the system for ensuring quality?

The system commonly adopted to ensure quality by many industrial companies in the US and the UK in the 1950s was that of 'inspection', which fell under the remit of the quality control department. Quality control involved checking the product as it came off the production line to identify any faulty goods, which were either rejected or 'fixed' by a group of staff especially employed for this purpose. Along with this approach arose the notion of 'acceptable quality levels'. These were laid down by managers, or the customer, who stipulated the accepted level of faulty goods. For example, 90% of chocolates produced would meet the specifications.

In recent years, many companies have identified several difficulties associated with inspection as an approach to managing quality:

- **It is retrospective.** This causes difficulties in managing quality, since errors are identified only *after* they have occurred.
- **It is expensive.** Extra expense is incurred in employing staff to check the product; employing others to fix it; and in the wasted materials.
- **It generates a 'fix it' approach to errors.** Fixing mistakes after they occur alleviates the symptoms of poor quality (in that they are not passed on to the customer) but does not tackle the root cause of why the problem arose in the first place.
- **It is threatening for staff.** Typically, the knowledge that the quality control team were coming on a visit to a division would be viewed with trepidation. As one member of staff observed, 'We put as much time and effort into hiding our mistakes as the Quality Manager does in trying to find them.'

The whole cultural climate created by such an approach is one based on fear of management. It also places the responsibility for detecting errors in the hands of those who have limited knowledge of the work process that is producing the errors, rather than with those who have the greatest insight as to why problems may arise, namely the staff involved in the process.

In view of these limitations, it can be appreciated that such an approach could have even greater difficulties when applied to the NHS, where the 'product' is not an inanimate object but a health service that is delivered to patients.

In spite of these weaknesses, many approaches to quality assurance in the NHS still retained these four weaknesses. In one respect, the rush for audit was putting the cart before the horse. The tools identified weaknesses in the service and where errors were made (such as in monitoring customer complaints), but no effective method for solving these problems had been established prior to such an audit. This undermined the usefulness of many of the quality assurance tools, with some staff dismissing them as a waste of time. In fact, it was not the tools themselves that were at fault. Audit is an essential part of quality management. The reason staff became disillusioned was because of the way in which quality assurance tools were implemented and used by management. There is absolutely no point in spending time and money on audit if nothing improves as a result.

Crosby's second absolute of quality management

The system for causing quality is prevention of mistakes.

This changes the focus from detecting mistakes after they have occurred to preventing them from occurring in the first place. Crosby believes this can be achieved by close analysis of the work process (by use of the tools and techniques) and building prevention into the process itself. Such an approach can be fully realized only by empowering staff to improve their work, as they are in the unique position of being able to identify weaknesses and offering solutions.

What is the performance standard?

In one of our workshops, staff were asked to consider the application of 'acceptable quality levels' in relation to three health service work processes: (a) amputating a patient's leg; (2) ensuring patients received the lunch they ordered; and (3) filling in forms correctly.

It was unanimously agreed that there was no room for error in the case of the patient having a leg amputated. It was expected that, in 100% of cases, the correct leg would be amputated, with all the necessary requirements for this process being met.

The process of delivering the correct meal to the correct patient created some debate. It was accepted that there were occasions when this did not happen. Some nurses raised the concern that this could be detrimental to the patient, for example a diabetic patient receiving a non-diabetic meal. In view of this it was generally accepted that, in 100% of cases, the patient should receive the correct meal.

The process of filling in forms was viewed as tedious, which staff rated as a low priority. Many felt that there were too many forms, and filling them in detracted from time spent in direct patient care. Staff were then asked how often they were on the receiving end of incomplete paperwork, which brought forth a flood of complaints. For example, the pathology and X-ray departments estimated that between

20% and 30% of the request forms they received were incomplete or inaccurate. On exploring the problem further, nursing and medical staff were largely ignorant of the 'hassle' (a word that was used frequently) they caused these areas when sending poorly completed forms. A common complaint was that parts of the form were perceived as irrelevant to the person filling them in. This illustrated the clear lack of agreed requirements on the form design. As staff began to appreciate the significance of various forms, the 'acceptable quality level' began to change. It was agreed that filling in the forms properly was not technically difficult, and there was no real excuse for not achieving 100% compliance.

In terms of the performance standard for staff when doing their work, and the impact not meeting these standards could have on the patient, it was agreed that staff should 'get it right first time'. An advantage to meeting this standard was identified in the reduction of hassle and time wasted doing things over again. It was noted that although people were often too busy to fill out forms properly, they always had to find time to do them again when returned.

Crosby's third absolute of quality management

The performance standard is zero defects.

Before completing the educational courses, staff found the wording rather Americanized. In spite of this, they grasped the concept when explored further, although 'Do it right first time' was felt to be a more acceptable alternative.

'Zero defects' is the most commonly misunderstood of Crosby's concepts. Deming categorizes it along with motivational programmes; others misunderstand it to mean 'perfection', and therefore view it as unachievable.

The educational material demonstrates that this is not the case. The purpose of zero defects is to create an attitude within the staff that no amount of non-conformance is acceptable. (Crosby uses the term 'non-conformance' when his first absolute of 'conformance to requirements' is not met, i.e. there is a mistake or an error. These are the requirements as defined in the process model work-sheet by the customers and suppliers of the process. They will therefore be both achievable and measurable.)

For example, staff have a zero defects standard on the prescribing and administration of drugs, in that it is appreciated that no amount of error is acceptable. This does not mean that drug errors never occur. However, there is an attitude that, if they do occur, appropriate steps are taken to decrease the likelihood of the same mistake being made again. This philosophy is expanded to all work processes (including filling in forms!). Many of us identified that we had the attitude that many of the things that caused us hassle were inevitable and insoluble. We constantly received 'non-conforming' equipment or services from other departments and fixed it ourselves, rather than discussing the problem with the department concerned. This seemed to be a cultural problem within our organization, as we tolerated things at work that would not be tolerated in our private lives. However, such an attitude is self-perpetuating, as the problems that caused us hassle were never solved. We needed to work at making sure things were done correctly the first time.

How can quality be measured?

There were other consequences of not identifying and meeting requirements, not building prevention into our work processes and not 'getting it right first time'. Apart from the hassle, there was also a cost in terms of time and money. Staff were asked how much of their time was spent sorting out problems that arose because things had not been done right the first time, or 'fire fighting'; estimates ranged from 10% to 90%. Ward sisters and middle managers typically stated the highest figures. We built up a picture of what we called 'the Monday morning syndrome'.

The Monday morning syndrome

It is Monday lunchtime. The doctors are stressed because the ward round was delayed for 20 minutes waiting for some X-rays to be found; theatre is running late, which means cancelling cases; there are no empty beds and an hour was spent ringing round to try and find one for an acute admission.

The charge nurse is stressed because there were not enough breakfasts for the new admissions and it took 20 minutes to get some sent up from the kitchen; stock items on the drug trolley had run out and it took an hour to complete the drug round as a result; there was no clean laundry and a nursing auxiliary had to go and borrow linen from other wards.

The staff nurse is stressed because two admissions arrived that no one had told her were expected; and an ambulance arrived to transfer a patient, but a chair had been booked instead of a stretcher. As a result it took 45 minutes to rebook another ambulance. The enrolled nurse is annoyed because she had an appointment with the unit manager at 10 a.m. and waited 30 minutes outside her office before being told the manager was too busy to see her today.

The auxiliary is tired because she has made three trips to the kitchen, two trips to pharmacy, searched the ward and department for missing X-rays and been round all the wards borrowing linen.

Staff caught up in such a scenario are, for a significant proportion of their time, not doing the job they are employed to do. Staffing is the largest single expenditure within the hospital budget and yet, as a result of things not happening in the way they are supposed to, this resource is not used to its full potential.

Financially, this wasted staff time can prove expensive. One hospital calculated that, owing to the pharmacy not being able to meet its requirements, nurses regularly had to 'nip down' to pharmacy to collect urgent drugs or drugs for patients who were awaiting discharge. These 'nips' equated to two whole-time equivalent nurses when they were multiplied up for an average week (mean times taken to walk backwards and forwards to pharmacy in a large hospital multiplied by the total number of nurses 'nipping').

Many managers cited examples of meetings starting late. If one considers the case of ten managers waiting 12 minutes for a meeting to start, this represents two hours of management time that is wasted per meeting. If this is multiplied by the number of late meetings over a year, it can be appreciated that there is a significant cost to the organization.

There are other financial costs in the Monday morning scenario. Cancelled theatre lists evoke costs because, in the majority of cases, the patients are occupying a hospital bed in anticipation of their operation, and many will have had X-rays, blood tests and other preoperative routine procedures. This is on top of the daily cost of keeping a patient in an NHS bed. Some of this money is wasted in the event of a cancellation. Then there is the added cost of readmitting the patient at a later date. Mistakes made on ambulance bookings, particularly in the event of an ambulance having to leave without a patient, are also wasteful.

Crosby's fourth absolute of quality management

The measurement of quality is the price of non-conformance.

Crosby stresses that for every error there is a cost, either in rework, waste (either of time, materials or both) and often a knock-on effect in other areas. He estimates that such error costs can be as high as 40% of the annual budget in service industries. Preliminary surveys in the NHS show this to be between 23% and 30% of the annual budget. The purpose of calculating a price for these errors is two-fold.

First, it is an effective method for gaining a manager's attention. In terms of impact, nurses constantly voicing concerns about the contents of Central Sterile Supplies Department (CSSD) packs generates less response than a report showing the amount of CSSD waste, with supporting data, calculated as costing £25,000 per annum.

Second, it acts as a baseline measure that helps to determine how the quality improvement process is working. It is also important to build on measurement techniques currently being utilized within the hospital, such as clinical audit and the various quality assurance tools. The cost of quality should be viewed as an adjunct to such tools, not as a replacement. In practice, we also found the tools and techniques outlined in Chapter 2 helpful in developing clinical audit.

Preliminary summary

Crosby's four absolutes of quality management are:

- The definition of quality = conformance to requirements.
- The system for quality = prevention.
- The performance standard = zero defects.
- The measurement of quality = the price of non-conformance.

Underpinning these is the concept that 'All work is a process, a series of actions that produces a result.'

The integration of these concepts into the culture of an organization is managed through an implementation framework, as shown in Figure 6.4. Here, the concepts

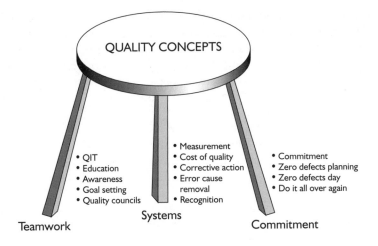

Figure 6.4

The Crosby approach to quality management (adapted from Crosby (1989))

are supported by commitment, teamwork and systems, which are divided into 14 steps. These are, in turn, supported by the tools and techniques, some of which are outlined in Chapter 2.

Crosby views his 14 steps as essential to establishing a successful quality improvement process, in conjunction with his other concepts. In practice, we found the term 'steps' misleading, as it implied that they be done in sequence and, although the educational material stressed this was not the case, it confused some staff. Eight of the steps are addressed initially, and, as demonstrated through the theories of change in Chapter 5, they need to be considered in relation to their influence on other steps. These steps, and the practical aspects of implementation, will therefore be discussed in the order in which we tackled them, rather than Crosby's numbered sequence. For each step we define the purpose, discuss how it was approached and implemented, and identify specific examples of what worked well and what presented problems.

In order to implement the steps, a structure for managing quality within the organization needs to be established. General guidelines for doing this, based on our experiences, are outlined below.

ESTABLISHING A STRUCTURE FOR QUALITY IMPROVEMENT

In spite of the success of some of our earlier attempts at initiatives with quality as a central theme, such as quality assurance, quality circles, setting standards and 'personalizing the service', there were several common problems that we identified with these approaches. Our frustrations at such problems were as follows:

- Many of them started well, but seemed to run out of steam after a while.
- Many of the staff involved in these projects had a great deal of enthusiasm and commitment but were disadvantaged by having little personal power within the organization. The role of the manager was therefore crucial in realizing the aims of their particular initiative. There were examples of management commitment not being demonstrated, with resultant disillusionment and loss of morale.
- Medical staff seldom got involved in these initiatives.
- Funding to support such initiatives was limited.
- There was little central coordination, hence different areas often worked on similar problems and work was duplicated rather than shared.

Quality circles, standard-setting and clinical audit tended to reinforce departmental and professional boundaries because they were predominantly interprofessional or interdepartmental. In practice, realization of these initiatives was dependent on factors outside the control of these groups. For example, nurses could spend months developing a superb discharge standard, but if the medical staff give only five minutes' notice of a patient's discharge, this standard can never be met. Similarly, clinical audit may dictate that discharge summaries should reach the patient's general practitioner within seven days of discharge, but this cannot be met without cooperation from the medical secretaries.

There was no forum where staff could raise problems identified through such initiatives, or for senior management to learn what these were to enable them to take action.

These problems arose from the traditional approach (or lack of one) to the process of managing quality in hospitals; it was just accepted that 'quality' would happen. Hence no clear direction was given from senior management, there was no budget allocated for it and there was no one individual with a responsibility to coordinate these initiatives.

This changed slowly owing to a combination of initiatives. Political pressure was pushing quality as an important issue against a backlash of criticism of cost cutting, and growing waiting lists, culminating in the White Paper *Working for Patients* (Department of Health, 1989) and latterly *The New NHS: Modern Dependable* (NHS Executive, 1997). Hospitals were encouraged to prepare 'quality strategies' and a number of individuals suddenly found themselves with 'quality manager' added to their title. Many of these were disadvantaged by the fact the new role was not integrated into the hierarchical structure of the hospital, and had therefore to rely purely on personal power, as the post had no position or financial power (i.e. a budget). The post holder, therefore, was totally reliant on the support of senior managers and consultant medical staff in implementing any quality initiative. With such posts being new within the health service, many post holders were unsure exactly what was expected of these roles.

Crosby recognized the difficulty of such a structure for managing quality. Like the other authors in this field, he stresses that management commitment to making quality happen is absolutely essential. Quality should be led by example, from the top of the organization. This includes having the quality manager on the executive board. As he points out, quality is as serious an issue as finance, therefore both need representation on the board.

There were some general guidelines we found useful when developing an organizational structure for managing quality. These were as follows.

Identify the structure

The structure for managing quality should align as closely as possible to the current hierarchical structure. This is important, as it is essential that line managers take responsibility for quality in their area. At first we expressed concerns about the latter proposal, as there were individuals who we knew would be unhappy with this arrangement. However, the alternative (which is to give interested individuals lower down the organization responsibility for quality) is fraught with difficulties. Essentially, the end result is a series of poorly coordinated initiatives, of the kind outlined above. In our experience, the most resistant line managers have more difficulty subverting the efforts of quality improvement if they are given an active part in its implementation and it is included among their objectives. Furthermore, staff look to management involvement for an example that things are changing. A common criticism by staff of many of the initiative-led approaches to quality was that if it was really that important why weren't there any managers or senior medical staff actively involved?

Convene a steering committee

The steering committee guides the quality improvement process. Ideally, this should be driven from the top of the organization as a demonstration of management commitment, and chaired by the chief executive. Another alternative is that a subgroup of executive board members joins with other individuals from within the organization who have significant influence within it and those with any specialist knowledge in quality to make up the steering group.

It is vital that the steering committee has sufficient authority to allocate funds and make decisions. Initially, owing to the volume of work involved, senior managers may be tempted to create a steering committee of middle managers who report directly to them. This creates problems, as staff view lack of executive involvement as a lack of commitment, resulting in the quality improvement process being perceived as a low priority. Second, if the steering committee has to refer continually to another group to authorize its decisions, things take longer to implement and the group may be regarded by many as a toothless watchdog.

Devise an implementation structure

The steering committee devises the structure for implementing the quality improvement process throughout the rest of the organization. The structure recommended is shown in Figure 6.5, which is a modification of the model used in practice in the case study. This was altered owing to some of the difficulties of the original structure. Here it can be seen that a number of quality improvement teams (QITs) are the functional unit for implementing the quality improvement process within

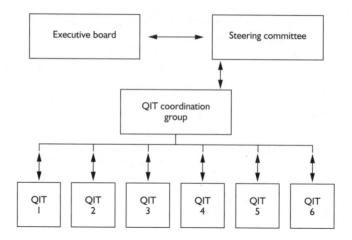

Figure 6.5

A structural framework for the quality improvement process (adapted from Crosby (1989))

a given area. The steering committee needs to decide how best to divide up the organization, defining the areas to be represented by each QIT. In our experience, a manageable unit for a quality improvement team is roughly 400 whole-time equivalent staff.

Dividing the organization into quality improvement teams
There are several ways to divide the organization:

- **It can be split through professional groups.** For example, a QIT consisting of medical staff is responsible for all the medical staff in the hospital. We would not recommend this approach because it reinforces the professional boundaries that the quality improvement process is trying to overcome.
- **It can be split through geographical location.** Such an approach can be advantageous in a large organization, particularly if divided into different blocks or working across several sites.
- **It can be split through clinical specialities.** For example, the medical unit, surgical unit, X-ray unit, etc. all had their own QIT. This can help break down professional boundaries because the QIT will be multidisciplinary. However, care needs to be taken not to emphasize departmental boundaries, such as, for example, creating barriers between the surgical unit and theatres. One way of overcoming this is to have cross-speciality QITs that are heavily dependent on each other in solving work-related problems, as in the case of surgery and theatres or medicine and coronary care.

Once the split has been made (advisedly with consultation with the heads of department and senior members of the professional staff), the senior managers identify members of the QIT. The role of the steering group is then to provide guidance and support for the QITs.

Coordinating the quality improvement teams

Within a larger organization, we found there was a need to coordinate the efforts of the quality improvement teams and provide a forum where they can share experiences, report on progress and identify problems that require resolution at steering committee level. This should be coordinated by the quality manager. Monthly meetings of the chairs of all the QITs are recommended as an effective approach (this group is therefore also identified in Figure 6.5).

Initially, we baulked at what appeared to be another bureaucratic structure, and the amount of work involved in creating it. In practice, it is difficult to manage a cultural change of the magnitude of TQM without a structural framework.

CASE STUDY 6.1   A CASE STUDY OF THE IMPLEMENTATION OF THE CROSBY APPROACH TO TQM IN AN NHS SETTING

Following the identification of the roles and responsibilities at the most senior level in the organization, the next stage is to establish the functional units whose role is to plan the implementation of the quality improvement process at a local level. The actions necessary to achieve this aim are outlined below. The steps that follow are the practical aspects of implementation and we have discussed them in the order in which we tackled them, rather than in strict numerical order.

The application of Crosby's 14 steps in practice is explored based on the experiences of one quality improvement team (QIT). This team was responsible for a general hospital with approximately 160 beds, offering a broad range of services to the local population, including acute medical and surgical beds, rehabilitation wards, casualty and outpatients. Staffing levels were approximately 400 whole-time equivalents. Although significantly smaller than most general hospitals, this hospital offered a microcosm of many of the functional units into which larger hospitals are divided, in that within it were a wide range of professional disciplines and different services. It was managed as a discrete unit, although it was ultimately accountable to a body of management elsewhere.

Thus, many of the practical aspects used as part of the implementation process could be applied in a larger hospital, in the presence of extra coordination via a structure such as that outlined in Figure 6.5.

In the structural diagram in Figure 6.5, the quality improvement team used in the case study is shown as QIT 1. It is accountable to the steering committee, and the chair has access to this committee via the structural framework devised for implementation. The other QITs are on a separate, larger site, all within one hospital.

Step 2. Quality improvement team

Crosby's 14 steps for total quality management

1	Commitment
2	Quality improvement team
3	Measurement
4	Cost of quality
5	Awareness
6	Corrective action
7	Zero defects planning
8	Education
9	Zero defects day
10	Goal setting
11	Error cause removal
12	Recognition
13	Quality councils
14	Do it all over again

Purpose: to run the quality improvement process

The QIT is the group of staff who are given the responsibility of running the quality improvement process. Based on our experiences, the following guidelines are recommended when selecting the appropriate individuals for the team and running the quality improvement process.

Action 1

Senior managers, in conjunction with heads of department and senior members of the professions, need to identify all the individual staff who fall under their sphere of responsibility. In this case, it meant everyone employed at the hospital. This is important, because ideally the quality improvement team should consist of a broad cross-section of the staff it is supposed to represent.

Action 2

The QIT members are selected on the basis of fulfilling one or more of the following criteria:

- They are a member of senior management, whose support is crucial. On this basis, the Unit General Manager, Director of Nursing Services and the two Clinical Managers became QIT members.

- They are a head of department or senior member of a professional group that represents a significant proportion of staff employed by the hospital (or, in a larger hospital, a unit). On this basis, the Consultant Physician, Acting Superintendent Physiotherapist, Catering Manager, Operational Services Manager and Medical Records Manager all became QIT members. At a later date, following a management restructuring, the Clinical Director also joined the QIT.
- They have a specific skill or expertise that is useful to the team. On this basis the TQM project coordinator and Acting Senior Nurse for Service Development (which included a responsibility for quality assurance and the nursing workload dependency system) became QIT members.

The rationale for selecting such a seemingly top-heavy group was that it is essential that the QIT has authority to act, i.e. that decisions can be taken within the meetings without needing to be approved by more senior managers at a later date. It was also essential that these key individuals are involved in, and committed to, the process, as they are in the key positions to be able to cascade the quality improvement process throughout the organization. Resistance at this level could potentially undermine the whole implementation process. Finally, it was a way of demonstrating to staff that this process was sufficiently important for these individuals to devote a significant amount of their time to it.

Three months into the process, the QIT felt that more grassroots input would be useful to help with the implementation process, as at this stage the team was heavily involved in Step 5 (quality awareness). Two ward sisters and a staff nurse who had undergone the educational course also joined the team. The sisters adapted well to their new role; the staff nurse experienced difficulties in fulfilling some of the roles and responsibilities of a QIT member, in spite of her initial enthusiasm. A key factor for this was in her lack of hierarchical authority to implement QIT decisions back in her area. This reinforced the need to retain authority as one of the selection criteria for QIT members. Provision for grassroots staff to access the quality improvement process is made through some of Crosby's other steps.

Action 3
The QIT members need to undertake the relevant education to equip them with knowledge needed to implement and manage the quality improvement process. Details of this are given under Step 8 (employee education).

Action 4
The terms of reference need to be agreed between the QIT and the steering committee.

Action 5
The roles and responsibilities of individual QIT members need to be determined. This was done by having a facilitated 'QIT start-up day'. In practice, we found

we needed a significant amount of time set aside to give the QIT a clear sense of purpose and direction. Participants generally felt it was helpful to have a facilitator with extensive experience in this approach offering support and advice, as many were unsure of what was required in the beginning, and concerned about the logistics of how to tackle such a large project.

Responsibilities of QIT members

QIT members had two key areas of responsibility. These were:

- To be the link person between the QIT and an allocated group of employees, external customers and suppliers (e.g. the ambulance service, general practitioners, Community Health Councils, etc.). The hospital employees were divided up equally and logically between all QIT members. It was decided that managers for certain areas would always be the link persons for their own staff. Very small staff groups, such as occupational therapy, were given a link person who commonly had communication with them, in this case, the physiotherapist on the QIT; the Consultant Physician acted as the link person for all the medical staff. Every employee therefore had a QIT member to represent their interests. The communication was two-way, with information on QIT progress and decisions being passed on to staff by the members and staff feeding back their opinions and problems via the QIT member. Much effort was put into informing staff of these new arrangements (as described in Step 5 (quality awareness)).
- To be a 'step sponsor' for one of the 14 steps. The steps were allocated to the individual QIT members on the start-up day. This was done as fairly as possible, with members agreeing to take on the sponsorship. The step sponsor is responsible for planning and coordinating this particular step. The selection of step sponsors was found to be important for two reasons. First, it cut down the amount of time spent planning and discussing each step. Each step sponsor would draw up an action plan for the step, circulate it to the team a week before the meeting, and make a five-minute presentation at the next meeting. QIT members then had the opportunity to make further recommendations or alterations to the plan before approving it. This was much more effective than the whole team planning each step from scratch. It was then the responsibility of the link person to ensure that actions regarding this step were completed in their area. For example, if the step sponsor for education identified that 20 staff from each area would be allocated a place on a course in the next three months, it was the responsibility of the link person to ensure that 20 of their staff attended. Each step sponsor would report regularly to the QIT on progress and difficulties made with implementing their step. Again, this cut down on meeting time, as it prevented the necessity of each link person reporting on the progress of all the steps in their specific area.

Second, it generated an action-orientated approach to the QIT meetings. Many of us had expressed reservations that we already spent too much time in meetings, and were anxious this should not become a group that sat around debating the philosophical points of quality. This was enhanced by the use of the meeting techniques outlined below. It also ensured that none of the steps was overlooked, and that they were reviewed constantly.

Another advantage of adopting the step sponsors approach was that it placed the onus for action firmly with specific individuals, and the workload was shared equally. This was in contrast to many other meetings we attended, where some members contributed significantly less than others in forwarding the various committees' objectives.

There were two other roles to be assigned, those of chair and administrator. Both were selected by the QIT itself, which was felt to be important.

The role and responsibilities of chair included chairing all the meetings, using the techniques identified as important for effective management of meetings through the educational courses. This also involved representing the QIT via the steering group. The QIT selected the Consultant Physician as the chair. This worked extremely well, both because of the skills of the individual concerned and because it secured the active involvement of the medical staff; something many other TQM pilot sites appeared to have difficulty doing.

The role of administrator was more wide-ranging than that of the traditional meeting secretary. This individual should have considerable expertise in the quality improvement process and should be able to act as an adviser to step sponsors in planning their steps; the Quality Coordinator was selected for this role.

Action 6

Create a set of clearly agreed requirements for QIT meetings
We were conscious that it was important that QIT team members were seen to practise what we preached with regard to 'getting it right first time', and that the meetings were an example. Drawing on the techniques learned from the educational materials, the following requirements were found to be useful. It was agreed to meet once a week for one hour and:

- All meetings will start and finish on time.
- Timed agendas and relevant papers will be circulated to all members one week before the meeting.
- Agenda times will be adhered to.
- Except for annual leave and sickness, members will attend all meetings.
- Minutes from the meeting will be distributed to all members within 24 hours.
- All action assignments will be marked with a name and completion date in the minutes, and reviewed by the QIT members who will inform the

administrator of any errors in minutes within 24 hours of receipt. Corrections will be circulated before the following meeting.

These rules may seem draconian, but the important factor in meeting these requirements was that everyone had agreed the list above.

Most of the team were frustrated by other meetings they attended that started late and ran way over time, had poorly thought-out agendas (or no agenda at all) with one item taking up the whole meeting time, a pile of essential papers being circulated in the same meeting as a decision on their content was expected, key members not turning up to meetings or sending apologies and then spending the subsequent meeting disagreeing with all the decisions agreed at the meeting they had missed, minutes from the previous meeting not distributed or circulated in the next meeting for approval, some individuals taking up most of the meeting time by arguing over the accuracy of previous minutes, and action assignments not documented or completed.

In practice, these new guidelines proved effective. An audit was established to examine if guidelines were conformed with, and within 4 weeks the score had altered from one of 45% to one of 100% on all items. It was interesting to note the change of attitudes over this time. Initially, many were sceptical that these standards could be met. Once it was agreed that these were things the team was serious about, and they were seen to be achievable, everyone worked hard to meet the requirements.

For example, circulating the minutes within 24 hours may seem an impossible achievement. In practice, it was agreed that the minutes should be a brief factual record of decisions taken, with actions arising marked as specified. They did not necessarily need typing, provided they were legible. This made it possible to meet the requirement.

Once the team was established, the first 18 months of work was concentrated on the introduction of eight of the 14 steps, all of which needed to be considered in relation to each other. For example, there is little point setting target dates for staff to start measuring work processes or establishing groups to solve problems if they have not completed an educational course to equip them with the relevant skills.

General learning points concerning coordinating these first eight steps of the Crosby approach are discussed at the end of this chapter. In practice, the establishment of a project management team of this kind was found to be an extremely effective way of managing a project of this scale. It was felt to be completely unrealistic to expect one individual with a 'quality' remit to their job to undertake the implementation of TQM on their own. Moreover, by encouraging local ownership of the process and involving key individuals, many of the factors important to effective change management were incorporated. Once established, the QIT offered a useful vehicle for implementing other associated projects. It was also found to be a useful method for breaking down interdepartmental and professional barriers.

This is not to say there were not some difficulties. Initially there were reservations as to the effectiveness of adopting this approach. Some people were put off by the amount of jargon, although this was largely overcome once the education was completed. Others were sceptical of the motives for adopting such an approach, as its implementation coincided with that of applying for NHS Trust status. A general comment was that it seemed a lengthy way of solving problems that could be resolved by individuals 'just chatting' about them. However, it was generally conceded that, although problem solving in a systematic way seemed logical, it was not something that happened as a matter of routine. This was highlighted by the significant number of ongoing problems within the organization which had been resistant to unfocused problem-solving efforts. Some individuals were more enthusiastic and supportive of the process than others but, nonetheless, every member contributed. As the process progressed, visible improvements started to occur and the support for this approach increased.

Step 1. Management commitment

Crosby's 14 steps for total quality management

1	Commitment
2	Quality improvement team
3	Measurement
4	Cost of quality
5	Awareness
6	Corrective action
7	Zero defects planning
8	Education
9	Zero defects day
10	Goal setting
11	Error cause removal
12	Recognition
13	Quality councils
14	Do it all over again

Purpose: to make it clear where managers stand on quality

The initial activity involved in this step was the drafting and agreement of a quality policy. This was important for two reasons. First, it created a debate at the most senior level in the organization regarding senior managers' views on the quality standard for the service they were managing. It also created the opportunity for them to discuss this issue with their staff.

Second, it had to be followed by clear management action to support the policy. Staff are quick to question management actions that undermine such policies.

Crosby (1979, p.176) defines the policy as 'The state of mind held by the company personnel concerning how well they must do their jobs'.

It therefore needs to be short enough to remember, clear enough for all staff to understand and unambiguous. These were criteria the team found it very hard to fulfil. Writing the policy so early in the project meant many of us were still shackled by the traditions of the old culture. The sort of policy recommended by Crosby is 'We will provide error-free services, on time and within cost.' Many were anxious at the implications of adopting such a policy and displaying it publicly throughout the hospital. There was a concern that it might render us legally liable to comply with such a promise. The difficulty in being less definitive is that lots of weasel words creep into the policy, making it ambiguous. For example, 'We will endeavour to provide an error-free service, most of the time, and as close to our budget limits as possible.'

The other difficulty is that many staff confused the idea of a quality policy with that of all the other trendy organizational statements that seemed to be creeping into the NHS, referred to by clinicians as 'management-speak' – for example, 'visions', 'mission statements' and 'philosophies' – and were trying to compose the latter, rather than a quality policy.

Once the policy has been agreed, the question of how to communicate it to staff was raised. It was agreed that it should be printed on posters, signed by senior managers and displayed throughout the hospital.

Key learning points were:

- The policy should not be distributed until the quality improvement process is well underway. Displaying it too soon would mean that the initial impact was lost and it would be viewed with cynicism.
- It should be ready before the educational courses for staff. Course facilitators found it a useful way of starting the process of convincing staff that management was really serious in its commitment to the quality improvement process (a fact that some staff were extremely sceptical about).
- It needs to be launched in conjunction with other activities that demonstrate to staff that the quality policy is not just words but is about positive actions to improve. They needed to appreciate that something different was happening.

The launching of the quality policy was planned as part of Step 5 (quality awareness), and is outlined below. Once the policy has been launched, staff invariably scrutinize management actions and behaviour and are quick to point out any disparity between the two. As part of the educational courses, managers list actions that they can undertake personally to demonstrate their commitment to quality to their staff.

Management actions to demonstrate commitment

These actions included:

- Agreeing requirements with their customers and suppliers, and then meeting these every time. This proved an effective method for both improving professional relationships and identifying and resolving problems.
- Undertaking the educational courses and meeting all the requirements for these. This was important because if managers were seen to miss sessions, or not complete action assignments from the workshops, it implied that they were not genuinely committed to the quality improvement process. It also put the facilitator in a difficult position, as staff would argue that they should not be expected to fulfil the course requirements either.
- Talking to staff about their problems with work processes, and empowering them to solve them. This was found to be much more effective than trying to solve them for them. It meant setting time aside for 'management by walking about', and observing first-hand the difficulties staff encountered. Initially, managers were concerned about the amount of time they would have to devote to the quality improvement process. When asked how much time they could afford to devote to it, many stated they would be pushed to give 5%. As the project progressed it was realized it was necessary to devote 100% of their time to it. Everything they did in their daily work needed to be done in a 'quality' way, and meet the requirements right the first time; from answering the telephone to compiling a report. In practice, by doing this, more management time was made available because less time was spent on fire fighting or rework.
- Attending awareness sessions, at times outside office hours, to meet *all* staff.
- Making resources available. It was felt to be important to allocate funds to areas where finance was found to be the final barrier to effecting a solution to an ongoing problem. Lack of such support had the potential for staff quickly becoming disillusioned and losing faith in management commitment. A key factor here was honesty. If a large investment of cash is needed and is unavailable, then this needs to be explained, but with the manager exploring temporary solutions and agreeing to fund it in the future budget. For example, one ward identified that it required new mattresses for all the beds. This was not possible in the current financial year. Funding was made available for a proportion of these, with a commitment to start a yearly mattress replacement programme. In the interim period, those that were condemned were replaced by other mattresses from elsewhere in the hospital, which, although not new, were still functional.

It was our experience that problems that could be resolved by only a financial solution were in the minority. The majority required no more than improved communication and more effective use of current resources by improving work processes.

It is also essential to ensure adequate funding for the initial training and materials. It was a major setback when external funding for this project ceased after two years, when there had been an expectation that the funding was for three years. The staff, course facilitators and quality improvement team were demoralized, and resultant modifications to the project plan were perceived by some staff as lack of managers' commitment to the quality improvement process.

The QIT also initiated a communication survey, circulating a questionnaire to staff to ascertain their views on the way the hospital was managed. Following data collection and analysis, workshops were held with staff to discuss results and invite their suggestions on how to act on problems identified. A list of management actions was made, circulated and undertaken.

The management commitment step was one of the most difficult to draw up plans for, because it is largely reliant on senior management and professionals ensuring their behaviour is congruent with the written exhortations in the quality policy. However, peer support and the use of measurement were both useful in commencing this change. Such changes were slow and impossible to measure objectively, but as many of us internalized the concepts explained in the education, it was a common observation that there were changes in both attitude and behaviour.

Step 5. Quality awareness

Crosby's 14 steps for total quality management

1	Commitment
2	Quality improvement team
3	Measurement
4	Cost of quality
5	**Awareness**
6	Corrective action
7	Zero defects planning
8	Education
9	Zero defects day
10	Goal setting
11	Error cause removal
12	Recognition
13	Quality councils
14	Do it all over again

Purpose: to provide a method of increasing the personal responsibility felt by all employees in ensuring the conformance of the product or service and maintaining the quality reputation of the hospital

The process of raising staff consciousness on quality issues, promoting the vital contribution that all individuals had to offer in the quality improvement process and demonstrating how this could be achieved, was a key objective of Step 8 (employee education). This was also reinforced by other steps.

The QIT decided to tackle the awareness step fairly early in the planning stage. There had been some publicity in the local press about our selection as a pilot site for total quality management, and staff were starting to question what this would involve.

The initial decisions that had to be taken were on what and when to communicate with staff. It was agreed the information needed to be presented clearly and to have some kind of local flavour to it. There was also concern that previous attempts at communicating information through distributing leaflets had not been particularly effective, and it was felt this was owing to the impersonal nature of such an approach. The QIT was keen to talk to staff and provide a forum that allowed staff to ask questions and voice their concerns. It was felt this was another way in which managers could demonstrate their commitment to the quality improvement process.

The timing of the initial communications was also important. It was agreed this should not happen immediately because the team had not yet drawn up the implementation plan for the 14 steps, and it was felt that clear statements needed to be made on how this plan would affect individuals. Eventually, a date four months into the process was selected. This had the advantage that all the team members would have completed their educational course and would, therefore, be more knowledgeable about the tools and techniques when questioned by staff. The planning process for all the steps would be completed well before this date, and it also allowed sufficient time to prepare the supporting literature and make adequate preparations to ensure that we got this exercise 'right first time'.

In view of the large numbers of staff that needed to be involved in this exercise, coupled with the problem of reaching shift workers, it was decided a good way to meet the objective of enabling all staff to participate would be to hold an 'awareness week'. A number of sessions were arranged throughout the week, rotating between breakfast, lunch, tea and supper times, which meant that all shift workers had a slot occurring at least twice that week which they could attend. The format agreed for each 45 minute session was:

- An introduction and welcome from a senior manager.
- A video starring the chair of the QIT, explaining the potential benefits of the quality improvement to staff and the importance of everyone's role.
- An exhibition consisting of poster presentations by each of the step sponsors explaining the plans for their step. This would enable staff to walk

round and discuss these with individuals, enabling those who felt unable to ask questions in front of 30 or 40 other participants to do so on an individual basis.

- A short Crosby video of an American hospital, with interviews of staff who were two years into the quality improvement process, explaining what was involved, and what had been achieved.

In view of the amount of information available to staff, it was felt to be important to give them a summary of the key points presented in these 45 minute sessions. A considerable amount of work went into designing a folder, which was handed to staff personally when they arrived at the session. Learning from previous experience, the QIT avoided both glossy pamphlets with photographs of members beaming forth from the pages and cheap, photocopied, poorly presented materials. Staff tended to be critical of the former, viewing them as a waste of money that could be better spent elsewhere; and of the latter because they were seen as being done on the cheap. The appropriate combination was felt to be a printed A3 folder, folded so that a cartoon of the distinctive hospital main doors opened out to show the information inside, with the caption 'Opening the door to quality' underneath. On the inside two leaves were the four absolutes of quality, and the quality policy. In the centre was the logo the QIT had designed with the slogan 'Total Quality Improvement: Putting the "U" in Quality'. This had been arrived at after a brainstorming session, which had ruled out 'Putting the "Y" in Quality' and 'Knocking the "L" out of quality'. Coming up with a slogan was felt to be a good way of getting the essence of the quality improvement programme across in a short snappy phrase. The '"U" in Quality' stressed that this process was aimed at everyone, whether 'you' are the patient receiving a better service or the staff providing this. Nonetheless, it was something that was alien to many of us and, in the beginning, many felt self-conscious about coming up with ideas.

The folder held information on what the quality improvement process involved and why it was important to the hospital. On the reverse of the folder were cartoons of all the QIT members, with the staff groups they represented on the team printed underneath. This gave the message a local flavour. In the event, staff received the folder with interest, and found it helpful. We also seemed to have hit the right balance between it looking as though it was being done on the cheap and it looking like a waste of money.

The poster exhibition also featured cartoons from a local artist, with the accompanying text printed by the graphics department. This kept costs down, although the exhibition itself was clear, eye catching and professionally displayed. The chair of the QIT made an introductory video for the session, explaining why the hospital was embarking on this process. This was useful for the sessions, as clinical commitments meant he could not attend them all, and it ensured staff all got the same information.

The QIT debated how best to ensure good attendance at the session throughout the awareness week. In view of the fact it was intended to demonstrate commitment to the new culture, many felt it would be inappropriate to 'instruct' staff to come. It was agreed that all QIT members would approach their staff groups, tell them a little about the sessions and invite them to sign up to attend one on the quality notice board, which was placed in a strategic position on the way into the staff dining room. Managers also agreed to pay for the food at all these sessions. The team would like to think this had only a marginal influence on the subsequent pleasing attendance rate, with 320 attendees at the sessions over the week; approximately two-thirds of the staff. At the request of others who had been unable to attend, the exhibition remained up for a further week to allow the remainder of the staff to attend.

A short questionnaire was distributed for staff to fill in at the end of the session. This showed that the staff had found all aspects of the session useful, rating the poster presentation as most useful, closely followed by the locally produced video. Although the majority felt the Crosby video of some use, many did not like the 'Americanisms'. It also showed that the majority of staff felt positive about the concepts of the quality improvement process. Some cynicism was expressed in the form of comments from staff about senior managers' and professionals' ability to make it work. There were some individuals who felt the whole exercise was a waste of time, but these represented less than 1% of respondents.

The overall conclusions drawn from the questionnaire results were that the awareness week had fulfilled its objectives, and had been successful. Another benefit was that it had been the first time that many individuals on the team had worked together in this way, and a good feeling of camaraderie built up over the week.

The second stage in planning this step was in maintaining the initial momentum, and ensuring that the quality improvement process was given a continually high profile. This was achieved in the following ways:

- By continually updating the quality notice board. This included displaying lists of staff attending courses, measurements currently being made in different departments and results so far and details of problem-solving activities.
- By QIT members keeping their staff groups informed of developments.
- By printing articles written by staff about their quality improvement activities arising from the educational courses in the hospital newspaper.
- By planning the zero defects day (outlined as Step 9). This served to focus the efforts of the team on ensuring that effective communication occurred with staff. The approaches adopted above were an innovation, in that traditional approaches such as meetings and memorandums tended to be the norm.

A lesson learned was that it is not just the efforts of a team working on a project of this kind that is important; effective communication of the impact it will have on those who will be affected by it must also be given equal priority. This was crucial when the quality improvement process was cascaded throughout the hospital because if staff had a preconceived negative view then they were unlikely to become actively involved.

Step 8. Employee education

Crosby's 14 steps for total quality management

1	Commitment
2	Quality improvement team
3	Measurement
4	Cost of quality
5	Awareness
6	Corrective action
7	Zero defects planning
8	**Education**
9	Zero defects day
10	Goal setting
11	Error cause removal
12	Recognition
13	Quality councils
14	Do it all over again

Purpose: to define the type of education all individuals need in order to carry out actively their role in the quality improvement process

The Crosby system offers a variety of educational courses aimed at meeting the educational needs of all the individuals within the organization. Although this case study examines only one specific approach, there are some generic guidelines learned from our experiences that can be extended to others wishing to establish TQM within an organization.

First, the educational needs will differ for different levels of the organization, and this is determined by the role taken in relation to the quality improvement process. These fall into the broad categories outlined below.

An executive-level course

This is required to focus on the role of those at executive level, and the actions needed to lead the quality improvement process in their organization. The course should incorporate the writing of a quality policy, the implementation process (in this case study this was the 14 steps), the establishment of a structure for managing quality, and the tools and techniques.

Quality improvement for managers

There is a need for a course aimed at QIT members. This will need to outline the implementation process in detail to prepare team members for their new role. The workshops in the course used at the hospital in this case study facilitated consideration on adopting and implementing these steps at a local level. The final workshop involved drawing up an implementation plan for all 14 steps for the first year.

Quality education for the individual

It was identified by the QIT that there was a need for a comprehensive course aimed at senior individuals within the hospital, who were a vital component in implementation of the quality improvement process. The course used by the hospital in the case study included Crosby's four absolutes of quality, the use of the process model work sheet, measurement, calculating the cost of quality, teamwork and problem-solving techniques; in essence, all the tools and techniques that will help individuals understand and manage their work processes. Individuals were given action assignments that enabled them to introduce these in their workplace.

Quality education for the work group

To start the process of resolving work-based problems, teams of staff need to work together. This process can be introduced through mixed educational sessions aimed at work groups. Such courses need to cover the basic tools and techniques, which (in the case study) the group apply in their workplace – and then return to the next session with the results for discussion.

Introductory course

To fit in with the concept of TQM, all staff should be involved in the educational sessions. For some, this will require a basic introduction to the concepts of quality. There is therefore a need for a less intensive course than for those with the different roles and responsibilities above. Such courses are also useful as part of the staff induction process.

Cascading the education through the organization

It is the role of the quality manager to commence the whole process of education, although this responsibility is delegated to the QITs once they are established. The logistics of planning an educational initiative that involves everyone in the organization involved significant time and effort. From our experiences, the following approach is recommended.

Those at the top of the organization must attend the appropriate courses first. This is important, as without detailed knowledge of the implementation frame-work and the tools and techniques, it is difficult to lead the quality improvement process in the organization. It also gives the opportunity to review the educational packages and ensure they are suitable for use within the organization, and demonstrates commitment to the process.

STAFFORDSHIRE
UNIVERSITY 301
LIBRARY

All QIT members should attend the appropriate educational courses. This provides them with the knowledge needed to implement the process (in this case study, the 14 steps). This enables them to start functioning as a team from the outset. It also provides the team with the tools and techniques for individual participation in the quality improvement process. This prepares them for when their staff attend the courses, and come to them to discuss their activities and work processes.

The QIT should select at least one member (usually the education step sponsor) to be a 'master trainer'. They take responsibility for training a number of individuals within the organization to enable the courses to be cascaded to all levels. The education step sponsor will need to develop a training plan for all the employees represented by the team. This process ensures that everyone attends the appropriate course.

Cascading the educational process at a local level

The QIT tackled this by attending the initial courses as a group, combined with three other staff members. This had the advantage of developing the team and enabling them to begin to develop a multidisciplinary approach to problem solving. Having grassroots representation also had the advantage of beginning to break down some of the hierarchical barriers. With hindsight it is recommended that a good mix of staff, in terms of position, as well as discipline, creates the most productive sessions. It enables all staff to appreciate the roles and difficulties of others, often for the first time.

After completion of the quality course aimed at the individual's role in the quality improvement process, it was agreed by the QIT that each member needed support from someone else from the area they were representing on the team, who had the same insight into managing the quality improvement process. The second course therefore consisted of nominees recommended by QIT members.

Because of a few misunderstandings, clear requirements were set for following courses regarding selection and attendance, which vastly improved the whole process:

- Each QIT member would discuss the course with individuals from their area, and offer the opportunity to attend.
- Nominations were sent to the education step sponsor, with any dates or time when the individual was unable to attend a course (for example, because of annual leave or a busy time in the area).
- The nominees were allocated a place on a course that matched availability, and this information was returned to the QIT member who nominated them.
- It was the responsibility of the QIT member to ensure the individual was informed of course details, and to ensure attendance on the course.

This approach worked well for the following reasons. First, the education step sponsor had little hierarchical authority in areas that fall outside their normal managerial patch. By placing the onus on the manager, it prevented the situation arising where staff were not given permission to go. This put the responsibility for staff education firmly with the manager, rather than the education step sponsor.

Second, it was a clearly agreed requirement that places allocated to an area must be filled. This ensured that, if an individual was unable to attend, the manager would allocate the place to a substitute. This prevented the frustrating situation of running underattended courses.

Finally, it offered an effective way of ensuring staff and management communicated about the quality improvement process. Staff knew the manager had also done the course, and were shown the educational materials. This approach was found to reduce the complication of staff turning up claiming they had been 'sent' by their manager, but did not know why they were there.

It was agreed as part of the education step plan that each area should have a local quality course facilitator. This was seen as a good way of having resource people, spread throughout the hospital, to whom staff could go for help and advice. Therefore if the QIT member was unwilling or unable to become an instructor, it was important that the 'support' person they nominated for the educational course was willing to fulfil this role. In practice, this did not quite work out as planned, owing to a combination of staff leaving and some inappropriate nominations.

However, a lesson learned was the importance of not making assumptions about how specific individuals might receive the course, and who might make good instructors. In the event we were surprised by a number of individuals who proved to be excellent instructors, some of whom had skills of which managers were previously unaware.

Nominations for quality courses were sent to the education step sponsor by the QIT members, and courses were planned using the new facilitators who had attended the preparatory trainers' course.

General conclusions regarding implementation of this step

In terms of sheer scale, the education step is the one that involves the greatest amount of work. This led to some serious questioning of the need for all the different courses, and whether it was worthwhile providing education for every employee.

Once the QIT became familiar with the course content, the need for the different courses was appreciated. The key factor in selecting staff for courses was to consider the role they played in the quality improvement process. Early difficulties arose because staff attended an inappropriate course. For example, some staff struggled with the quality education aimed at the individual, because they were not in positions that required them to become managers, and another course would have been more appropriate. Some staff struggled with the technical elements in the work group course, but would have benefited from a simpler, shorter course, such as the introductory course. Interestingly, we estimated a much higher number as needing the work group course than recommended by the Crosby method. This is probably owing to the fact that the levels of accountability are pushed much lower in the NHS than in industry. For example, enrolled nurses, although appearing low down in the management structure, make important decisions about patient care.

The Crosby courses used by the hospital in the case study provided a comprehensive insight into the concepts and tools and techniques of quality management. There were some criticisms of the courses, predominantly about the Americanisms, the industrial bias and the 'soap opera' style videos. Some staff found the courses too easy, and others found them too hard. With hindsight, this was partly owing to bad planning and to some staff attending the wrong course. Medical staff in particular frequently commented it was long-winded, and it probably would have been more appropriate for them to do the shorter *Quality for the Doctor* course that has been developed recently. The disadvantage of this dedicated doctors' course is that the opportunity for them to mix in with the rest of the staff is lost; something that both doctors and staff rated as valuable.

The course evaluations from the work groups' educational sessions were positive, and the QIT was encouraged by the high standard of project work produced by participants. Other problems arose as a result of the way the educational process was cascaded throughout the organization. There was a management restructuring five months into the start of the implementation of the quality improvement process. This meant that those at executive level did not attend the course until many of their subordinates had done so. There were some instances of staff approaching managers to discuss their action assignments without the manager having done the course. This situation is to be avoided at all costs, as it compromises both individuals.

Another difficulty arose as a result of some of the early attempts at educating potential QIT members. The initial consultancy firm selected by the steering group used (unbeknown at the time) a Crosby-style approach, although it did not use the Crosby training materials. This meant that instead of the four-day quality improvement process course for QIT members, a two-day course was run on site. Although this provided an insight into some of the concepts of TQM, it was not until four staff attended the Crosby quality improvement process course at the Crosby Quality College, that the limitations of the two-day version were realized. The main problem was that too little time was spent on the 14 steps, or on the practicalities of implementation, which created difficulties for those expected to fulfil this role. By the time the decision to switch to the wholesale Crosby approach was taken, the next stage of the educational cascade had begun. Hence the majority of original QITs did not have any members who had completed the full Crosby course. The QIT mentioned in the case study was fortunate in that three of its members had attended the four-day course, and it was agreed that this was beneficial both for these individuals and to the team, in terms of their increased knowledge on how to manage the implementation.

For these reasons it is impossible to draw general conclusions about the success or failure of the Crosby educational materials, as two of the essential elements advocated – implementation cascaded from the top of the organization, and use of the course designed specifically to enable the QIT to function effectively – were never realized.

What became apparent to the QIT members cited in the case study was that, in spite of the difficulties of coordinating such an educational exercise, it was a crucial part in beginning the culture change previously mentioned. For many staff, it was the first time they had the opportunity to contribute to the organization in this way. As one member of staff said, 'I've worked here for 20 years, and it's the first time any one has asked my opinion on anything.'

The 'common language' used in the courses, combined with the tools and techniques, enabled staff to work with their peers at improving the work processes in which they were involved. It moved the focus away from the finger-pointing culture of looking for people to blame when things went wrong to one that looked at identifying and agreeing requirements to ensure things went 'right first time'.

As more staff attended the courses, the purpose of the other 13 steps in supporting their efforts to improve became more apparent. Quality improvement education alone is not enough; staff also require support and direction from a QIT through the setting of goals, a clear demonstration of management commitment, measurement charts and a system to enable problems identified through measurement to be solved, a framework to enable individual employees to communicate work problems to management, a continual awareness of their role in the quality improvement process, and recognition of their efforts. These other steps, and the practicalities of implementation, will now be examined.

Step 3. Measurement

Crosby's 14 steps for total quality management

1   Commitment
2   Quality improvement team

STAFFORDSHIRE
UNIVERSITY
LIBRARY

3	Measurement
4	Cost of quality
5	Awareness
6	Corrective action
7	Zero defects planning
8	Education
9	Zero defects day
10	Goal setting
11	Error cause removal
12	Recognition
13	Quality councils
14	Do it all over again

Purpose: to provide a display of current and potential non-conformance problems in a manner that permits objective evaluation and corrective action

Practicalities of implementation

The key responsibilities outlined by the step sponsor to ensure successful implementation of this step by the QIT members were:

- to pilot measurement charts and ensure they were printed in preparation for staff to use as part of the educational courses;
- to measure one work process as a method of demonstrating the importance of measurement to their staff;
- to act as a resource to staff by helping them to commence measurement of their own work processes;
- to promote actively the use of measurement in each area;
- to make staff aware of measurement being conducted throughout the hospital, and of actions arising as a result.

Staff were taught how to identify aspects of their work processes for measurement, and techniques for collecting and quantifying such data, as part of their education. An advantage of the use of measurement was that it changed the terminology of the identification of problems from the subjective (which under the traditional culture tended to blame specific individuals) to the objective (which described the problem in quantifiable terms that focused on deficiencies in the work process). For example, 'The linen room staff never supply us with enough linen at the weekend' becomes 'Over a one-month period, sufficient linen to meet the ward's requirements for the weekend was not supplied for 53% of the time.' This is important in promoting meaningful dialogue between the individuals involved in the process (in this instance, the nurses, the porters, the linen staff and the laundry), as it focuses the attention on the problem, rather than jumping to conclusions about the cause. Further measurement may show that there is insufficient linen in circulation to meet the weekend demand, that the stocks ordered by nurses are insufficient or that there are insufficient porters on duty at the weekend to deliver the linen.

Staff were encouraged to display their measurement charts in the work area, which served as a focal point for discussion between staff and managers, as well as identifying clearly the impact of methods being used in an attempt to solve the problem. There were exceptions to this rule if it was felt patients may misconstrue data presented; for example, a study to identify the number of errors on a prescription chart, which focused on drugs not signed for by the doctor, and start and stop dates not completed. Staff felt unhappy about displaying this 'prescription error' measurement chart in case patients thought the data implied they had received a wrong medication.

A number of key lessons were learned in implementing this step. These were as follows.

Guidelines when implementing measurement

Staff education
Staff education was essential for reducing the threatening nature of measurement. Staff asked to measure aspects of their work, before attending the quality educational courses, feared and mistrusted the task.

Positive attitude to measurement
It was crucial for managers to be positive about the use of measurement, even if this identified deficiencies in the service. Using the results of data collected in this way as a method of chastising staff for their performance was a short cut to guaranteed failure of the quality improvement process, as it undermined the whole philosophy of the culture change it was attempting to achieve.

Full knowledge and cooperation
No measurement of another department or profession should be carried out without staff's knowledge and cooperation. There were initial concerns that this would skew the results, as it would be likely that extra effort would be made to ensure requirements were met if staff knew these were being measured. In practice, in the case of genuine failure of specific work processes, this was difficult to maintain over the extensive period that the data were being collected. The benefits of including other areas in this way were two-fold. First, including more areas ensured that the data collection was done in a way that was accepted by those being measured as valid, and that the part of the process being measured was a reliable indicator of how the process was working. For example, ward staff may be unhappy about the quality of the patients' meals. The nurses measure the number of 'errors' (such as patients receiving food they did not order, items missed from the plate, etc.). Ward staff may have a

preconceived idea that this is because of inadequacies in the catering department. They present the 40% non-conformance rate of the catering staff as
evidence of their 'failure'. The catering department has also been concerned
about the problems with the same process. They use a different criterion and
measure the number of incomplete or illegible menus that are returned to the
kitchen. They present the 60% non-conformance rate to the nursing staff as
evidence of their 'failure'. Here, measurement creates barriers between the
departments. A more effective method is to convene a group of representative
individuals from all the disciplines involved in the process and, using the tools and
techniques such as the process model worksheet, look at ways in which they can
work together as a team to improve the process. In this instance, measurement
is used to identify deficiencies in the process, rather than to assign blame to
specific individuals.

As a result of using the staff to measure their own work processes, with the
specific objective of identifying an area in need of quality improvement, the data
collected tended to be more accurate than under the traditional 'hit squad' style
of quality assurance. For example, if staff know there is to be a health and safety
check, then they tend to tighten up on all the factors they know will be audited
and the data collected do not necessarily present a true picture of normal
practice.

Conversely, a member of staff who is concerned about the severe lack of
storage space in the ward may choose to audit the number of occasions when
items were found to be blocking the fire escapes. It is probable that the number
of instances would not reflect the findings of the health and safety check. This is
because the presence of the staff member on the ward would not be seen as
intrusive, and it is more difficult to fool staff who are based permanently in the
ward in this way. The people who understand where the non-conformances
commonly arise are those most closely involved in the work process.

Staff involvement

The staff themselves should determine which aspects of the work process to
measure. Staff who selected an area of measurement because it was something
that was causing them problems at work produced markedly more accurate and
better presented data than a minority of staff who had been instructed to
measure things in which they had little interest. The course facilitators were able
to recommend appropriate ways of collecting data once the staff had selected
the work process that they felt required improving.

Staff were encouraged to pick one or a maximum of two things to measure,
using the measurement guidelines in the above section. They were supported by
their course facilitator and QIT member in carrying out their measurement. It
was quickly identified that staff at all levels working in this way on a number of
small-scale projects could, collectively, have a significant impact on improving the

service. There were instances where staff measured processes that were perceived by them to be a problem, yet measurement proved that this was not the case. This was in itself important, as some areas had been branded with the label of not meeting requirements when in some cases this was unwarranted. The types of requirements measured crossed a huge range in both diversity and scale. Examples include:

- waiting time for outpatient clinics
- consultants not arriving on time to start clinics
- incorrectly addressed mail
- the number of incorrectly completed forms
- meetings not starting and finishing on time
- requests for directory enquiries via switchboard
- wheelchairs not conforming to requirements
- patients' personal laundry returned to the wrong ward
- wasted items in CSSD packs
- nursing time spent on clerical duties
- menus not returned to the kitchen by the required time
- inappropriate GP referrals to physiotherapist
- medical records lost or mislaid
- urgent requests not met on time

The results from such measurements gave a clear indication of the scale of the problem and also provided a useful baseline against which to compare the impact of actions subsequently taken to resolve it. The measurements themselves often provided the staff with essential information needed to present their case for the need for improvement to occur. For example, it was found that over half of the hospital wheelchairs did not conform to requirements (i.e. tyres pumped; all footrests and armrests present and functioning; wheelchairs clean and stored in the correct areas). This presented a powerful case for the purchase of some new wheelchairs, and for staff to agree requirements for maintaining wheelchairs in good working order. Under a traditional hierarchical culture, many staff would have resented an extra task such as wheelchair maintenance being added to their job. In this instance, because the staff themselves had identified that they were wasting a significant amount of their time fixing wheelchairs and that there was a risk to patients, and because they had identified the solution for themselves, the process could be improved. A crucial part in this was in management accepting this measurement and purchasing some new wheelchairs as part of the solution.

The final item on the list posed some interesting debates, as it was realized that no one had established a definition of 'urgent'. Hence, portering staff were constantly told a job was 'urgent'. In practice, only a proportion of these required immediate attention; for many others, a clear requirement such as 'within one hour' or 'before midday' would enable them to plan their work more effectively.

General conclusions regarding the implementation of this measurement step
The introduction of widespread, systematic measurement throughout the hospital is an essential part of quality management. There was also some sound theoretical underpinning in introducing it with the support of some of the other steps outlined in the Crosby approach. Consistent with the theories of effective management of change in Chapter 4, measurement proved to be an extremely effective method of 'unfreezing' or helping staff to perceive the need for change. The fact that they 'owned' the data they were collecting was an important part of the data's being accepted as valid. The biggest obstacle to measurement's introduction was in overcoming the mistrust of the way in which the data might be used. There was a strong initial suspicion that there was some hidden, ulterior managerial motive. It was therefore essential that staff believed in managers' commitment to the quality improvement process, and were convinced that measurement would not be used to staff's detriment.

Two other crucial steps in changing the culture to enable measurement on this scale were the education of all staff and the establishment of a corrective action system. Education equipped everyone with the knowledge and skills needed to measure their work, as well as helping them to appreciate its benefits to them personally. The corrective action system made it possible to resolve the problems raised through measurement.

Step 6. Corrective action

Crosby's 14 steps for total quality management

1	Commitment
2	Quality improvement team
3	Measurement
4	Cost of quality
5	Awareness
6	**Corrective action**
7	Zero defects planning
8	Education
9	Zero defects day
10	Goal setting
11	Error cause removal
12	Recognition
13	Quality councils
14	Do it all over again

Purpose: to provide a systematic method of conclusively resolving the problems that are identified through other action steps
Tackling this step fell into two broad categories: first, the education of all staff in the principles of problem solving; second, the development of an infrastructure

that supported them in this process. A mechanism was necessary to ensure that problems that could not be resolved at a local level reached the appropriate level for action to occur. If nothing changes as a result of measurement, staff motivation to continue quickly diminishes.

The five-step problem-solving method

This technique involves five stages which participants on the educational courses apply to their work-related problems.

Stage 1. Define the situation

This stage draws heavily on the measurement step. The situation that is causing the difficulty must be measured, both to establish the size of the problem and to enable it to be expressed in objective, rather than subjective, terms.

For example, the medical photography department may identify that 12 out of 24 pictures do not come out. When they are asked to define this situation, typical answers include 'the camera was faulty', 'they weren't developed properly' or 'the photographer made a mistake with the exposure'. Such responses illustrate the traditional approach to problem solving we have identified in the health service. The definition of the medical photographer's problem is that '12 out of 24 pictures did not come out'. The other answers do not define the situation; they make assumptions about the cause of the situation. In doing this, there is a danger that the assumption about the root cause of the problem is incorrect, and therefore the subsequent action taken to resolve the perceived (rather than the actual) causes of the problem is ineffective.

Stage 2. Fix

This stage involves introducing a temporary solution to the problem in order to enable the process to continue to function. In practice, we found that this is the stage at which many of the organizational problems had remained static. The hospital was full of evidence of quick fixes which quickly became the norm. These included wheelchairs, cot sides and other equipment held together by strapping tape; an extra checking stage built into many processes, such as forms being checked and authorized by up to three different managers; overordering or overbooking in the expectation that the process will not deliver as expected (for example, assuming a 25% non-attendance rate in the outpatients clinic and holding a month's instead of the required two weeks' worth of stock because of lack of confidence in the delivery system).

Stage 3. Identify the root cause

This stage involves further measurement and analysis of the problem to ascertain the underlying cause. For example, the medical photographer may have the camera serviced or check on the stages of the development process to analyse what the root cause of the problem is.

Stage 4. Take corrective action
This stage involves taking action to eliminate the root cause. For example, if the medical photographer finds that the developing agents are past the expiry date, they should be discarded and new ones bought.

Stage 5. Evaluate and follow up
The final stage involves the evaluation of the solution using further measurement to establish whether the problem has been resolved. In the above example, the medical photographer would inspect subsequent batches of photographs to ensure all 24 come out, and review this periodically to ensure the process is working properly.

The five-step problem-solving method enables individuals to solve problems related to their work processes. However, there will be occasions when they are unable to resolve these problems alone. A system to ensure they receive the appropriate support is necessary; this is described below.

Creating an infrastructure to coordinate and support problems
It is estimated that approximately 80% of problems identified can be solved at a local level. The remaining 20% require the involvement of other individuals, either for the purpose of effecting a solution, or in order to release some funding (Crosby, 1991). In practice, we found this figure to be extremely accurate.

Based on our experiences, it is recommended that the planning and implementation of this step are tackled in the following way. First, the steering group, in consultation with the corrective action step sponsors from all the QITs, designs and process-proves a corrective action system for use throughout the whole organization. This should be fully functional before the education of the staff. This is important, both so that the documentation supporting such a system can be introduced to course participants and to ensure that the system is ready to support staff immediately they require to use it. Confidence in management commitment fades quickly if significant efforts on the part of staff are not met with the support promised. An example of a corrective action system is shown in Figure 6.4.

How the corrective action system works
In the event of a problem that requires actions outside the scope of the individual, the member of staff identifying the problem and their QIT member complete a 'corrective action form'. This has two benefits. First, it promotes dialogue about the problem, which can often be resolved by the manager and staff member as a result of this meeting alone. Second, it prevents misuse of the system by individuals who have not carried out the initial stages of problem solving themselves (i.e. define the situation, fix, and identify root cause) and are attempting to dump the problem onto their colleagues.

If the problem does require entry into the system, the QIT member will pass it on to the corrective action step sponsor, who will present it at the next QIT meeting. The role of the QIT is to discuss which individuals need to form a 'corrective action team' to resolve the problem. These should consist of the individuals who are closely involved in this work process, and able to contribute to an effective solution.

The corrective action team is then formed and uses the tools and techniques learnt during the quality educational courses to resolve the problem. The corrective action team leader communicates the progress of the team via the appropriate documentation to the corrective action step sponsor. This is important, as once a large number of teams are established, there is a need to maintain a central focus on all the various projects. It also ensures that corrective action teams do not just sink without trace.

If the team reaches a point where it does not have authority to act (although this should not be a problem if membership was considered carefully in the first instance) then the corrective action step sponsor raises the difficulty at QIT level, and the QIT will pass the information on the problem and progress to date to the appropriate manager for action and a progress report within a specified period of time.

When the problem is resolved, all the details are retained by the corrective action step sponsor as a central record, and the QIT member responsible for Step 12 (recognition) ensures that the efforts of the team are recognized in an appropriate way. The corrective action team is then disbanded.

General conclusions regarding the implementation and use of this step

The five-step method of problem solving proved logical and useful, and was adopted quickly by staff. Although initially dismissed by some as 'pure common sense', the large numbers of unresolved problems that were identified as the quality improvement process was implemented were a clear indication that, in spite of some claims to the contrary, there was no systematic approach to solving problems within the hospital. These were traditionally tackled on an ad hoc basis, with no mechanism for monitoring and coordinating these efforts.

A crucial element in the successful implementation of this step is to establish a culture that recognizes and values the contribution of all staff and empowers all individuals within the organization to contribute actively to solving problems. This often involves delegation of responsibility, which can prove extremely threatening for some managers, who feel their position of authority is being undermined. It requires different skills from those of the traditional line manager, demanding the ability to empower staff and support and develop individuals to enable them to make their own contribution to the quality improvement process, rather than for problem solving to remain exclusively within the domain of management.

The corrective action system, as outlined in Figure 6.4, was initially viewed by the QIT as bureaucratic, cumbersome and too complicated. In the event, corrective action was not given high priority, and left until much later in the implementation process. Resistance to the system was exacerbated by the terminology used. 'Corrective action' sounded rather draconian. Early attempts to rename this step failed miserably, as this simply seemed to replace one type of jargon for another. In practice, most of the course facilitators referred to this step as 'problem solving'.

As the implementation of the quality improvement process progressed, four major problems became apparent. These were as follows:

- Staff were working on problems of which the QIT was completely unaware. This had profound implications when evaluating the impact of the quality improvement process, as there was no record of either the impact of these projects, or an identified price of non-conformance that needed to be incorporated into Step 4 (the cost of quality). It also meant that work was being duplicated, and some areas were subject to extraordinary stresses, which led to friction between departments rather than bridge building as intended. For example, large numbers of staff expressed an interest in working on projects requiring a considerable amount of input from the catering department. The QIT needed to intervene to ensure no further projects were started until the current corrective action teams were disbanded. The reasons were explained and accepted by staff, some of whom assisted individuals who had started work in this area, whilst others selected equally worthwhile projects.
- If staff were unable to resolve problems at a local level, they had no mechanism for seeking help once all the normal channels were exhausted. The difficulty here was the lack of a system to ensure that problems reached the level in the organization where someone could help. Typically, many projects were floundering because of the lack of a decision from a level sufficiently senior to authorize a change in work processes. On other occasions, significantly large problems were not being resolved owing to the inability of individuals to secure the financial support needed to effect a solution.
- The QIT digressed into a corrective action team. For team members who thrived on solving difficult problems, the temptation to provide instant solutions was too great to resist. This was detrimental for two reasons. First, it detracted from the real role of the QIT in managing the implementation of the 14 steps, and meant valuable meeting time was spent discussing a myriad of organizational problems. Second, it contravened the underlying philosophy of the culture change we were attempting to implement, in that we were imposing our solutions to problems within work processes that the staff involved were far more qualified to deal with. Furthermore, such imposed solutions bypassed all the essential mechanisms imperative in gaining staff ownership and acceptance of the required changes.

- A number of problems that were common to the whole organization, and not unique to our QIT, were identified. This created the potential difficulty of ten QITs working on the same problem with no central coordination.

These four problems threatened to reduce the quality improvement process to a series of uncoordinated quality initiatives. However, it was a useful learning experience, as it led to the appreciation of the need for the corrective action step, which offered a solution for the first three problems.

The fourth problem, namely lack of coordination of quality improvement projects, was resolved by forming a corrective action subcommittee, chaired by a senior member of the organization, and consisting of the corrective action step sponsors from all the QITs. The subcommittee's initial role was to establish an effective corrective action system that could be adopted uniformly throughout the organization. The role of this committee would later change to one of monitoring the large numbers of diverse projects, and coordinating the efforts of all the QITs. It also provided a forum for introducing problems that could not be resolved at QIT level and needed raising at steering group or executive level.

A number of the problems raised through this step were found to be causing a significant financial cost to the organization. This will now be explored.

Step 4. Cost of quality

Crosby's 14 steps for total quality management

1	Commitment
2	Quality improvement team
3	Measurement
4	**Cost of quality**
5	Awareness
6	Corrective action
7	Zero defects planning
8	Education
9	Zero defects day
10	Goal setting
11	Error cause removal
12	Recognition
13	Quality councils
14	Do it all over again

Purpose: to define the ingredients of the cost of quality and explain its use as a management tool

The 'cost of quality' was an unfamiliar tool for those of us within the Health Service, although one that was relatively easy to grasp and utilize once the concepts had been explained during the educational courses. Put simply, the annual budget can be divided as illustrated in Figure 6.5 (Crosby, 1991).

The price of conformance is the cost of doing business right the first time. For example, checking stock expiry dates in pharmacy, calibrating equipment, storing food at the correct temperature.

The price of non-conformance is the cost of not doing things right the first time. Hence every time a requirement is not met there is a knock-on cost in terms of time, money and human costs, from the set of medical notes going missing (causing extra work for the clerks) to the patient receiving the wrong operation. Often, the smaller errors are regarded as inevitable and are tolerated by staff and patients. The error-free cost is the normal cost of doing business, for example heating, lighting, staffing, etc.

The advantages of calculating the price of non-conformance are as follows:

- **It is an effective tool in directing managers' attention to a problem.** For example, dressing packs in the casualty department often have blunt scissors. This necessitates opening another pack, which is wasted. Staff measured these instances and calculated the cost of the wasted packs; it was £7000 per year. To replace all the scissors would cost £400. Such information is useful when prioritizing expenditure.
- **It can act as a catalyst for problem solving.** For example, 9% of patients coming for routine surgery in one area either did not arrive or were cancelled as unfit for theatre. The cost to the hospital (calculated by adding the cost of admission, administration and lost revenue) was £96,000 per annum. A multidisciplinary team was established to examine ways for reducing this problem.
- **It can redirect resources for more appropriate use.** For example, following the reduction in portering staff, an extra nurse was needed on the surgical ward to take patients to theatre. This had resulted in excessive overtime payments when theatre overran; it was calculated these would pay for a part-time porter. Furthermore, the nurse was then able to use her skills more appropriately.
- **It can act as a useful baseline measure.** This enables managers and problem-solving groups to compare the price of non-conformance from year to year and monitor progress.

Potential problems identified in using the tool
Some disadvantages were:

- Some managers may view it as a cost-cutting exercise.
- Staff may find it extremely threatening.

These problems can be avoided if cost of quality is introduced within a planned framework for implementing TQM. Managers and staff, therefore, will all have attended educational courses. This step is most powerful and accurate when all levels within the organization use it.

Conducting the cost of quality exercise

The collection of data on the price of non-conformance is divided into two phases. Phase 1 is the initial organizational exercise undertaken when starting the quality improvement process, which is designed to give a very broad overview of the potential scope for improvement. This exercise can be repeated on an annual basis to monitor the impact of the quality improvement process. Phase 2 involves the collection of more specific data by those actually involved in the work processes, and the collation of such data to create a more accurate organizational cost of quality profile.

The phase 1 cost of quality exercise gathers data on the key areas where requirements are not being met the first time. It was commonly found that, for many work processes, there were no set requirements, particularly at interfaces between different departments or different professions. With the help of the unit accountant, a cost was then put on this data to estimate the overall price of non-conformance.

These data were collected over a two-day survey, during which a representative sample of senior staff from all disciplines and areas within the organization was interviewed.

Typical findings from a cost of quality exercise

Studies carried out in a number of NHS units show similar problem areas arising.

Bed utilization problems

Examples typically include doctors spending a significant amount of time locating a bed for a patient, 'sleepers out' staying in hospital for longer than necessary, 'bed blocking' and acute beds used for 'social' admissions because of insufficient community back-up.

Retreatments

Before the introduction of medical audit there was little information on the extent of retreatment of patients (because of either incorrect initial diagnosis or patient non-compliance). Also falling into this category are iatrogenic complications, with hospital-acquired infection and treatment of pressure sores costing the health service millions of pounds per year (Hibbs, 1988).

Workflow problems

This is a knock-on effect of the interface problems outlined above. Examples include theatre teams waiting for up to 40 minutes for the porter to bring a patient, porters arriving to collect patients who are not ready and clinics running late. These problems are not the fault of the individual, but result from unrealistic or unclear job requirements.

Fire fighting
This is a common complaint from nursing and managerial staff. They seem to spend a large proportion of their time (up to 30%) repeatedly solving the same problems arising from work processes that are unable to meet service demands, or are not done right the first time. For example, forms filled in incorrectly, searching for lost items (ranging from medical notes to patients' false teeth), trying to obtain laundry at weekends, and what is commonly referred to as 'nipping' to other areas to deliver or collect things (such as drugs or equipment).

Wasted materials
In spite of efficiency savings in recent years in the NHS, we identified that there was still wastage of materials. Examples included drugs expiring because of poor rotation and overstocking, and poor stock management overall.

Unnecessary tests
Medical audit has, in many areas, identified a significant number of unnecessary or inappropriate tests.

Poorly run meetings
This is a common area identified by staff, i.e. that they start late, important people are not present (or others are present who get no value from the meeting), they do not produce positive actions and they overrun.

The results from the phase I cost of quality exercise are fed back to senior management at the end of the second day. This was found to be an important part in helping senior management appreciate the potential benefits in embarking on quality improvement. Such improvement cannot occur under the traditional management culture outlined earlier. It requires a significant amount of resources both in time and money to reach the point where the cost of quality is reduced. Most authors with experience of this approach advocate between three and five years to reach the point where significant financial savings are seen as a by-product of the quality improvements that result. It is important to stress that any costs reduced in this way are a beneficial consequence of the quality improve-ment process, rather than the underlying key objective. These benefits can be realized only by introducing a change in management culture, which needs to be supported by education, recognition and a firm management commitment.

General conclusions regarding the introduction of this step
There was little doubt that this cost of quality tool was viewed as extremely threatening by the QIT. At the time of implementation there were simultaneous widespread changes in management structure as a result of the White Paper reforms, occurring against a backdrop of rumours about financial difficulties. The QIT accepted that such information could prove useful to them, but there were widespread concerns at all levels within the hospital regarding the way in which this information would be used. The primary concern was that staff would

'improve' themselves out of a job. Two factors were identified as important if the tool was to be accepted:

- that some of the savings made as a result of improvement should be made available to the QIT to plough back into the quality improvement process;
- that potential savings identified would not be subtracted from the budget allocation for the following year.

The second point was particularly important once the phase I cost of quality was completed. The data collected in phase I are intended to give a very general picture of areas that could benefit from improvement, rather than areas where budgets can be cut. Although some of the savings identified will fall back to the bottom line, there are also a significant number of others that cannot be realized in this way as they are not cash releasing.

We likened it to an approach to shopping, when we may, for example, have a budget of £100 to spend on clothing. On spotting a bargain that is reduced from £100 to £50, we spend the remaining £50 on shoes, also reduced from £100. We are delighted because we have 'saved' £100, even though the money is never liquidated. The important thing is that we get much better value for our money. Similarly, in the case of staff time wasted on dealing with ineffective work processes, such as the example of the two whole-time equivalent nurses walking backwards and forwards to the pharmacy, improving this process does not mean that two nurses are no longer needed. However, the proportion of all the nurses' time that went to make up the figure of two whole-time equivalents can now be devoted to other, more appropriate, activities.

In practice, the majority of staff undertaking the work group educational course were far less sensitive about the use of the phase 2 cost of quality tool than had been previously imagined. It did prove to be a major factor in helping them to identify many of their processes that were not functioning well. As many commented, 'We'd never considered how much time/money was wasted, we just considered it as inevitable.' They also found the calculation techniques taught as part of the course useful when demonstrating to managers the financial implications of deficiencies in work processes that required minor financial investment to correct.

For example, medical records did not have an industrial paper shredder, and the £2000 required to purchase one was not a high priority for the budget holders. This necessitated clerks tearing the records manually. Calculating the average time spent by all the clerks tearing notes, on a pro rata basis, came to approximately £6000 per annum. This did not mean that the purchase of a shredder would mean the loss of a part-time member of staff owing to time saved, but that the considerable backlog of work in this department could begin to be cleared as a result of extra time available. Having identified and realized savings in this way, most staff had no objection to these being publicized.

The other advantage of developing the phase 2 cost of quality is that it is a way of illustrating the financial return on the initial investment made in staff training and problem solving. With hindsight, it would have been advantageous to complete the planning and implementation of this step far more thoroughly than was done in practice.

The financial figure identified as the 'cost of quality' was high enough to cause grave reservations about expressing it in terms of cash, in case this was misconstrued in some quarters. Managers were more comfortable to express the figure in terms of a percentage of the annual budget. Surveys of this kind of wastage or opportunity costs conducted in the NHS show figures ranging from 23% to 30% of the total budget.

This may paint a depressing picture but, in fact, it is not significantly worse than many other organizations in both the public and private sectors. What is illustrated is the scale of opportunity that exists if staff work positively together to solve these problems.

The benefits will not be realized through a conventional cost-cutting approach, with all its negative implications. The key is to empower the staff to talk in a constructive manner about the problems they have, and to give them the time and resources to tackle them systematically through a structured approach to quality improvement.

It is essential to recognize the efforts of staff who contribute in this way to the quality improvement process. Methods that can be used to achieve this are explored below.

Step 12. Recognition

Crosby's 14 steps for total quality management

1 Commitment
2 Quality improvement team
3 Measurement
4 Cost of quality
5 Awareness
6 Corrective action
7 Zero defects planning
8 Education
9 Zero defects day
10 Goal setting
11 Error cause removal
12 **Recognition**
13 Quality councils
14 Do it all over again

Purpose: to appreciate those who participate

The purpose statement for this step was an accurate phrasing of what many QIT members acknowledged was something that was lacking in the traditional NHS culture. The word 'appreciate' is used in the same context as when referring to art or antiques; it refers to acknowledging the value of something. There were widespread complaints from both ends of the hierarchy about being undervalued and unappreciated. Many cited examples of extra efforts made, for which they were never thanked. Many managers admitted that they were overloaded with sorting out everyday problems, that they spent more time pointing out what was wrong with the system than what was right with it. Although they acknowledged there were individuals who were reliable, hardworking and putting in extra effort, many felt unsure how to demonstrate their appreciation without seeming patronizing or insincere. They themselves also felt unappreciated.

The QIT addressed this by discussing with their staff groups what forms of recognition would be considered appropriate. The two key areas of enquiry were: (1) what sorts of actions required recognition; and (2) how such actions could be acknowledged. The key recommendations presented to the team as a result of these discussions were as follows:

- Staff felt that actions involving extra effort over and above their normal job role warranted recognition. Many commented that a simple 'thank you' or occasional 'well done' would be much appreciated. It was also felt that those attending courses should receive some kind of recognition on successful completion.
- Staff felt the selection of individuals for recognition would have greater value if they were nominated by their colleagues rather than by managers.
- There was a strong feeling that financial recognition for efforts was inappropriate. Although a minority felt that if their contribution saved the hospital significant amounts of money then they should receive a proportion, the majority stated they would prefer to see it reinvested in patient care. Many stated they would like to see some of it invested in their project or area.
- There was a strong feeling, particularly among QIT members, that there needed to be a sum of money set aside specifically for the purpose of recognition. This was seen as an important way of demonstrating management commitment.

As a result of the discussions and planning, the following suggestions were implemented as part of this step:

- All staff who completed any of the educational courses received a certificate of attendance, signed by the chief executive and presented by a QIT member, at the end of the course. Staff valued the certificate as something they could add to their curriculum vitae, and in spite of reservations about the presentation of these at the end of the course, the majority of staff appreciated marking the end of their course in this way. The fact that senior members of staff had taken the trouble to attend the final session and had taken an interest in staff's projects curbed initial scepticism about the extent of management commitment. Many senior managers were far more self-conscious about presenting certificates than the staff were receiving them, which was perhaps a reason why this suggestion was not originally well supported.

- Each educational course chose to have a group photograph taken on completion, which was framed and displayed. These were received in good humour, and helped to illustrate the number of staff who had successfully completed these courses.

- Completed quality improvement projects, measurements being undertaken and other quality improvement efforts were displayed on the quality notice board with the names of those involved. This had two benefits: (1) it was a useful method of sharing ideas among staff, some of which were then implemented elsewhere; and (2) it facilitated peer recognition, as many individuals were contacted by other staff for further information about their efforts. A number of these were also reproduced in more detail and printed in the hospital newspaper.

- There was a concerted effort on the part of QIT members to be more active in seeking out staff and praising them for their efforts. This was made much easier once the mechanisms for coordinating the corrective action step were established, as all QIT members were kept informed of the efforts of staff. It also included the acknowledgement within the QIT of the efforts made by its members both verbally, in terms of thanks from the chair, and documented within the QIT meeting minutes.

- Approximately three months after completing the educational course, participants attended a follow-up session. The session was designed to be informal and was coordinated by one of the course facilitators. Each individual gave a brief summary of the process they had selected for improvement, the results from their measurement, and their progress in using the five-step problem-solving method. Each session was attended by at least two QIT members, who were responsible for feeding back the progress to the QIT. These sessions proved successful. First, staff were supportive of their peers' efforts, and gave them a great deal of encouragement. In instances where projects were experiencing setbacks, many came in with offers of help, and it proved an effective way of breaking down professional and hierarchical barriers. Second, the fact that staff outnumbered the managers seemed to give them the confidence to identify areas in which they required more help and support. These comments were then raised at QIT level, with specific QIT members being actioned to help remove any roadblocks identified by staff. Actions taken were reported to the individual member of staff, as well as the QIT. All staff attending these days received a personal letter of thanks for their efforts, with confirmation in writing of any actions promised as a result.

- One year into the process, a conference was arranged with a lunchtime exhibition featuring poster presentations of all the project work completed during the educational courses. Over 60 projects were submitted for presentation. This forum provided an excellent opportunity for senior managers and peer colleagues to acknowledge the efforts of these staff. Two of the completed projects were selected for special recognition, and these staff were presented with a book token by the Chair of the Health Authority. These projects involved the establishment by an enrolled nurse and a registered nurse of a counselling service for women admitted for breast surgery, and the introduction of teaching sessions and a resource pack aimed at increasing staff knowledge on the system for ordering stores. This was the project of a member of the office staff, who identified a large number of non-conformances when measuring this process.

General conclusions regarding the implementation of this step

There was a consensus of opinion that it was absolutely crucial to recognize the efforts of those who contributed to the quality improvement process at all levels within the organization. The way in which this step was implemented took account of local opinion and tailored the approach to meet this recognition step. Recognition was an important part of the success of this step, as this was accepted by staff as genuine and sincere, rather than too much management hype. It was also an important step in changing the culture of the organization to one that visibly valued the efforts of its staff.

The initial eight steps for planning and implementing the quality improvement process using the Crosby approach have now been outlined and illustrated by the practical actions necessary to effect these as taken by the quality improvement team in the case study. As identified earlier, the term 'steps' is a misnomer, as they need to be coordinated with each other. This process will now be explored.

Coordination and planning of the first eight steps of the quality improvement process

The above eight steps took the QIT 18 months to plan and partially implement. There were some difficulties, as outlined under the specific steps, but one of the biggest factors that was underestimated was the importance of synchronizing the introduction of the different steps in an order that enhanced, rather than inhibited, the corporate impact. This difficulty in coordinating the implementation of TQM can be overcome by drawing up a comprehensive action plan that considers the timing of different actions in relation to each other.

The rationale for planning steps in this order is based on a number of factors identified in response to difficulties experienced in practice. These are outlined below:

- Establish management commitment before any public declarations of the implementation of the quality improvement process in the area covered by the QIT. Staff were quick to point out examples of what they perceived as lack of management commitment to the process.
- Conduct a general awareness exercise before commencing educational courses for staff. Course facilitators were greatly disadvantaged by staff turning up for courses with no idea why they were there.
- Ensure staff have attended the appropriate course before any involvement in measurement or problem-solving activities. Problems arose when 'new-style' problem-solving groups fell back on 'old-style' methods of subjective arguments and finger pointing due to some members not having the necessary skills and knowledge, such as problem solving and measurement.
- Conduct a cost of quality exercise (or similar baseline audit) early on in the implementation process, and repeat at regular intervals. When funding becomes scarce, clear facts and figures to demonstrate benefits are needed.
- Ensure that mechanisms for recognizing the efforts of individuals are established in good time. Staff were critical that certificates for the initial courses were not ready before completion, and that their efforts were not always acknowledged by senior managers.
- Maintain the momentum of the quality improvement process over a sustained period of time. After 18 months, the QIT experienced difficulty in maintaining momentum. At this time, it is advisable to change some of the team members and relaunch the QIT using the format of the initial start day. It was acknowledged that guidance from an experienced facilitator would be extremely beneficial, as many team members felt they had lost direction. A key objective for this day is to produce an action plan for the 14 steps for the following year. At this time, it is appropriate to consider the other steps, which are designed to be introduced at a later stage in the quality improvement process. These are outlined below.

Step 10. Goal setting

Crosby's 14 steps for total quality management

1 Commitment
2 Quality improvement team
3 Measurement
4 Cost of quality
5 Awareness
6 Corrective action
7 Zero defects planning
8 Education
9 Zero defects day
10 Goal setting
11 Error cause removal
12 Recognition

13   Quality councils
14   Do it all over again

Purpose: to turn pledges and commitments into action by encouraging
individuals to establish improvement goals for themselves and their groups
The need for this step was apparent following the use of the cost of quality tool,
widespread use of measurement and the introduction of the corrective action
system. These steps identified areas for improvement, but there was a need to
set goals against which progress could be measured. In some areas, in spite of
deficiencies identified, nothing further happened after measurement was
completed. Goal setting is required to provide staff with a target which can be
reached through the application of tools and techniques from other steps.

Steps 7 and 9. Zero defects planning and Zero defects day

Crosby's 14 steps for total quality management

1   Commitment
2   Quality improvement team
3   Measurement
4   Cost of quality
5   Awareness
6   Corrective action
7   **Zero defects planning**
8   Education
9   **Zero defects day**
10   Goal setting
11   Error cause removal
12   Recognition
13   Quality councils
14   Do it all over again

Purpose (Step 7): to examine the various activities that must be conducted
in preparation for formally launching zero defects day

Purpose (Step 9): to create an event that will let all employees realize,
through a personal experience, that there has been a change
At the initial QIT educational sessions, concern was expressed over the Crosby
anecdotes regarding the baton-twirling, brass-and-parading, balloon-releasing
events popular with American companies using this approach. These steps
therefore lay dormant for a considerable amount of time. They were reconsid-
ered after the success of the follow-up days for course participants, and the
poster presentations in the recognition event. Apart from the advantages of these
events in recognizing those who participated, they were also a beneficial way of
demonstrating to staff who were still waiting to attend the courses the scale of

improvements that had arisen as a result of the quality improvement process. Without these, many of the projects would never have been heard about by large groups within the organization. These events also rejuvenated many flagging projects when staff appreciated what had been achieved by many of their peers, and the advice and support offered by these individuals was a far greater motivating force than any management pressure could ever achieve. Although the term 'zero defects day' was consigned to the archives, there was an acknowledgement for the need of some kind of event that fulfilled the same purpose.

Step 7 (zero defects planning) was important because an inappropriate or badly planned range of activities could potentially do more harm than good. It was established early in the quality improvement process that any activity or individual linked directly with the implementation was scrutinized closely by all for evidence of 'quality'.

Step 11. Error cause removal

Crosby's 14 steps for total quality management

1	Commitment
2	Quality improvement team
3	Measurement
4	Cost of quality
5	Awareness
6	Corrective action
7	Zero defects planning
8	Education
9	Zero defects day
10	Goal setting
11	Error cause removal
12	Recognition
13	Quality councils
14	Do it all over again

Purpose: to give the individual employee a method of communicating to management the situations that make it difficult to meet the pledge to improve

This was another step that was regarded initially as an unnecessary bureaucratic venture by the QIT and disregarded in the initial stages of implementation. At this time, problems were commonly being identified through the training courses, and the corrective action system ensured these were dealt with. As time progressed, two major problems of using only these methods were identified.

First, the problems being identified and resolved tended to be small scale, of the kind that could be resolved within a discipline or department. These were extremely important but there was a notable lack of the organization-wide problems that we all intuitively knew existed (e.g. the inability of the portering and pharmacy service to meet demand, lack of car-parking space, waiting list length and times, and so on). As a result, there was a noted absence of corrective action teams at a senior level, and a paucity of success stories in comparison to those arising from lower down the organization.

The second problem was that once the educational courses stopped there was no method to enable staff to refer problems to the quality improvement team. The corrective action system is designed to involve staff in solving work problems for processes that they can influence. Staff identified numerous hassles in their daily work which were not appropriate for them to feed into this system, as they were not involved personally in the specific process that was creating the difficulty.

The error cause removal system is designed to address these problems. It involves the completion of a simple form, which states, 'The following situation is making my job difficult because . . .' or 'The following idea could improve the quality of service in the hospital . . .'.

This form is then sent to the error cause removal step sponsor on the QIT, who initiates the series of events necessary to resolve these. This enables every individual within the organization to raise problems that will be directed to the appropriate individuals who can effect a solution.

Major reservations were expressed about the ability of the QIT to deal with the potential workload of such a system. A visit to an industrial company ten years into the quality improvement process showed one team dealing with up to 100 suggestions in one week, and a requirement that all slips received were acknowledged and action arising cited to the initiator within 48 hours. Key factors identified in achieving these requirements were: (1) commitment from senior managers (i.e. they allocated time and resources to make the system work); and (2) the effective establishment of the other steps in creating the culture where such a system can work.

Parallels were drawn with the 'suggestions box' initiative that had been tried in a number of areas with limited impact. Traditionally, two things would typically happen if such a system was introduced without the support of the other 13 steps identified by Crosby. One option is that nothing would happen, because staff will not use a system in which they have no confidence. The other is that a few staff will try the system to see what happens. The absence of a clearly thought-out method for dealing with the forms when they are received leads to two scenarios. One is a defensive exercise to identify either the initiator of the form to argue that no such problem really exists; the other approach is characterized by the manager acknowledging the problem and seeking out the individual who they perceive is responsible for it arising in the first place. Both send negative messages to staff and preclude the use of such systems.

The introduction of error cause removal is the final step in the jigsaw in the quality improvement process. For it to work effectively, the other steps must be firmly in place. When working effectively, it offers something no other quality initiative can – the ability of every employee to access the quality improvement system, with the knowledge that appropriate actions will be taken to resolve the problem.

Step 13. Quality councils

Crosby's 14 steps for total quality management

1	Commitment
2	Quality improvement team
3	Measurement
4	Cost of quality
5	Awareness
6	Corrective action
7	Zero defects planning
8	Education
9	Zero defects day
10	Goal setting
11	Error cause removal
12	Recognition
13	**Quality councils**
14	Do it all over again

Purpose: to bring together the appropriate people to share quality management information on a regular basis

Crosby cites the need for individuals with expertise in the quality improvement process to meet regularly to review the approach and generate new ideas. He notes the contribution many former QIT members can make as a result of their experience. In practice, this step was never implemented because in the initial stages all those with quality management information were heavily involved in the implementation process.

Step 14. Do it all over again

Crosby's 14 steps for total quality management

1	Commitment
2	Quality improvement team
3	Measurement
4	Cost of quality

5 Awareness

6 Corrective action

7 Zero defects planning

8 Education

9 Zero defects day

10 Goal setting

11 Error cause removal

12 Recognition

13 Quality councils

14 Do it all over again

Purpose: to emphasize that the quality improvement process is continuous
This step is self-explanatory but nonetheless essential. It was important that the quality improvement team created a new action plan on a yearly basis to develop previous work, and maintained the momentum of the quality improvement process. In a rapidly changing sociological/political/economic climate, the requirements of the service are in a constant state of flux, and therefore in need of continual review. From this perspective, the quality improvement process is never-ending. Such constant change differentiates this approach from that of other initiatives or 'flavour of the month' approaches to managing quality – it is not a project or a programme, but a never-ending process.

General observations and key learning points from the case study

As a result of close involvement in the implementation of the quality improvement process, the following observations are made, based on a personal perspective of the impact of introducing such an approach into a hospital environment. There are several important factors to consider when reaching conclusions for this specific approach. First, although the framework adopted followed the Crosby 14-step process, this was somewhat anachronistically applied, which undoubtedly created many difficulties. There is a clear recommendation that the whole process should start at the top of the organization and be cascaded down. In practice, a major management restructuring several months into the process meant this did not occur. This posed difficulties for the QIT in the case study, predominantly a lack of clear direction from the steering committee, the constitution of which also changed several months into the process. This meant that systems such as corrective action and error cause removal were not ready at the point when the QIT needed to begin to use them.

The second deviation from the Crosby approach occurred in the use of their educational courses. In this QIT only three out of the eventual 13 members attended the Crosby quality improvement course to prepare them for their role in the implementation process. Approximately 40 staff attended the 'individual' educational course and 120 attended the work group course, at which point the external funding for the pilot site ceased. The percentages in the other QITs were significantly lower than these. It is impossible to draw specific conclusions about the overall impact of educational materials, since two of the key implementation methods were never realized.

It also raises a sombre message about securing adequate funding at the outset of the implementation process. In the case study, the loss of funding created a serious dip in morale for both the team and the course facilitators. It occurred when many of the initial hurdles had been overcome, and benefits were just starting to be realized. What was encouraging was that the team were sufficiently convinced of the benefits of this approach to resolve to continue, and to explore ways of circumnavigating the funding difficulties. This would have been inconceivable 18 months previously, because commitment to the approach and the knowledge base of staff were lacking.

Key learning points for particular steps are outlined in the text. Although these are derived from the use of the Crosby approach to TQM, many can be extended to the wide range of approaches outlined at the beginning of this chapter.

The need for an overall implementation framework

It is common for those charged with the task of implementing TQM within an organization to feel overwhelmed by the scale of the process. A major problem identified in the case study was that many texts explore TQM concepts, but very few give definitive ideas about practising TQM within a healthcare setting. As a result, there is a danger of falling into the 'paralysis by analysis' trap in the initial stages of implementation. In our experience, this was typified by long debates over terminology and 'refining' some of the tools and techniques before using them.

The major advantage of creating a structure for implementation, be it the 14 steps or another framework, is that it offers those with the responsibility of introducing TQM a clear path to follow. The quality improvement team in the case study proved to be invaluable in focusing the thoughts of members on actions rather than philosophical debates.

It is strongly recommended that whatever framework is adopted, the best course of action is to begin it and, if necessary, to modify the approach while going along. In the early stages of the project, there was strong pressure to cut out certain aspects and add in others. The key lesson learned in our attempts to customize the approach is not to take out any of the bricks before being clear on why they are there. For example, prior to understanding the process there were suggestions that some of the steps (notably corrective action and error cause removal) were unnecessary and could be dropped. It was not until we were much further into the process that the importance of these was recognized, necessitating a hasty implementation, after a break in the continuity of implementation.

It is important to incorporate a local flavour to the approach and, in practice, we found this was best managed at QIT level rather than further up the organization. There was a marked difference in teams' views on steps such as recognition, based on their local knowledge.

The need for a comprehensive educational programme

In our experience, the educational step, once cascaded throughout the hospital, was an essential factor in generating the desired cultural change. One problem was the tendency for managers to make assumptions about the ability of their staff to understand tools and techniques. In practice, many of these staff used these tools far more than the managers, as they found them a useful method of identifying and resolving problems in a new way.

Time spent on piloting and modifying courses, training local facilitators to a high standard and on staff education reaped dividends. Attempts to cut costs by modifying this step would inevitably cause problems.

The need to evaluate the TQM approach

Faced with a project of this scale, methods for formal evaluation may fall low on the list of priorities. The difficulty arises when funding is restricted and objective measures of improvement would prove beneficial. Evaluating such a sizeable project, and attempting to control the myriad of variables, is something that defies the bounds of a traditional clinically controlled trial. Faced with all these pressures, the offers from external sources to help in the evaluation process can appear extremely inviting. Based on our experiences, we recommend caution in adopting these offers without careful consideration of the following factors. First, establish the motives for the offer, which may not always be explicit in the initial contact. Some of the 'surveys' that were circulated to us promising feedback on various approaches were, in fact, generated from rival consultancy firms with an interest in TQM. Apart from the danger of bias in such studies, it is worth considering that information supplied is likely to be more lucrative to the recipient (the rival company) than feedback to those who partook in the initial questionnaire.

Second, it is worth critiquing the proposed research design and the amount of time and effort required by local staff before becoming involved in external evaluations. Some of us were disconcerted by the use of what were, quite clearly, shorthand-style notes being taken throughout personal interviews in one study, rather than tape-recording or writing out the interview verbatim. If staff are to be released for such interviews, it is important that a robust method is used to make participation worthwhile. Another difficulty can arise if researchers are travelling considerable distances. In one instance this led to a request for a large number of a representative cross-section of staff to be interviewed in one day. Given the clinical commitments of the majority of staff, this was very difficult to organize and, in retrospect, the use of staff who could attend, rather than those who should attend, did not give a representative sample.

The timing and appropriateness of interview schedules or questionnaires used by researchers is also worth reviewing. In one study it was not apparent until after staff had been exposed to questioning that the researchers were seeking staff views on benefits seen as a result of using the Crosby method. Many of the staff interviewed had only very recently become involved in the TQM project; many had not completed the relevant courses; and the QITs had only recently been formed. It was therefore inappropriate for staff to be expected to contribute meaningful material at this stage, as it was too early for any objective benefits to be appreciated by staff who had yet to be involved in the work.

Several advantages and disadvantages were observed while implementing the quality improvement process. These were as follows.

- **Advantage: breaking down professional and hierarchical barriers.** The multidisciplinary nature of the quality improvement team did much to improve communication and understanding between the different disciplines. This was particularly noted as part of the educational courses throughout all levels of the organization, where staff gained insight into colleagues' roles and responsibilities, often for the first time. This undoubtedly helped to break down barriers, as staff tended to become more sympathetic to the difficulties of other groups and endeavoured to help them solve their work problems.
- **Advantage: beginning the process of changing from a finger-pointing culture.** The major advantage in adopting the tools and techniques in this approach was that it focused the staff's attention on aspects of the work process where requirements were not being met (or were not established) rather than on the traditional approach of blaming errors on specific individuals. This process of depersonalizing problems proved a useful method of reducing the conflict when staff attempted to resolve them.
- **Advantage: providing a 'common language' for communicating quality.** This original claim, by those advocating the Crosby approach, was met with some scepticism by many staff. However, as more staff undertook the course, it was noticeable how the phrases initially criticized as jargon had slipped into the general vocabulary. The advantage of terms like 'non-conformance', 'requirements', etc. is that, once staff have been educated as to their meaning, they are understood by all. The widespread use of the same tools (such as the process model worksheet and measurement charts) by all departments and professional groups also provided a valuable uniform approach to addressing problems. In an area such as healthcare, littered with confusing terminology, it is interesting to note the amount of resistance that exists to 'non-health' terminology. The important lesson learned was that the term itself was less important than its universal interpretation. For example, one would not refuse to use 'computerized axial tomography' purely because the name of the tool is complicated. The important thing is to understand what the machine is used for. The name may be shortened to 'CAT scan', as this is more user friendly, but this does not detract from the staff's

understanding of its purpose. So it is for terms such as 'zero defects'. The important thing is the benefit of the tool, rather than the term itself. The latter can be changed to suit local needs if necessary, but it would be foolhardy to discard a useful tool on the basis of its name alone.

- **Advantage: providing a systematic approach for managing quality.** This approach offered an umbrella under which to pull all of the different quality initiatives and ensure they were managed in a systematic way. This is the big advantage of using the quality improvement process, as its ability to encompass all the activities and individuals within an organization offers far-reaching benefits for all customers and suppliers.
- **Disadvantage: threat of change.** The implementation of the quality improvement process can prove threatening because it implies criticism of traditional management methods. The implementation structure requires those most sensitive to these criticisms to throw their full weight behind the changes. The whole process of empowering staff can also be interpreted as an undermining of the position power of the line manager, and it is a power some are unhappy to relinquish. It can, therefore, prove an uncomfortable process for some individuals.
- **Disadvantage: raising customer expectations.** Going public on the organizational commitment to TQM undoubtedly raises the expectations of internal and external customers. This can be a disadvantage if the mechanisms are not in place to ensure they can be met.
- **Disadvantage: substantial initial investment before returns are realized.** All the authors in this field emphasize that TQM is a long-term investment. Full implementation can take up to five years, and the process must be ongoing if the benefits are to be sustained. Those who view this as a short-term initiative and expect immediate results will be disappointed. In consequence, a significant initial financial investment is required, with no visible financial returns for several years.

CONCLUSIONS REGARDING THE USE OF THE CROSBY METHOD OF TQM

Our intention was not to critique the finer philosophical points of one approach to TQM over another. This would be unfair in the absence of hands-on experience of more than one approach. For this reason, conclusions can be drawn on only the Crosby approach.

From a purely practical perspective, as a result of using this method, we believe it to be a comprehensive system that is flexible enough to be adapted for use in hospitals. However, using the expertise of committed personnel from within the hospital is a key factor in adapting it to a healthcare environment.

On re-reading the works of other leaders in this field (notably Deming, Juran, Koch and Shaw) we find some common themes:

- the need for management commitment and leadership;
- the need to empower workers;
- the need to establish clear requirements or specifications, and meet these every time;
- the value of breaking down the work process into a number of identifiable steps and using the increased understanding gained during the process to find and eliminate quality problems;
- focusing on the prevention of problems or errors;
- utilizing statistical techniques;
- recognition that quality is a never-ending process.

These similarities (and other clear differences) can be confusing to those attempting to select one system, or a combination of several, for implementation. A framework for evaluating and selecting a quality improvement process has been developed by Fine and Bridge (1987), based on three dimensions:

- **Decision rules and decision tools.** These examine the three issues: (1) cost of quality; (2) direct (physical) measures of quality; and (3) revenue and cost of quality and their value in specific type of organizations.
- **Managerial style.** This is defined as 'the philosophy behind the management of the human resources of the firm'. In essence, this is divided into authoritarian and participative styles. It explores the underlying management theories of Deming, Crosby and Juran, and their adaptability under different organizational styles of management.
- **The management of the transition to TQM.** This examines the theoretical basis of the specific approach by referring to the theories of organizational change.

Using the above framework to analyse the Crosby approach, its creators drew the following conclusions:

- First, that the Crosby approach presents a management style that is predominantly authoritarian but has some participative elements. All employees are told what is expected of them, but they have input into identifying and solving problems. Because of this, the Crosby process can accommodate a range of management styles.
- Second, that the Crosby process could be viewed as 'a classic example of how to manage transition' (Bridge, 1984). The 14-step programme meets almost every criterion set by Beckhard and Harris (1977) for managing complex changes in organizations.

The purpose of utilizing the above framework is to allow the selection of an approach that best meets the specific individualized need of the organization. For example, it has been observed that organizations that are predominantly authoritarian may have difficulty in adopting the managerial style advocated in some of the TQM approaches (Fine and Bridge, 1987).

In conclusion, by far the most important factor in adopting this whole process is the realization by senior managers that TQM is worthwhile, and their decision to commit themselves to adopting its principles. Once this has been decided, the selection of the methods used becomes an essential, but nevertheless academic, argument about which specific approach (or the decision to use an eclectic model) offers the best method for their organization.

TQM in context

In the introduction to this chapter, we introduced total quality management as an organizational framework for improving quality. As health professionals, we found much of the jargon confusing when it came to reviewing organizational frameworks for supporting healthcare professionals in improving their clinical work. This was not assisted by the fact that many approaches are launched as a wonderful new solution or radical new approach. This has had the misfortune of causing many such initiatives to be labelled as 'flavour of the month' and has generated a considerable amount of cynicism. Having reviewed a number of organizational approaches to quality improvement, we conclude that many are less about radical reinvention than a natural evolution of what has gone before. We find it easier to understand them in context by viewing them along a spectrum, as shown in Figure 6.6.

Using the industrial models, in the early days of production, particularly in the post-war era, the emphasis was very much on *produce, deliver and react*, i.e. the goods were made with little attention to quality assurance. They were delivered, and if things went wrong then the company would react retrospectively to put it right. As competition increased, customers became dissatisfied with such an approach and it became necessary for companies to address the problem. They did this through quality control, which is essentially about monitoring the endpoint of production. A great deal of effort therefore went into inspecting the finished product or service before it went to the customer but after it had been made.

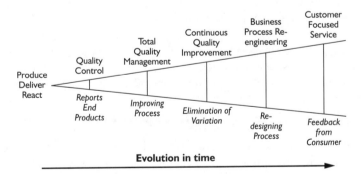

Figure 6.6

The development of approaches to quality in industry (used with the permission of Philip Crosby Associates II, Inc. All Rights reserved, www.philipcrosby.com)

335

For many years in industry, quality control and quality assurance systems based on this kind of inspection and revision were common. Even now, they form the basis of quality management in many companies. However, although quality control has some advantages, it also has some important limitations, namely:

- It is retrospective, so it does not stop mistakes being made; it finds mistakes only after they have happened and then corrects them, which is less efficient and more costly than preventing any mistakes from occurring in the first place.
- It creates a culture within the organization which says that mistakes are an inevitable part of the manufacturing or service process, and that a certain level of mistakes is acceptable. This does not encourage people to try to do better.
- It puts responsibility for ensuring the quality of the product on those inspecting the work, not on the people who actually make the product or provide the service. This makes people think that mistakes do not matter too much because the inspectors will always pick them up.
- There is a tendency to end up with more inspectors, although this does not necessarily mean they are any more effective at detecting mistakes. There is a danger that each quality inspector assumes that any mistakes they miss will be picked up elsewhere.
- Quality control by inspection creates a 'them and us' culture in which the inspectors are the quality police out to detect and punish mistakes. In this kind of atmosphere, mutual trust and good morale are difficult or even impossible to create and maintain.
- Quality control and quality assurance are very expensive. Not only are there costs of fixing the mistakes (which could have been prevented), there are also the costs of employing quality inspectors.

This is not to say there is no place at all for quality inspection in healthcare. However, it is only one of a number of ways to approach quality improvement. There are significant disadvantages if used in isolation. Primarily, of course, in healthcare, once a mistake has been made the fact that we are dealing with people rather than products means that our mistakes are much less easy to put right. Interestingly, as in industry, any attempts at quality assurance focuses on the quality control element. Emphasis is placed on managing complaints, into which considerable health service resources are diverted. There are no available figures for comparison with preventative activity.

'Prevention' is the key word of the total quality management approach. Hence, the emphasis shifts from just looking at fixing things when they have gone wrong to seeking to understand what is problematic about the way in which work is organized but can be improved. The emphasis of TQM is, therefore, on understanding work processes and identifying and resolving problems within them.

Fast on the heels of total quality management came a new buzzword, 'continuous quality improvement'. This builds on many of the principles of TQM, and many of the tools and techniques are similar. There is a subtle distinction in the two approaches: we would observe that TQM is about *doing the same things better* (normally by identifying and reducing variation in the process) whereas CQI builds on this slightly by focusing not just on organizational problems and reducing error but on seeking new and creative ways of working which will be of benefit to the customer. In CQI, all processes (even those working well) are believed to be capable of further improvement. Indeed, new processes that have previously not been thought of may be needed.

It is perhaps inevitable, therefore, that the next evolution of organizational approaches to quality improvement shifts from *doing the same things better* to *doing different things*. In the new high-tech industries such as computing, with their rapid rate of change, the incremental approach was clearly insufficient. For many organizations facing massive turbulent change, equally dramatic approaches were required to ensure they retain their commercial edge. It could be argued that in healthcare, too, change is now so rapid that slow and incremental approaches to improving services are no longer sufficient. Indeed, the White Paper *The New NHS: Modern, Dependable* (NHS Executive, 1997, p. 11) places emphasis on forging new partnerships across health, social services and other organizations as a way of 'doing things differently'. In industry, business process re-engineering is the latest of such organizational approaches to evolve. Business process re-engineering has been defined as 'the fundamental re-thinking and radical design of business processes to achieve dramatic improvements in critical, contemporary measures of performance, such as cost, quality, service and speed' (Hammer and Champney, 1993).

This definition contains three key words:

- **Fundamental.** In undertaking re-engineering, managers must ask the most basic questions about their organization and how it operates, namely: 'Why do we do what we do?' and 'Why do we do it the way we do?' Asking these questions forces people to look at the underlying assumptions about the way in which they organize and carry out their work. Often these assumptions turn out to be obsolete and inappropriate. Re-engineering begins with no assumptions; in fact, organizations that undertake re-engineering must guard against the assumptions that most processes already have embedded into them. For example, to ask 'How can we improve a centralized admissions service?' assumes we *need* a centralized admissions service. Re-engineering first determines *what* an organization must do; then *how* to do it. Re-engineering takes nothing for granted, it ignores what *is* and concentrates on what *should be*.
- **Radical.** The word 'radical' is derived from the Latin *radics* meaning 'root'. Radical redesign means getting to the root of things, not making superficial changes or fiddling with what is already in place but throwing away the old. In re-engineering, radical redesign means disregarding all existing structures and procedures and inventing completely new ways of accomplishing work. Re-engineering is about organizational process *re-invention*, not organization improvement or organization enhancement.

- **Dramatic.** Re-engineering is not about making marginal incremental improvement, but is about achieving quantum leaps in performance. If a hospital underperforms by a small margin (e.g. measurement of quality standards show 3% underperformance), the hospital does not need re-engineering. More conventional methods, from motivating and encouraging staff to establishing incremental quality programmes, can facilitate the limited improvements needed. Re-engineering should be brought in only when a need exists for 'heavy blasting'. Marginal improvement requires fine tuning; dramatic improvement demands blowing up the old and replacing it with something new.

Re-engineering can be summed up in two words: starting again. Re-engineering is about beginning again with a clean sheet of paper. It is about rejecting the conventional wisdom and assumptions of the past and about inventing new approaches to process structure which bear little or no resemblance to those of previous eras (Hammer and Champney, 1993).

Hence, it can be appreciated that such organizational approaches have evolved from each other, with many of them using common tools and techniques. As with the differing frameworks for documentation outlined in Chapter 2, it is important to pick the right one for the purpose for which it is intended. Hence for health-care organizations seeking a small increase in performance, business process re-engineering would be like using a sledgehammer to crack a nut. Conversely, an organization seeking dramatic improvements and radically new ways of operating would not get the results it requires from quality control. Some healthcare organizations have used such approaches as an attempt to provide an organizational framework for improving the quality of the service they provide. The next chapter explores one geared specifically to health rather than derived from industry – explains the theory and uses a case study of an application in an NHS Trust.

REFERENCES

Beckhard, R. and Harris R.T. (1977) *Organisational Transitions: Managing Complex Change*, Addison Wesley, Reading, MA.

Berwick, D.M., Glanton, G.A. and Roessner, J. (1990) *Curing Health Care: New Strategies for Quality Improvement*, Jossey Bass, San Francisco.

Bridge, D.E. (1984) The role of managerial accounting in quality improvement programmes. Master's thesis, Sloan School of Management, MIT, Cambridge, MA.

BS 4778 (1987) *Quality Vocabulary: Part 1 – International Terms (ISO 8402 (1986)*, HMSO, London.

Crosby, P.B. (1967) *Cutting the Cost of Quality*, USA Quality College Bookstore, Orlando, FL.

Crosby, P.B. (1972) *The Art of Getting Your Own Sweet Way*, McGraw-Hill, New York.

Crosby, P.B. (1979) *Quality Is Free*, McGraw-Hill, New York.

Crosby, P.B. (1984) *Quality Without Tears*, McGraw-Hill, New York.

Crosby, P.B. (1986) *Running Things: The Art of Making Things Happen*, McGraw-Hill, New York.

Crosby, P.B. (1988) *The Eternally Successful Organisation: The Art of Corporate Wellness*, McGraw-Hill, New York.

Crosby, P.B. (1989) Quality Education System for the Individual, The Creative Factory, Crosby Quality College, London

Crosby, P.B. (1990) *Leading: The Art of Becoming an Executive*, McGraw-Hill, New York.

Crosby, P.B. (1991) Quality Improvement Process Management College (course material), The Creative Factory, Winter Park, FL.

Deming, W.E. (1982) *Quality, Productivity and Competitive Position*, MIT Center for Advanced Engineering Study, Cambridge, MA.

Deming, W.E. (1986) *Out of the Crisis*, MIT Center for Advanced Engineering Study, Cambridge, MA.

Department of Health (1989) *Working for Patients*, HMSO, London.

Feigenbaum, A.V. (1983) *Total Quality Control*, 3rd edn, McGraw-Hill, New York.

Fine, C.H. and Bridge, D.H. (1987) *Quest for Quality: Managing the Total System*, Institute of Industrial Engineers, Industrial Engineering and Management Press, New York.

Hammer, M. and Champney, J. (1993) *Reengineering the Corporation: A Manifesto for Business Revolution*, Nicholas Brealey Publishing, London.

Hayward, J. (1996) Promoting clinical effectiveness. *British Medical Journal*, 15, 1491–2.

Hibbs, P. (1988) *Pressure Area Care for the City and Hackney Health Authority*, City and Hackney Health Authority, London.

Ishikawa, K. (1976) *Guide to Quality Control*, Asian Productivity Organisation, Tokyo.

Ishikawa, K. (1985) *What is Total Quality Control? Tthe Japanese Way*, Prentice-Hall, Englewood Cliffs, NJ.

Juran, J.M. (1988) *Juran on Planning for Quality*, The Free Press, New York.

Juran, J.M. and Gryna, F.M. (1980) *Quality Planning and Analysis*, 2nd edn, McGraw-Hill, New York.

Koch, H.C.H. and Chapman, E.H. (1991) Planning for high quality care. *International Journal of Health Care Quality Assurance*, 4(6), 10–18.

Koch, H.C.H. (1991a) Quality of care and service. *Managing Service Quality*, July, 1–5.

Koch, H.C.H. (1991b) Obstacles to total quality in health care. *International Journal of Health Care Quality Assurance*, 4(3), 30–2.

Mortiboys, R.J. (1990) *Leadership and Total Quality Management: A Guide for Chief Executives*, Department of Trade and Industry/Moore & Matthes Group, London.

NHS Executive (1997) *The New NHS: Modern, Dependable*, Department of Health, London.

Oakland, J.S. (1986) *Statistical Process Control*, Heinemann, London.

Oakland, J.S. (1989) *Total Quality Management*, Heinemann, London.

Shewhart, W.A. (1931) *The Economic Control of Quality of Manufactured Products*. Van Nostrand,

Shingo, S. (1986) *Zero Quality Control: Source Inspection and the Poka-Yoke System*, Press, Stamford, CT.

Taguchi, G. (1979) *Introduction to Off-line Quality Control*, Central Japan Quality Control Association, Magaya, Japan.

Taguchi, G. (1981) *On-line Quality Control During Production*, Japanese Standards Association, Tokyo.

Wilson, C.R.M. (1987) *Hospital-Wide Quality Assurance: Models for Implementation and Development*, Harcourt Brace & Co., London.

7 PATIENT FOCUSED CARE

The previous chapter outlined total quality management and described a case study applying this approach to a hospital in the UK. However, there are a number of other organization-wide approaches to quality improvement in the literature which have been applied in industry and more recently in the health service. These appeared to us to be less about a new and radical approach and more about developing ideas along a continuum where each successive approach drew heavily on elements of its predecessors. This chapter describes one such approach, patient focused care, in more detail and provides a case study of its application in a UK hospital. We have selected patient focused care for further exploration because it has been used extensively in healthcare institutions in the US and was introduced into four UK hospital pilot sites in 1992.

PATIENT FOCUSED CARE: WHAT IS IT?

Patient focused care is a model of healthcare delivery based around the needs of the patient. Its proponents are critical of traditional models of healthcare delivery, which they cite as being geared more to the hospital structures and convenience of the professional groups than to the needs of the patient. The literature abounds with examples of patients confused by the 'sea of faces' (Langan, 1993a) as they meet up to 60 different staff for a short episode in hospital; delays in service delivery as a result of processes that seem unnecessarily complex (e.g. 62 process steps and 12 staff involved in one patient X-ray); and a bewildering bureaucracy for those attempting to secure healthcare across institutional boundaries as they move between primary, secondary and social care.

The term 'patient focused care' is attributed to the pioneering work undertaken at the Lakeland Medical Centre in Florida from 1988 onwards. This established decentralized operational units with their own support services, refocused services closer to the patient and established multiskilled care teams who were responsible for small numbers of patients. Patient care pathways were developed and unitary patient documentation (i.e. one patient record used by all professionals) was also central to this approach.

There are a number of definitions of patient focused care (PFC) from various parts of the globe, predominantly the USA, UK and Australia, where PFC has been implemented. These include Booz-Allen and Hamilton's (1990) description of 'involving moving clinical services closer to patients, the creation of small autonomous work teams, refocusing the hospital to support and empower staff providing clinical care'.

What is the difference between TQM and PFC?

It is helpful to pause at this point and examine whether there are similarities and differences between TQM and PFC, to clarify understanding of what each approach entails. This may interest those who followed the TQM route who are now looking with bemusement at the PFC approach, as well as those who took the latter approach and who may have viewed TQM as passé. The comparison of PFC and TQM may also be useful for those seeking some kind of organizational framework to develop quality who, after wading through the myriad of different approaches to organization-wide methods purporting to offer radical solutions to managing quality in healthcare, are confused (as we were) by the jargon, and wonder whether the latest flavour of the month (as many of us cynically viewed such initiatives) could really be the panacea they seek.

Some writers compare the different perspectives of initiatives such as TQM and continuous quality improvement (CQI) against business process re-engineering and patient focused care as follows (Moffit and Galloway, 1992):

> *Four blind men were walking through the country one day when they confronted a large object. The first, feeling that it was long and round, said it was a snake. The second felt it was very large and round and rough. He claimed he had stumbled upon a tree. The third said the object must be a vine because it was very narrow and long. The fourth described it as a fan that waved in the air. Finally, the guide, who could see the whole picture, arrived and told them they had found an elephant.*

They make a distinction between one kind of approach which concentrates on a study of the parts (TQM/CQI) and seeks to continuously improve current processes, and other approaches (BPR/PFC) which examine and radically redesign the whole. Others blur this distinction by arguing that TQM is also about whole systems rather than a sum of the parts. For example, Deming's approach to TQM, outlined in the previous chapter, stresses that the overall system rather than individual functions must be optimized. Some functions may even need to be suboptimized for the greater good of the whole system. The raison d'être of both TQM and patient focused care is to satisfy customers by optimizing the whole system. However, Deming suggests, the latter is impossible to do if an organization attempts to do this 'one bit at a time'.

Moffit and Galloway (1992, p. 3) observe that in highly compartmentalized organizations (such as hospitals) the culture and reward systems encourage empire building. Staff can be disinclined to adopt a solution that suboptimizes or reduces the size of their functional areas of responsibility. This (they say), coupled with the hierarchy inherent within and across professional groups, can mean that anything that threatens professional identity is met with resistance. They argue that functional importance takes a back seat to customer satisfaction and system optimization if the proposed change (although logical in terms of patient care) means that one area 'wins' and another 'loses', using the old methods of measuring power and value.

They cite key differences between TQM and PFC as follows. TQM attempts to 'eat the elephant one bite at a time', and this incremental approach leads to a problem focus rather than an improvement focus. Hence one concentrates on the tail or the trunk, rather than the whole elephant. They express concerns that with TQM, deep-rooted resistance to structural change and the achievement of its associated benefits can be cloaked in compromise for the reasons listed in the previous paragraph, which are inherent within the organizational culture. This is a slightly different perspective from Deming, who does, in fairness, stress the importance of examining the whole. However, it would seem that Moffit and Galloway's perception of TQM is based on their own observations of the application of TQM in practice, rather than the theory, i.e. whatever the textbooks say about the principles of TQM being a whole systems approach, their experience has led them to conclude that in practice it tends to address incremental improvement rather than a radical redesign of the whole system.

Moffit and Galloway believe that by implementing both TQM and PFC, synergies and opportunities not open to those adopting one or the other approach are opened up. PFC, through its restructuring of patients into new units and redesigning traditional approaches, advances past the problem-focused stage beyond which some TQM programmes never develop. However, if one views PFC as a one-time quick fix, there will be no infrastructure to support a cycle of continuous quality improvement, and it would be a rare organization that redesigns everything and does this right first time. Even if work processes were improved, inevitably there will be changes in service requirements which will necessitate the need for further review and change. This is where TQM and other continuous quality improvement and problem-solving programmes can help.

The purist view of PFC in the literature reviews does indeed emphasize radical restructuring as fundamental to this approach. There is overlap with business process re-engineering (BPR), outlined in the last chapter. At a simplistic level, patient focused care could, we feel, be described as the healthcare version of business process re-engineering. A number of hospitals in the UK have embarked on what they are describing as BPR programmes, including Leicester Royal Infirmary and Kings Healthcare (who call their initiative 'transformation') (Bevan, Cullen and Windess, 1997). In spite of the different terms used, many of these approaches share a similar philosophy, use similar tools and techniques, and work on similar issues (e.g. redesigning clinical care processes; reviewing and changing staff roles; and seeking to improve patient outcomes). The principles of PFC are outlined below, along with a commentary on the application of these principles into practice, based on the author's experience of implementing these in one of the four UK PFC pilot sites.

Central components of patient focused care

The literature highlights the following components of PFC:

- patient care groupings and operating units
- decentralization (process, physical redesign)
- multiskilling staff

- teamwork
- enhanced patient autonomy and decision making
- process redesign (including both clinical and non-clinical processes)
- reducing costs

These are explored below, along with a case study of how each of these were implemented in an acute NHS Trust in the UK. Demographic information about the Trust in the case study is outlined in Chapter 5.

Patient groups and operating units

A key principle of PFC is the structure of clinical units and the patients they house. This falls into two categories; first, the principle of decentralizing services, and, second, the characteristics of patients in the new units. These will now be examined.

Decentralizing services

In much of the literature from the USA, the evolving healthcare system was severely criticized for its centralist approach to service delivery. The forerunner of the patient focused care work at the Lakeland Regional Medical Centre identified that much of the difficulty in controlling costs and quality stemmed from the fact that hospitals have become highly specialized and fragmented (compartmentalized) organizations (Watson *et al.*, in Clouten and Weber, 1994). Although each of these departments is independently cost effective, a look at the entire organization showed a non-cost-effective system (reinforcing the allegory of the elephant looked at earlier – a case of the whole being less effective than a sum of the parts). They cite that (for example) staff spend a majority of their time scheduling, coordinating and documenting care, rather than actually delivering it. This results in less than ideal care and increases costs. Lathrop states that for each dollar spent on direct medical care, three or four more are spent on 'waiting for it to happen, arranging to do it and writing it down'. He estimates that 75% of staffing costs for simple patient procedure consists of structural idle time (Lathrop, in Clouten and Weber, 1994). The examples of decentralization in the literature vary, including the complete devolvement of pharmacy, radiology, pathology and other support services into smaller care centres so they are closer to the point of service delivery. The inpatient, outpatient and diagnostic and therapeutic services are therefore grouped together in one geographical location.

The second category for decentralizing services centres on the characteristics of patients in the new units. This is described below.

Patient groupings

A key principle of PFC is grouping together patients who have similar diagnoses and needs. For larger hospitals, Moffit and colleagues (1993, cited in Mang, 1995) suggest that the optimal size would be 75–100 beds so as 'to create enough critical mass to allow the units to be managed as stand-alone entities with a minimal amount of shared services'.

In the UK, there are conflicting recommendations in the literature about the size of patient focused care units. The optimum size seems to depend on the care group and the number of localized services. The literature does agree, however, that underoccupied patient focused care units are wasteful. Further empirical work in patient groupings and unit size is needed. The literature is also unclear about the space needed for patient focused care hospitals. Space depends on whether centralized diagnostic and treatment services remain alongside new satellite services (Hurst, 1995, pp. 3–4).

Reviewing patient groupings will challenge the way in which patients are currently grouped together, e.g. hospitals that group all patients over 65 into elderly care units on the basis of age rather than care needs; or grouping women together in units where some may be undergoing a termination of pregnancy while others are waiting for delivery, i.e. on the basis of gender rather than care needs. The importance of establishing the most appropriate patient groupings can be appreciated, although in reality they are often based on historical factors rather than sensitivity to patient needs.

Under the regrouped system, instead of having staff providing care for a range of patients with differing problems, the caregivers on each unit develop expertise in caring for the specific needs of that particular grouping of patients. The assumption is that this leads to higher-quality care as expertise develops (Mang, 1995).

Process for reviewing patient groupings in case study
The background summary of the NHS Trust used in the case study is outlined at the beginning of Chapter 5. It was one of the four original pilot sites for PFC which were funded by the Department of Health in 1992 (later expanded to nine). The Trust adopted the term 'integrated patient care' (IPC) in place of 'patient focused care', largely because the latter term invoked negative reactions from the clinical staff at the implied assumption that what they had been practising to date was not focused on caring for patients. The pump-priming monies from the Department of Health were used largely to employ management consultants to advise on the establishment of PFC in the pilot site, and latterly to employ an internal IPC team to take forward this work.

Reviewing patient groupings
The management consultancy held two workshops in early 1993, with a cross-section of staff to review how patients were grouped together for treatment. Following the workshops, 16 new patient groupings were defined. Although the groupings that emerged were discussed at length, it was clear that these remained controversial with clinical staff, and it would be misleading to pretend there was in any way full ownership or consensus for the groupings. By the time the consultancy was completed, the issue was unresolved; so although the roll-out of IPC started in the care centres where agreement was secured for a discrete care centre grouping (namely gastroenterology; obstetrics and neonates; renal and ophthalmology), the big picture of the final configuration and numbers of care centres

Table 7.1

IPC patient care groupings

Vascular	Oncology and Haematology
Cardiac	Respiratory
Digestive diseases	Infectious diseases
Urology	Dermatology and Plastics
Ophthalmic	Trauma, Orthopaedics, Rheumatology
ENT and Oral	Accident and Emergency
Elderly medicine	Paediatrics
Renal	Gynaecology
Endocrine and diabetes	Obstetrics, Midwifery and NICU
Neurosciences and rehabilitation	Breast

Reproduced with the permission of Brighton Health Care NHS Trust.

was put on hold. The groupings were revisited in 1998, with the clinical management team and the board finally agreeing the configuration (Table 7.1). At this point we had reached a critical mass at which it was impossible to proceed with other care centres without addressing the big picture of how the newly configured Trust would function.

In a purist PFC approach, agreeing the patient groupings should have been resolved much sooner. There were a number of reasons why this could not be achieved. First, the resources allocated to the project were insufficient to allow the big bang approach of setting up all the groupings simultaneously. (This was a common phenomenon in other PFC work outside the US, both in the UK and Australia (Hurst, 1995, pp. 3–4; Braithwaite, 1995).) We were fortunate to have secured significant funding for a capital redevelopment scheme which, although not originally linked with the PFC pilot bid, afforded a number of opportunities that enabled us to apply PFC principles to the areas of new development. In spite of the capital funding, this investment was insufficient to achieve the levels of redesign in other sites. Although there were a number of schemes (outlined below) that permitted greater integration, we were unable to develop stand-alone units with satellite radiology, pharmacy and pathology in each. Interestingly though, investment in a vacutube system provided an equally satisfactory alternative, with wards able to send specimens and scripts to the pharmacy and the laboratory. Coupled with developments in IT which enabled results reporting to be accessed on ward PCs, some of the principles and advantages of decentralization could be achieved without actual physical relocation.

Lack of money meant that only limited numbers of staff could be assigned to the IPC project team, and it will be seen from the description later in this chapter that to 'IPC' an area needs significant input from both clinical staff (requiring replacement costs) and a central team to provide support and expertise. Inevitably the speed of roll-out of the project is influenced by the amount of time staff can devote to its implementation.

Second, the principles of good change management are not wholly compatible with a radical change in the way services are delivered. Our approach has been to work alongside clinicians, staff and patients with a philosophy of 'doing with' rather than 'doing to'. There was a delicate balance between challenging the status quo, and risking losing the cooperation of the participants, versus 'going native' and having a good relationship but not retaining a degree of objectivity and challenge. When staff are involved in redesigning their practice, they inevitably bring with them the values and culture of their professions and organizational norms. Dictating radical new practices and imposing them in a top-down approach was an option rejected by the steering group as counterproductive.

Third, the fact that the key professional groups (notably medicine, and to a lesser extent nursing and professions allied to medicine) have a rich and long cultural history inevitably affected how radical any new patient groupings could realistically be. The respective Royal Colleges inevitably focus on professional boundaries and requirements for trainees. We therefore had to be cognisant of this fact when considering how we grouped patients together. Inevitably we were influenced by current medical specialisms. In involving the professionals in redesigning the groupings, it was perhaps not surprising that many advocated maintaining the status quo.

Decentralization

One of the key principles of decentralization is to create a single care centre based on patients with similar needs so that the patient can receive most of, if not all, the required care within the unit. This was achieved by two methods: by ensuring that IPC principles informed the capital redevelopment team and interior design group, and through the IPC diagnostic and design phases that plan and envision the 'ideal' environment in dedicated areas (outlined later in this chapter). The IPC team worked with local sponsors and groups of staff and patients to design the 'ideal' care centres, within the constraints of available resources, for these patient groups.

The groupings in Figure 7.1 created new challenges. Using the US recommendation of 75–100 bedded units as a size sufficient to stand alone, based on our bed numbers we should have been looking for around six or seven IPC centres. The final consensus model identified 22 care centres. The next stage was to review with the clinicians which centres seemed most logically to form natural alliances with others so they could be clustered together to share the decentralized manager, personnel, finance and other central support. Clearly, it was uneconomical to provide these to each individual care centre, as this would significantly increase our management and administration costs – something PFC was supposed to reduce. Work is now being undertaken to reconfigure all the budgets, activity and contracts from our current model of a clinical directorate structure supporting five clinical directorates down to four. Clearly this has significant implications for the current management structure, which at the time of writing is still under revision.

Although this has proved a lengthy, sensitive and very difficult process, there have been significant improvements for some client groups as a result of this

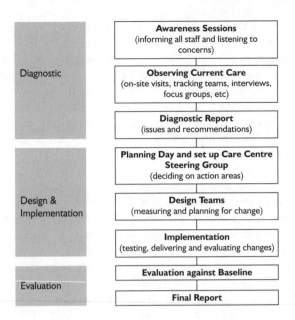

Diagnostic	**Awareness Sessions** (informing all staff and listening to concerns)
	Observing Current Care (on-site visits, tracking teams, interviews, focus groups, etc)
	Diagnostic Report (issues and recommendations)
Design & Implementation	**Planning Day and set up Care Centre Steering Group** (deciding on action areas)
	Design Teams (measuring and planning for change)
	Implementation (testing, delivering and evaluating changes)
Evaluation	**Evaluation against Baseline**
	Final Report

Figure 7.1

Phases of IPC (reproduced with the permission of Brighton Health Care NHS Trust)

approach, most notably for patients with gastrointestinal disease. A radical transformation of gastroenterology services will occur with the opening of the gastroenterology care centre in early 1999. The current service, which is delivered over three sites in 14 possible clinical areas, will be replaced. The new integrated care centre will incorporate both medical and surgical patients, outpatients department, endoscopy and one business centre, all within close proximity to A&E and theatres. There will also be some decentralization of pathology services, which will take place in the care centre.

Another group to benefit from the new care centres and IPC were women and babies requiring obstetric and neonatal care. Prior to IPC in the maternity and neonatology department, inpatient care was provided on the top four floors of a 14-storey tower block. The hospital antenatal clinic was situated on the southeast of the hospital site, a considerable distance away. The fabric of this building was poor. Ultrasound facilities were situated in the main X-ray department, which was geographically distant from the maternity service. The maternity and neonatology IPC steering group set out to design the ideal care centre within the constraints of available resources and space. The service was redesigned to house both antenatal care, labour and postnatal care in one area. Antenatal care was reconfigured to include the relocation of the early pregnancy assessment clinic from A&E, to develop a new foetal assessment unit and to provide decentralized ultrasound facilities on the same floor.

The benefits of these developments include reduction of inpatient stay for some antenatal women and minimizing the need for women to travel some distance to attend the main X-ray department. The incorporation of a birthing pool on the labour ward, en suite toilet facilities and high-dependency rooms has improved both privacy and choice. Additionally the neonatal intensive care unit has expanded, with substantive capital investment to improve the environment vastly. This includes an increase in the parent facilities from one to three bedrooms; increased storage and changing facilities have also been developed, and major refurbishment has been carried out.

Multiskilling and cross-training of staff in special care teams

The third principle of PFC involves multiskilling or cross-training caregivers. The aim of multiskilling is to improve the efficiency and effectiveness of patient care. By broadening and increasing staff responsibilities (e.g. nurses cannulating or undertaking protocol-driven prescribing), the assumption is that continuity of care will increase. One US study estimated that through cross-training 90% of the patient's care needs could be accomplished by the nurses on the floor, and that this led to a 75% reduction in the number of hospital staff the patient may see during his or her stay (Clouten and Weber, 1994, in Mang 1995). This approach challenges why, for example, three different people perform the tasks that one can accomplish: why have one domestic, one porter and one maintenance person, when by cross-training all could undertake cleaning, portering and simple maintenance functions? For example, in the diagnostic phase (outlined later) we found that, for many areas, changing a lightbulb for a patient's bed light required a complex series of process steps and could take days before it was completed. Simple instructions for all staff enable anyone around at the time of need to be able to change the lightbulb immediately.

Multiskilling and cross-training are the most controversial elements of patient focused care. Multiskilling health professionals is not new in the UK, yet many professionals have expressed concern. Some reject the concept of multiskilling despite accusations of protecting their own interests. Criticism from all professional groups is evident, with loss of professional identity being central to their concerns. Nurses, for example, feel that low-status jobs, unwanted by other professionals, will be delegated to them. Professions allied to medicine fear that cost cutting is the main agenda. Others believe that risk to patients and staff from multiskilling is unacceptable (Hurst, 1995, pp. 4–5). It also has implications for training; for example, if nurses undertake all venepuncture and cannulation, the opportunities for junior doctors to acquire these skills are reduced. The latter is a weak argument (Hurst, 1995).

An evaluation of PFC in the UK notes that the evidence supporting multiskilling and cross-training is compelling. Studies comparing staff and patient activity in conventional and patient focused care hospitals show significant financial and qualitative advantages. The way patient focused care enables some clinical staff to jettison administrative work is particularly welcome. Earlier 'before and after' studies in PFC units have generated important findings. They show that diagnostic testing, treatment and care in North American and United Kingdom patient focused care hospitals are transformed by multiskilling (Booz Allen and Hamilton, 1990 in Hurst, 1995, pp. 4–5).

Recognized advantages of multiskilling

Multiskilling and cross-training are cited as worthwhile because:

- many healthcare interventions are readily cross-trained;
- in-service education is efficient and effective;
- much hospital equipment is user friendly;
- integrated care paths suit this new style of care (Hurst, 1995, p. 41).

Cross-training is an important part of reducing the 'sea of faces' experienced by the patient. It is also instrumental in reducing the number of process steps, since staff can provide a broader range of services and/or care, rather than constantly referring to those with expertise. This reduces the time the patient has to wait. Consequently, the UK PFC pilot sites invested heavily in multiskilling educational programmes. Recent literature and survey data from pilot sites do not paint a picture of staff unhappiness in the UK. They do on the other hand suggest that staff are satisfied with patient focused care and do not wish to revert back from it (Hurst, 1995, p. 46).

Multiskilling in one case study

Our approach to multiskilling was to begin the process with a review of all professional roles in the care centre. No prejudgements were made about possible role reconfiguration; it was agreed at the start that the PFC roll-out needed to be grounded in an analysis of the patient's needs in the care centre. A role review involves examining the skills required to deliver a service and how the skills are best provided. With increasing demands placed upon service provision, we needed to re-examine how we did things to ensure efficiency and effectiveness. Role review offered the opportunity to examine and challenge traditional professional boundaries and grades of staff. The methods used in role review varied depending on the service being looked at. However, the following steps were usually undertaken:

- identifying all activities currently undertaken – the 'activity audit';
- identifying who does what;
- thinking about what activities could be undertaken elsewhere;
- identifying what external factors and technologies will affect service provision in future;
- regrouping current and desired activities to form new roles or job descriptions;
- deciding on how many levels of each new role are required;
- identifying and meeting the training implications/needs of new roles;
- auditing the medical legal implications of new roles;
- with reference to activity levels, deciding how many of the changed roles are needed to provide a service, i.e. the dependency ratio;
- identifying the 'best fit' working patterns.

Although this was facilitated by the IPC team (who also conducted the activity audit and analysis), it is important to stress that a high degree of participation from care centre staff was essential both to complete the skills analysis and to help redesign their jobs.

Teamwork
The establishment of small multidisciplinary patient care teams is closely linked with the principle of role review. The teams are created so that the patient has a group of primary caregivers who are 'responsible for managing their needs from preadmission to discharge' (Sidky Barrable and Stewart, 1993, cited in Mang, 1995, p. 429). Two authors report that 'physicians appreciate these teams because they enable them to relate to a small group of people who are well informed about the patient's condition' (Clouten and Weber, 1994, in Mang, 1995). Of greater importance (we feel, given the fundamental philosophy of putting the patient at the centre) was the finding from our research that the patients them-selves placed great importance upon having a team of caregivers who were well informed about their needs and able to deliver these (Hart, 1997).

Although we have undertaken role review in a number of areas, new roles were well developed and established in our obstetrics and neonatology care centre. Two groups of staff were most influenced by the role review exercise: the midwives themselves, and a new role that was developed – that of the care centre assistant.

Care centre assistant
The care centre assistant role was a hybrid of the old domestic, portering and some auxiliary duties. As part of the evaluation, the new care centre assistants were asked about their roles and how they were working in practice. This was done once the roles were well established. All care centre assistants had received a competency-based training programme. Care centre assistants report directly to the IPC care centre manager (a midwife).

Qualitative data were collected by an IPC team facilitator who had not previ-ously been involved with this IPC centre. An open invitation to participate in a focus group was given to all care centre assistants and participants were self-selecting. Two focus groups were formed involving 12 care centre assistants (CCAs) – nine female and three male. This was out of a total of 13 CCAs employed in the care centre and was therefore deemed to be representative. The following issues were raised at the evaluation.

Best features
CCAs particularly liked three key aspects of their new role:

- **Work variety.** The new roles offered a greater range of different duties. Comments included: 'we had set jobs previously and weren't allowed to do anything else' and 'more variety of jobs'. They found this more satisfying. Staff surveys before and after starting this new role showed an increase in satisfaction across a range of different criteria.

- **Working in the same unit.** Staff preferred being allocated to one specific area. It created a stronger sense of feeling valued. Comments included: 'Not being pulled out to work in areas and feeling more involved with the other staff in the unit.'
- **Increased individual responsibility.** Postholders preferred the greater sense of autonomy. Feedback included: 'There are no supervisors, we make our own decisions' and 'don't feel as if we are being watched'.
- **Teamworking.** CCAs felt that they were part of a cohesive team, that they worked well together and supported each other. The changes from the role review had resulted in the CCAs feeling they were now a part of the whole care centre team. 'Sisters and auxiliaries treat you as a person, not as a dogsbody.'
- **Role clarity.** All the CCAs felt they were working to their (up-to-date) job descriptions. They identified that there had been some initial problems when staff had originally taken on the new roles, but these had quickly settled and all were now happy and clear about their duties and responsibilities.
- **Management.** All the CCAs were pleased to have no supervisors. It was felt that most issues could be self-managed; however, there were some conflicts that could not be resolved within the team. All the CCAs knew their line manager and said they would go to them if there was a problem. They also felt the line manager offered good support when they needed it.
- **Training and development.** All CCAs felt they had sufficient training to carry out their roles. Participants had clearly valued initial training which gave them insight into the way a mother might feel following miscarriage or still-birth.

Worst features
The worst features identified concerned the supply of linen, which seemed to be a source of major frustration in CCAs' work.

Team midwifery
The implementation of IPC coincided with the national initiative *Changing Childbirth* (Department of Health, 1993a, b). It was agreed at the beginning of the project to pilot team midwifery. Three teams of midwives were created for a pilot scheme with a variety of geographical locations, caseloads and working practices. Additional training was given to prepare midwives for their new role within community-based teams. A qualitative and quantitative research study was carried out over a period of two years to evaluate the impact of team midwifery on mothers, practitioners and practice (Hart, 1997).

The research showed that the multiskilling facet of team midwifery brought job satisfaction to many midwives. As one participant noted, 'it is brilliant how we get to do so many different things. I never know quite what the day will bring. Nobody could ever say that my job was boring. A daily run of antenatal clinic after antenatal clinic got a bit dull. Now I am up to all sorts; it is the best way for a midwife, the most rewarding way of working you can have' (team midwife interview).

STAFFORDSHIRE UNIVERSITY LIBRARY

However, the research also identified that others felt their skills and experience were inadequate for working in the labour ward. These anxieties ranged from concerns about carrying out specific tasks to feeling unfamiliar with the physical environment, such as where things were and how equipment worked.

Enhanced patient autonomy and decision making

The fifth principle of PFC, enhanced autonomy and decision making, attempts to help staff work in partnership with patients and to get patients more actively involved in making decisions and informed choices about their care. This theme runs through much of the work in the pilot site. The diagnostic phase (explained later) seeks to ascertain from patients through a variety of methods (including questionnaires, focus groups, one-to-one interviews and tracking patients through the system) what they need from the service and how well current services are meeting that need. Patient information, both verbal and written, is reviewed and improved as part of the IPC process. Processes are redesigned to allow greater involvement of the patient and carer where it is found that improvements are needed. The Trust employs a patient's advocate to assist patients who may need help in articulating their needs. The patient's advocate supports them through this process, but (importantly) helps them to do it for themselves. The pilot in obstetrics and midwifery used an action research approach to ensure the views of service users were actively sought and utilized in redesigning the current service (Hart, 1997).

PROCESS REDESIGN: WHAT IS IT?

Process redesign is one of the building blocks for developing IPC (also referred to in the US literature as task simplification). It involves restructuring and redesigning every aspect of giving care, and making the process more efficient. Core processes of care are identified, analysed and redesigned to streamline the delivery of care by reducing the number of process steps and organizing the care around the needs of the patient in order that the patient is truly put at the centre of the service. (For example, analysis of one process identified an X-ray examination as taking 62 process steps and involving 12 staff in a chain of activities.) A variety of methods described later in this chapter are used in the IPC diagnostic and design phases to analyse and redesign core processes. The literature cites numerous examples of how process redesign and decentralization have demonstrated reduced process delays, made more efficient use of staff and created greater autonomy (Hurst, 1995, pp. 3–6). Both clinical and non-clinical processes are included in the review. The former are generally addressed through the development of clinical pathways, guidelines or protocols, detailed in chapters 1 and 2.

Process redesign in many ways afforded us more opportunities than physical redesign, as lack of capital and physical space meant we had to compromise on some of the more ambitious elements of PFC outlined in the American literature (e.g. local pharmacy, X-ray and other services).

Example of redesigning processes in the case study

An example of process redesign is the review of processes in ophthalmology out-patients department and medical records in the Eye Hospital. This review was set up in response to issues identified through the IPC diagnostic phase. In particular there were concerns about patients having to attend the Eye Hospital for post-operative dressings between 7 and 8 a.m.; a number of elderly patients experienced difficulty in getting to the hospital so early. There were also delays in clinics owing to late starts, and clinics were overrunning as a consequence. Medical records staff were suffering low morale and reported dissatisfaction with the way work was organized on a rota system. There were unsatisfactory working practices, with phones not being covered for incoming calls, delays in consultant coding of referral letters and poor tracking of referrals until appointments were made. The physical bottle-neck of patients at the main outpatient entrance resulted in patients frequently standing in a queue for up to ten minutes to be seen at the reception.

In response to these problems, a multidisciplinary redesign team designed and implemented the following changes. Clinic schedules were changed, referral letters were monitored and consultants coded the letters on receipt. If the consultant is absent, then the medical secretaries arrange for another consultant to do the coding. Postoperative patients now attend the ward in the late morning for dress-ings. Dedicated cataract clinics have been set up with one consultant taking the lead. Nurse-led glaucoma clinics are currently being developed. Working prac-tice for medical records clerks has also been examined in a role review exercise. Additionally, two staff are now allocated to the front desk to reduce patients' waiting time. Phones are being covered during working hours and patients are encouraged to phone for appointments after 10 a.m. Substantial investment has been made to expand and redevelop the outpatients department. The floor plans have been examined to identify the best possible flow of patients, materials and information. Signage was reviewed and has significantly improved the flow of patients through the department.

It can be appreciated that many of these changes are not radical, but they have improved patient care. Involving patients and staff in redesigning processes is key to success. It is the users and participants in the service who are best placed to spot where improvements can be made, and to work together to deliver these.

Protocols and integrated records

Care paths go under many names in the NHS. They are not unique to patient focused care but they are important. They are checklists of interventions for ill-nesses and procedures with a separate record indicating if, when and why care has deviated from the expected (Hurst, 1995, p. 5). The national evaluation of PFC sites states that the better care paths are home grown and some patient focused care sites are actively writing and implementing them. However, it is important these are based on empirical evidence and use nationally produced guidelines (such as those from the Royal Colleges). Evaluating care paths is more advanced than evaluating other elements of patient focused care at a national level. The findings

STAFFORDSHIRE 353
UNIVERSITY
LIBRARY

from these evaluations are interesting, not least the key stages for writing and placing care paths successfully (Layton and Morgan, 1994). Care path records that
require all professionals to prescribe and record their care in one document are an
important component of patient focused care. Integrated care paths aim to simplify
healthcare and allow consistency of treatment based on best practice. They link
with clinical audit through 'variance analysis' (i.e. variations in practice from the
care prescribed in the pathway). Integrated care paths facilitate the patient's
involvement in designing and monitoring care and contribute to cross-training and
multiskilling. They have been shown to reduce storage space and the risk of forgetting tests, treatment and care. The results from a national study evaluating integrated care pathways are encouraging. Patients' lengths of stay are shorter. The
staff spend less time writing. Questions are also raised about the appropriateness
of routine procedures (Hurst 1995, p. 6).

As with other elements of PFC, integrated care paths are not without their
critics. Some are sceptical of 'cookbook' medicine and argue that integrated care
paths limit clinical freedom. Others say they are inflexible. The language and
style of the records can deter patients. Although very few believe litigation is
likely, the medical legal implementations of integrated care paths are untested in
the UK. However, it is clear that integrated care paths are evolving. Computerizing
records and bridging acute and community care through common protocols are
two important developments in the UK (Hurst, 1995, p. 6).

Care pathways in case study

The first integrated care pathway (ICP) in the Trust was for cataract surgery.
The method used to write the ICP for cataract surgery was developed by the
IPC team. This is based on a review of the literature and practice from work
undertaken by other National Pathway User Group members (see Chapters 1 and
2). The process starts by convening a multidisciplinary project team which is
representative of the different staff groups who play a part in the patient's care.
Representatives are selected by colleagues within each of the staff groups. The
team is led by a senior clinician (for this project, an ophthalmic consultant). At
the first meeting the IPC facilitator presented the idea of ICPs, how they are
used and the pros and cons of using them. Terms of reference were then agreed
with clear objectives.

The Clinical Outcomes Coordinator undertook a literature search to identify current best practice as defined in guidelines, protocols or standards from the Cochrane
Centre, Royal Colleges and other sources (Royal College of Ophthalmologists,
1995, *Evidence Based Medicine Bulletin*, 1996). Existing local guidelines and standards, for example around extended nursing roles in preassessment clinics, were
identified. Team members gathered written ICPs for cataract surgery from three
other hospitals, although none was thought to be suited to local conditions.

Brainstorming produced a flowchart of the current pathway for patients listed
for cataract surgery. The scope of the pathway was agreed. This was to start at
'the patient being put on the operating list' and end at 'the two week postoperative outpatient appointment'. The flowchart enabled the pathway to be

broken down into manageable stages, and individual team members were given responsibility for comparing current practice with known best practice for each of these stages. Each stage of the pathway was closely scrutinized and discussed to ensure that each patient's care was safe, effective and efficient. A checklist with two axes was devised as a way of ensuring consensus on all the necessary elements required for each stage of the pathway. When consensus is reached across the checklist, the ICP is then piloted, amended and finally adopted for routine use. A variance-tracking sheet (to monitor compliance against the ICP and clinical outcomes) was developed by the department of clinical audit for use during the pilot phase. The pathway was then further developed into a stand-alone multidisciplinary patient record.

The unitary patient record reduced the time spent documenting care and eliminated duplicate information.

A number of changes were made to reduce delays to patients. For example, nurses and orthoptists were trained to lead preassessment clinics in line with protocols agreed by a lead consultant. Nurses were also trained to undertake first-day postoperative assessment of patients, a role previously performed only by doctors.

Benefits of this approach included:

- The ICP is designed and owned by the staff in the care centre.
- It is based on known best practice and is evidence based.
- It provides a way of identifying differences in practice and securing clinical consensus.
- External facilitation enables current practice to be challenged firmly and diplomatically.
- Facilitation from IPC brings tools and techniques for prioritizing, analysing and solving problems.
- Variance monitoring using electronically scanned variance sheets enables efficient and effective auditing of high-volume care processes:
  - Over 500 patients were monitored for variances during the pilot alone.
  - Results showed that 98% of operations resulted in improved eyesight. Audits have been targeted on those cases where vision did not improve.
  - Out of 62 patients who required more than two follow-up appointments, 40 had underlying conditions and 22 were experiencing complications. These complications are the subject of further detailed audit.

Some difficulties we have noted with the introduction of patient care pathways are as follows:

- Not all IPC areas are suited to ICP development (we have found ICPs are best suited to high-volume, high-cost, high-risk and routine care).
- Securing input into the development of pathways from patients is difficult. Reasons for this have included:
  - Difficulty finding patients whose views are representative.

- A proportion of patients want the professionals to take charge and do not wish either to be told about alternatives or to suggest alternatives for themselves (the 'you just do what you have to, doctor' syndrome). Clearly these patients have equal rights to have their views respected.
- Timing of patient involvement. It is inappropriate to involve patients when they are very sick, but whether their involvement is before or after intervention will also influence their perspective. Beforehand, some are worried that criticism may result in some kind of retribution; afterwards (as in the case of the cataract patients), patients can be so grateful for the outcome of the operation that they do not offer constructive suggestions for improvement.

- Variance analysis needs to be undertaken by those using the pathway but support and expertise are needed to set up appropriate systems. This requires adequate resourcing.

From our experience, there have been a number of factors that influence the success (or otherwise) of ICPs:

- Education and awareness of the purpose, use, development and evaluation of ICPs is essential for all team members involved in writing the pathway.
- The need for a respected senior clinician to lead the pathway development.
- External facilitation to assist team members in developing and piloting the pathway, to challenge current practice and to review and critique the literature for the best available evidence.
- All staff likely to be involved in following the pathway must be represented on the team designing the ICP.
- It is worth considering whether the diagnosis or clinical condition is better suited to protocol or guideline development (see Chapter 2).

Getting IPCed

Having explained the principles and key elements of IPC, it is also important to consider the mechanism for achieving IPC within a healthcare organization. The process for developing a fully functioning PFC hospital does not, according to a review of the literature, have a single unitary approach. Since many of the IPC sites in the UK were supported by consulting firms, the approach has often been dominated by the consultants. The NHS Executive (Hurst, 1995, p. 7) report identified from its evaluation of eight pilot sites a number of key success factors in bringing about the change to PFC:

- Commitment to the project from the chief executive and senior managers. The concept is radical to many and must have unswerving support from the top.
- A structured approach to managing the project, which is complex.
- A diagnostic phase of some sort to reveal whether change is needed and to convince the organization that restructuring will be of value.

- A dedicated project team and resources, including financial resources, to support that team.
- Visible values: be clear why you are doing the project.
- An incentive to do it – such as the need to change to maintain competitive position in the market; to focus the organization; to plan/design the optimum new facility.
- Champions on the front line. Champions at the top are key, but so too are champions at the operational sharp end and indeed throughout the organization.
- A recognition of the importance of communication, training and the human resources implications of the change programme.

It was our experience in the following case study that all of these factors were important in the implementation of PFC. The next section describes in more detail how we have progressed to date, what we did in practice, and reflects on lessons learned as a result.

CASE STUDY 7.1   IMPLEMENTING PATIENT FOCUSED CARE: A CASE STUDY*

Having identified the discrete IPC groupings, the next task was to ensure that the key success factors identified were fully implemented in practice. In this case study, we adopted three phases when establishing an IPC centre:

- the diagnostic phase
- the design and implementation phase
- the evaluation phase

Each of these phases will now be examined along with the structures put in place to support the introduction of IPC.

When establishing a PFC hospital and moving through the above phases, it is clearly important to identify responsibilities for implementation. In the UK pilot sites there have been a variety of different structures put in place to achieve a patient focused hospital. In our Trust the project was initially coordinated and facilitated by a consultancy company. Their brief was:

- to communicate the project goals to hospital staff;
- to assess the organization's readiness for change;

---

* NB – throughout the case study we shall use the term 'integrated patient care', as this was the local agreed term for PFC for reasons cited earlier in this chapter.

- to develop a vision for a patient focused hospital;
- to design and set up a pilot IPC care centre;
- to transfer the principles of multiskilling and documentation to the rest of the Trust.

Steering group

A steering group comprising the Trust chairman, chief executive, directors and management consultants was established in March 1993 to define the scope and steer the project. Initial work concentrated on identifying new patient groups according to clinical need, gathering the baseline indicators on current care delivery and identifying key success criteria against which to measure the impact of the project. This was funded from initial pump-priming monies from the Department of Health.

The key success criteria identified and agreed by the steering group were:

- reduction in length of stay
- increased proportion of time spent on direct care
- reduced unit costs
- improved patient satisfaction
- improved staff satisfaction
- higher rates of treatment success as defined by clinical audit
- reduced number of staff contacts in a patient's stay
- reduced number of bed moves in a patient's stay
- reduced time spent on documentation
- reduced turnaround time for laboratory tests

Groups involved

The key groups involved in PFC were:

- management consultants
- Trust IPC steering group (later to become the clinical performance improvement group)
- an internal Trust IPC team
- staff from the care centres (IPC project group)
- directorate management teams

As with any project, the benefits of reflection inevitably identify pros and cons of the approaches taken. Ours are offered here for the benefit of those wishing to develop PFC elsewhere. They are, however, the subjective and personal opinions of the authors, based on the experience of one case study.

Use of management consultants

At the inception of the project there was clearly limited expertise within the Trust for establishing care centres or a patient focused hospital. The expertise of an external consultant was advantageous. Other advantages included the 'fresh eyes' look at our organization from independent professionals, and having dedicated individuals who could work full time on the project. Some of the disadvantages of using external facilitators included (in some cases) the lack of acceptance of external facilitators by staff (particularly where some were perceived as having a poor understanding of health service issues), the high cost of consultancy and the fact that it can create dependency on external consultants rather than developing the skills of our own staff.

IPC steering group/clinical performance improvement group (CPIG)

The Trust-wide IPC steering group was effective in providing quality assurance and steering the project. This was largely owing to two factors: the small size of the group and the key players involved, e.g. chief executive and all executive directors, including those of finance and IT. This group reviewed and expanded its brief in 1994 when it became known as the clinical performance improvement group to steer implementation of the Trust's clinical performance improvement unit.

Integrated patient care team

At the start of the project, three whole-time equivalent (WTE) members of staff were assigned to the project. Following the departure of the management consultants, a full-time IPC manager was appointed in January 1994.

The composition of the team has changed, with the management category (M2) cost reductions having an impact on staffing in this department. The team currently have two whole-time equivalents working on the project, with 0.5 WTE administrative support. A Trust researcher was appointed in 1995 to evaluate the impact of team midwifery in the women and children IPC centre, but was made redundant in 1997. The smaller size of the team has affected the speed at which the project can be implemented across the organization.

Advantages of an internal IPC team

The advantages of having an internal IPC team include:

- It is less costly than external consultants.
- Trust staff have developed expertise in both IPC and facilitating change and are able to pass these skills on to care centre staff as they work alongside them.
- They are independent of the clinical directorates, bringing about a 'fresh eyes' approach with which to challenge care delivery when reviewing the care centres.
- Team members have a good understanding of the health service and professional issues because of their clinical backgrounds (which can encourage acceptance of their recommendations by clinical staff).
- The team devote a large proportion of their time to the implementation of

IPC. The latter point is important when considering the workload of clinical directorate staff. Although clinicians are closely involved in the IPC process, current feedback indicates that, on the whole, they do not feel they have the time or the expertise to drive this project without support from the central team.

- Team members are sensitive to the political, economical, technical and cultural nuances of the Trust, and their decisions and actions reflect their awareness.

Potential difficulties include the risk of 'going native' and, as relationships develop with care centre staff, losing a degree of objectivity. The small size of the team also tends to create a wealth of expertise in a few individuals which can be difficult to replace if they leave, making succession planning a significant consideration. The skills of the internal team are paramount in the development of the project, making recruitment and selection of those with the necessary skills an important task. Personal development plans for team members are essential to ensure frequent exposure to others working in this field elsewhere in order to share experiences.

IPC steering groups

As IPC care centres are established, a local steering group is developed to work in conjunction with the IPC team. The advantages of such a group have been:

- The clinical directorate steers the project, with support and advice from the central IPC team.
- The team contribute to setting the agenda of work and therefore are more likely to own and lead the project.
- The key stakeholders are involved.

A disadvantage of this approach has been the time commitment for key team members. Another difficulty was that at this stage of the project there was no identified care centre manager, hence no leader within the care centre to manage and lead the project.

Care centre manager

The women and children's directorate appointed a care centre manager in December 1994, well after the project started. The advantages of this appointment were soon apparent in terms of providing a focus for leading and steering the project in the care centre. The review of workforce structure in renal and ophthalmology also pointed to the need for the appointment of a care centre manager. On reflection, earlier appointment of the IPC care centre manager is recommended, since it gives the advantage of a strong local lead and provides the opportunity for the IPC team to pass on their experience to one individual. This enables the central team to facilitate rather than manage the IPC process, and ensures continual development and support of the IPC process. It is not desirable or realistic to get the central team to do the detailed work – this has to remain the responsibility of local managers.

The roll-out of IPC in the case study

The Trust Board sanctioned the design of a pilot gastroenterology care centre in September 1993. Considerable work was done with gastroenterology staff when designing the new care centre, examining current roles, developing unitary documentation and mapping work processes. Unfortunately, owing to space constraints, the implementation was postponed by the Trust Board until phase 1 of the capital redevelopment programme. This work is now being revisited in preparation for the opening of the new unit. A powerful lesson learned was the importance of working through the physical locations for all the proposed care centre groupings at the start of the work, particularly when it may mean other specialities are displaced. This was difficult because (for reasons outlined above) final agreement on the number and composition of care centres was not agreed at the start. The decision was taken, therefore, to proceed with a number of care centres to evaluate their impact before taking the definitive decision to roll this approach out throughout the whole Trust. Some early successful centres were therefore essential to convince those who were more sceptical about the impact of this approach.

IPC in obstetrics and neonatology

The women and children's directorate expressed an interest in developing the principle of IPC in the obstetrics and neonatology departments. This was agreed by the Trust Board in January 1994 and subsequently the central team concentrated their time working with staff in this area to apply the principles of IPC in the maternity and neonatology care centre. Work also at this time continued with gastroenterology. In December 1995 and August 1996 work began on two new care centres, ophthalmology and renal.

Lessons learned: advantages and disadvantages of this IPC roll-out approach

The impact that IPC had on the delivery of patient care in the Trust is outlined below. This is largely attributable to the amount of hard work that was undertaken by the care centre staff and managers; the local steering group; and the IPC central team. It is inevitable in a project of this scale that, with the benefit of hindsight, there are things that perhaps could have been tackled differently. The following observations based on our experience are therefore offered to inform others who are considering PFC.

The use of a pilot site

In reviewing the early IPC project proposals, significant emphasis was placed on the importance of a pilot site. It was intended that the pilot would be evaluated (including reference to cost benefits) before rolling out IPC throughout the Trust. There are two features of interest in what has happened in the pilot sites: first, the process used to implement IPC, and second the outcomes that have resulted from the establishment of care centres.

Process
In terms of process, having a pilot site where we can identify the best mechanisms for implementing IPC is helpful. What we learned in the pilot sites has proved useful, with a number of changes having already been made to the approach taken for work in subsequent care centres.

Outcomes
In examining the outcome of what IPC has achieved, the use of a pilot as a means of assessing future potential for IPC has presented some difficulties. What is clear is that outcomes are unique to the care centre studied and are not generalizable. This is perhaps inevitable, since each care centre has very different patient groups, there are different people involved in the project and different external constraints. It would be easy to say that a women and children IPC care centre was not a 'typical' area. However, in reality there are no 'typical' areas that could provide a blueprint of the exact impact and cost of a project of this magnitude.

Following the gastroenterology experience, a decision was made to apply the principles of IPC to discrete units or specialities with close geographical locations. The fact that gastroenterology has proved more challenging reinforces the need for a detailed diagnostic phase. Establishing care centres that fall outside traditional current patient groupings, or attempting to merge areas that are geographically disparate (such as, in our experience, gastroenterology), must be carefully considered. Clearly, much more time will be needed to work on these more complex projects.

Replication of outcome
When considering the conclusions from evaluation of the women and children pilot sites, caution is needed in assuming that the advantages and disadvantages (in terms of what IPC does or does not achieve in our pilot sites) may be replicated elsewhere. However, from the overall progress, some assumptions can be made about the impact IPC has had and could have in future.

A difficulty with the roll-out plan to date is the speed at which it can occur. The slow-down in pace has been exacerbated by a reduction in the size of the central team, and work pressures, which make it difficult for clinical staff to be released to work on IPC development. At the inception of the project, the amount of time needed was vastly underestimated. However, this has been a helpful and important lesson for planning the development of future care centres. Although the process has now been streamlined, it is anticipated that the IPC team will need to work with care centres for around a year if the current approach to implementing the project continues. The IPC team has developed a critical path that enables them to work with two care centres simultaneously. It can therefore be appreciated that with approximately 20 care centres still outstanding, the process of getting the whole of the Trust IPCed would take approximately ten years. Further work, therefore, is now examining alternative methods to speed up this process. The incremental approach to roll-out has been imposed by the resources available to support the project. The benefits of a radical, hospital-wide approach outlined in the PFC literature have not been realized at this point.

Planning

Much effort has been put into developing detailed start-up plans for IPC care centres. The IPC team have recognized that a weakness in the current approach has been the lack of similar detailed plans for withdrawal from IPC care centres. Although working with new care centres, the team have continuing commitments with all the established care centres to date. This raises two issues:

- At what point (if any) should the IPC team sever links with the care centre?
- What are the ongoing responsibilities for the care centre in continuing the IPC process?

Although unlikely, there is technically nothing to stop an IPC care centre reverting to previous ways of working once the care centre team has withdrawn. More clarity needs to be given to the withdrawal process with identified responsibilities for continuing with IPC. This has been identified as a central role for the care centre manager at the maternity and neonates care centre. What has become clear from the pilot sites is that there will not be an endpoint to the IPC process. If we accept that IPC is a vehicle for ongoing organizational development (albeit within a specific framework) for all the components within this framework, then an improvement in the review process needs to occur. For example, patient care pathways will need reviewing and updating in line with contemporary practice. The same can be said for reviewing roles; the latter two elements will require continuous review of the way we organize and deliver care. Experience in designing unitary documentation indicates a need to review and improve it continuously, and to ensure that the professionals responsible for completing this are doing so in an appropriate and timely manner.

Corporate issues

Another potential weakness in the current roll-out of IPC is the incremental 'care centre by care centre' approach. This does not encourage rigorous examination of the structures and processes that transcend care centres. For example, if we proceed with 20 or more IPC centres, all with a care centre manager, then how does this fit with the current directorate structure? As well as the central functions and services, there are also organizational aspects that need to be considered corporately, such as, for example, bed management. A balance needs to be struck between the desire to decentralize services and the cost of maintaining some central functions. In reality, however, we have recognized that the purist approach of having satellite pharmacy, X-ray, pathology services, etc. within each care centre is too expensive to be viable. Also with the implementation of new technology such as the vacutube, continued centralization does not always compromise efficiency.

Now that we have examined the advantages and disadvantages and lessons learned about the process of rolling out IPC within the Trust, a more detailed review will now be carried out of the discrete phases used to implement IPC in the Trust: the diagnostic, design and implementation, and evaluation phases. Since November 1995, plans for implementing IPC have followed an adapted version of the PRINCE (Projects in Controlled Environments) project management method. Figure 7.1 illustrates the key phases used in the case study to establish IPC centres.

Key phases in case study

Diagnostic phase

The diagnostic phase is used both to benchmark and to review critically the way services are currently organized. It enables the IPC team and care centre staff to develop an understanding of how the service operates and how well different aspects of the service are integrated around the needs of the patient. Lessons learned from the first two pilot areas of IPC in gastroenterology and maternity and neonates changed the method used in this phase significantly. The current approach is outlined below.

Before the diagnostic phase was undertaken, a series of staff awareness sessions were arranged to explain what IPC is and how the project could be developed within the area concerned. These sessions provided an opportunity for staff to ask questions and discuss concerns. The phase examined four main aspects of care: physical environment, organization of care, roles, and documentation. A wide range of tools and techniques were used to develop an accurate picture of the services provided. These included on-site observations, patient-tracking teams, process mapping, collection and analysis of activity, finance and staffing data, audit of clinical documentation, and surveying staff and patient views through SWOT analyses, interviews and focus groups. Every aspect of the service which affected the patient's experience was reviewed during the diagnostic phase. This included information gathered through semi-structured one-to-one interviews and focus groups with patients and relatives.

Involvement in diagnostic phase

The bulk of the diagnostic review is undertaken by the IPC manager and the IPC facilitator, workforce planning manager, unit manager, unit accountant, clinical audit officer, nurse information coordinator and staff from the clinical performance improvement unit, where, under the direction of the director of nursing, a matrix management system has been developed to pull in staff with appropriate expertise as required. We have also used clinical staff patient 'trackers', observing what happens to patients in different areas of the department and using a proforma to record these observations. All of this additional staff input was coordinated by the IPC team and carried out according to specific briefs.

Timescale of diagnostic phase

The time required for the diagnostic phase depends upon the scale and complexity of the service and the patient group. It also depends on the extent to which an area is already integrated around the needs of the patient. The most recent diagnostic phases covering ophthalmology and renal services were undertaken over a 12 week period (excluding planning time and staff awareness sessions).

The diagnostic phase culminated in an in-depth written report which included recommendations for change. The report was circulated to care centre staff. A planning day was then held with a cross-section of staff to provide an opportunity to discuss the findings and prioritize the key issues; and a steering group was established to take the project forward.

Reflection on approach to date

Some advantages of the above approach include:

- It enables patients and staff at all levels help to set the agenda for change.
- It provides strong evidence for the IPC team to challenge current practice effectively.
- It provides in-depth knowledge and evidence, which enables the team to challenge traditional perceptions and assumptions.
- It allows time to build confidence and trust among staff – essential to implementing the change process.
- It enables problems of implementation to be put into context using a PEST (political, economic, social and technical) analysis.
- It allows the central team to make comparisons with similar services elsewhere.

Some difficulties with this approach include the fact that it is a relatively lengthy process. Timescales for completion often mean that changes in service delivery are made before the presentation of the final report, which is then out of date. It can also raise expectations that cannot be met because of cost implications (e.g. structural changes). Finally, the limited involvement of many care centre staff can occasionally mean limited ownership of the report findings. It also requires much time building relationships to overcome suspicion and fears. Consequently, we have now streamlined the diagnostic phase to make it sharper and shorter.

Design/implementation phase

Following the diagnostic report, the IPC team facilitate a planning day when issues are prioritized and project structures and reporting mechanisms are determined. A project steering group and six or more design teams are then set up with terms of reference and objectives. Membership of these multidisciplinary teams is drawn from across the care centre and includes all grades of staff. The steering group is responsible for driving through changes. It includes managers and clinicians with the authority to authorize major changes. Design teams are led by a member of staff from the care centre and are supported by either the IPC manager or the IPC facilitator.

The purpose of the project teams is to find solutions to the issues identified in the IPC diagnostic report. Staff involvement is critical to the success of the projects (Hurst, 1995, p. 7). The style is facilitative rather than directive, with the aim being that the teams develop solutions, where possible, through a creative consensus. An important role of the IPC team is to challenge any plans for change in order to ensure that the patient's perspective is fully considered. The team also acts as a resource by providing facilitation skills and methodological expertise (e.g. the role review, integrated care pathways).

An information leaflet, *Care Centre Bulletin*, is used as a briefing tool, and staff on the project steering group have responsibility for cascading plans to staff in their own areas. Elements of design and implementation overlap, as different projects will work to different schedules. Examples of the achievements that have come from the current pilot sites are shown in Table 7.2.

Some advantages of this approach have included:

- Proposed changes are based on patient need, following consultation with focus groups.
- The involvement of staff increases the sense of ownership and encourages involvement in changes.
- The solutions are not imposed upon, but are generated from within, the care centre.
- The change is incorporated into contemporary practice.
- IPC can be used as a vehicle through which to tackle long-term issues and problems.

One difficulty with the above approach has been the problem of securing patient participation in the redesigning of services (as opposed to commenting on current service provision). Moreover, active participation increases staff time spent in meetings and away from clinical practice. Organizing meetings with clinicians has been difficult. It is impossible to improve quality in some areas without initial investment (e.g. structural changes), for which funding is not always available. Finally, there is the danger that IPC is seen as a way to make difficult management decisions (e.g. seeing role review as a way to deal with poor performance).

Table 7.2

Examples of IPC design team project key achievements

	Physical environment	Organization of care	Roles	Documentation
Gastroenterology	Concept, design and commissioning of purpose-built IPC centre for all inpatient and outpatient activity including endoscopy suite.	Integrated care pathway for oesophageal cancer being facilitated by clinical outcomes coordinator.	Review for all roles for new care centre. Multiskilled health care assistant roles. Cross-training of out-patients, endoscopy and ward nurses.	Unitary patient notes. Step-by-step patient information for care pathway.
Maternity and neonatology	Developed new integrated care centre with antenatal clinic, foetal assessment unit and early pregnancy advisory clinic.	Established team midwifery and team nursing. Redesigned antenatal clinic processes.	Streamlined management structure. Designed new care centre assistant role. Skills training for midwives to work across community and hospital.	Unitary documentation for maternity. Protocols and procedures updated.
Ophthalmology	All signage developed to RNIB standard. Voiceovers used in the lift. Review of children's services: play areas upgraded and theatre recovery separated from adults.	Integrated care pathway for cataract. Redesign of outpatients and appointments processes.	Role review leading to consultant-based clerical teams. Nurse-led preassessment and postoperative clinics for cataract patients.	Unitary document for cataract pathway. Electronically scanned variance sheet. Audiotape for cataract patients.
Renal	Capacity and resources review: establishment of satellite dialysis units.	Medical secretarial and clerical processes redesigned. Computerized system introduced for test results.	Streamlined management structure. Review of nursing and renal technician roles.	Patient literature review and new booklet. Clinical standards established for all modalities. Protocols and procedures updated.

Reproduced with the permission of Brighton Health Care NHS Trust.

Evaluation phase

The evaluation phase of IPC aims to compare the effect of changes against the baseline information contained in the original diagnostic report about the care centre. The evaluation covers changes in the key areas of physical environment, organization of care, roles, and documentation. The evaluation should also include an analysis of changes in cost.

Maternity and neonatology

The evaluation of IPC in maternity and neonatology predominantly focused on the impact of team midwifery and *Changing Childbirth*. Here, the Trust researcher has carried out an extensive and in-depth evaluation of one major process redesign, that of team midwifery. Additional to this focused and rigorous evaluation, a final report has been compiled by the general manager, care centre manager and IPC manager to describe the changes brought about by the IPC project in this area. The final report therefore consists of a number of separate surveys carried out on satisfaction levels of staff and service users, and detailed audits on service standards.

Methodology

Following the evaluation in the first phase, we have reviewed the whole evaluation process. More rigorous analysis was clearly required in the first evaluation to establish whether the benefits were significant enough for the Trust Board to extend this approach throughout the Trust. The board took the view, on the presentation of the final report, that the whole Trust would adopt IPC as its philosophy of care. Future evaluations, therefore, will be less detailed and results will compare changes made against the original diagnostic report. It is fair to say that we have experienced methodological problems in isolating variables. These methodological difficulties are not confined to our organization, but are evident in all nine of the UK pilot sites for IPC (Hurst, 1995, p. 14).

Some advantages of the current approach include the following:

- It enables comparisons with baseline information and diagnostic reports.
- It identifies what worked well and what could be improved in terms of process and outcomes.
- It enables exploration of the impact of IPC on complex concepts such as culture and hierarchy.
- Some discrete elements of IPC can be evaluated in depth (e.g. team midwifery).
- The research can be validated by those involved in the study.
- The robust method used by the Trust researcher means that the research stands up to external scrutiny.
- It encourages debate about the effectiveness of IPC.

The difficulties we have experienced have included the fact that the complex variables make it difficult to isolate the effect of IPC from other influences; the depth and detail of the IPC methodologies mean that reports are time consuming to write and lengthy; it is difficult to identify cost savings except in terms of staff costs (pricing mechanisms are not sophisticated enough in areas of process); the final report is a self-evaluation by care centre staff and IPC team members responsible for the project, and as such could be accused of bias; some cost savings may not be declared if it is felt that this will reduce the budget allocation to the area; and the differences in patient groups and local circumstances make it difficult to generalize findings to other areas.

The cost of patient focused care

Costing patient focused care is the greatest challenge facing the patient focused care evaluator. There is uncertainty whether PFC saves money, is cost neutral or increases costs. Evidence from a review of PFC sites in UK is thin and contradictory (Hurst, 1995, p. 14). Two main reasons for the cost savings achieved in the US are cited. First, patients' length of stay shortens as carers' autonomy increases. Second, test processing speeds up care and treatment. This uncertainty is not surprising when issues like patient satisfaction have to be considered in a cost benefit analysis. Amounts and uses of money for developing PFC vary from site to site in the UK. Buildings, management consultancy, staff salaries and education programmes are the biggest predicted PFC cost items.

The cost of localizing services in patient focused care units is complicated. Buying and maintaining extra equipment and building works increase costs. Space reduction, as centralized services and corridors are decommissioned, lowers costs. It is not clear whether these issues apply to the UK to date (Hurst, 1995, p. 28).

Staff savings through multiskilling are predicted to offset the increased capital and maintenance costs (Hurst, 1995, p. 59). In the early days of PFC, the requirements were that staff numbers will fall and that grade mix will dilute. Additionally, the number of managers is expected to fall (Hurst, 1995, p. 59). These changes have materialized in some UK PFC units. Staff education in the PFC units on the other hand is costly, although a good investment. Simplified healthcare as a result of integrated care paths reduces costs as staff time is shifted to direct care. The costs of computerizing records and linking patient care paths with continuing care protocols are, as yet, unclear (Hurst, 1995, p. 59).

Cost analysis

In the maternity and neonatology pilot it was considered necessary to obtain a financial baseline of the current service in 1994 before the implementation of IPC principles. This enabled a financial evaluation to be carried out in the future. A range of developments and changes to the organization and service delivery have subsequently been made. The key focus of the financial evaluation was the maternity service. The variance in budget between 1994 and 1997 was established and adjusted to account for known additions to the baseline during this period, for example pay awards and changes to junior doctors' hours.

It is important to emphasize that major changes were made to the services without unplanned additional expenditure. Indeed, the implementation of team midwifery, which has placed greater emphasis on community-based midwifery, is in line with IPC and *Changing Childbirth* principles, which has resulted in a reduction of income to the Trust. This reduced income was attributed to the increase in home birth rates and home assessment of women in early labour, both previously counted as finished consultant episodes and which are now not formally recognized within the current contract currencies. The home assessment of women led to major increases in quality of services, and has reduced inappropriate admissions, hence improving the service the women receive.

Additionally the original agreed business case was based upon an assumption that the Trust would increase its market share through the predicted transfer of maternity services from another Trust. This transfer did not take place during the present evaluation and, as a consequence, the Trust did not realize the extra income. Therefore, the actual reduction in income to the Trust was £162,500; although the Trust has not made a major saving through this process, the demand for health authority funds has decreased, thus giving a saving direct to the purchaser.

This is an important lesson when reconfiguring services in the community. It is essential that securing income for this work delivered in new ways is captured in the contract negotiations. This will ensure that the financial gain that accrues to the health authority is reinvested in the Trust, or in part of the contracted service from which income is derived.

A summary of the other savings includes:

- rationalized and streamlined management structure with the inception of a care centre manager replacing the previous director of midwifery services and the patient services manager for paediatrics;
- establishment of care centre assistants, demonstrating a cost saving of £15,000 for 1996–97;
- an anticipated cost saving of £25,000 at the end of phase I due to a saving on the additional doctor hour payments.

Progress against critical success factors
The critical success factors as agreed at the inception of the IPC project were:

- reduction in length of stay
- increased proportion of time spent on direct care
- reduced unit costs
- improved patient satisfaction
- improved staff satisfaction
- higher rates of treatment success as defined by clinical audit/outcomes
- reduced number of staff contacts in a patient's stay
- reduced number of bed moves in a patient's stay
- reduced time spent on documentation
- reduced turnaround time for laboratory tests

Examples of progress against each of these in relation to maternity and neonatology and ophthalmology IPC centres are briefly detailed below.

- **Improved patient satisfaction.** A substantial piece of work has been undertaken in this area into the effectiveness of pilot team midwifery as part of the IPC and *Changing Childbirth* programme (Hart, 1997). There is evidence of increased patient satisfaction. A series of patient focus groups and semi-structured interviews are currently being repeated in ophthalmology.
- **Improved staff satisfaction.** Qualitative evaluations through interviews and focus groups with Trevor Mann Baby Unit (TMBU) nursing staff, care centre assistants, midwives, consultants and managers demonstrated increased staff satisfaction. Improved teamwork is a common theme that emerges from the focus groups. The care centre assistants identified that the changes following the role review had resulted in them feeling they were now part of the team. Similar results are emerging from the IPC project in ophthalmology. In addition to the qualitative evaluations, a quantitative survey was carried out at the start of the ophthalmology IPC project and repeated at the close. Results from the staff satisfaction questionnaire showed improvements in 25 out of 30 criteria, with significant positive changes around communication, teamwork and role clarity. It also identified a shift in the culture of the service, with a 19% increase in the number of respondents agreeing with the statement 'This hospital puts patients first' and a 28% increase in those who agreed that 'We are encouraged to provide extra services to patients and staff.'
- **Higher rates of treatment success as defined by clinical audit.** This key success criterion is not directly related to the practice of midwifery. However, the changes made to the maternity services in terms of the rise in home births and other quality improvements such as home assessment in labour are regarded as a hallmark of good practice demonstrating flexibility of the service (Audit Commission, 1997). In ophthalmology, analysis of the variance against the cataract pathway enabled clinicians to measure clinical outcomes and compliance with evidence-based practice as documented on the pathway. This also allows accurate measurement of treatment success, as the variance tool can target audits on those cases where treatment is not successful. In cataract care, audits of extended nursing roles in preassessment, postoperative assessment and outpatient follow-up clinics have shown no adverse impact on treatment. Developing the pathway also helped to streamline service delivery.
- **Reduced number of staff contacts in a patient's stay.** A continuity audit undertaken in maternity and neonatology shows a reduction in the number of different members of staff dealing with the mothers. Hence we have been successful in reducing the 'sea of faces'.
- **Reduced number of bed moves in a patient's stay.** Audit showed this was not found to be a problem in maternity and neonatology or ophthalmology. However, the opening of the care centre, which incorporates antenatal clinic, foetal assessment unit, early pregnancy assessment unit and decentralized ultrasound facility, significantly reduces patient movement throughout the hospital. Similarly, in ophthalmology, the extension of nurse

and orthoptist led preassessment clinics reduced the number of visits for patients.

- **Reduced time spent on documentation.** An audit of the time nurses, midwives and doctors spend on documentation in both care centres shows a significant reduction of time spent making records after the implementation of unitary documentation.
- **Reduced turnaround time for laboratory tests.** This objective was less of an an issue to address in the maternity and neonatology or ophthalmology care centres, as these were not high users of clinical pathology services and so turnaround times were less of a problem.
- **Reduction in length of stay.** Reductions in length of stay are not directly relevant in maternity and neonatology. However, baseline measures have been re-audited, showing a reduction in inappropriate hospital attendances.
- **Increased proportion of time spent on direct care.** Through the use of the Nursing Information System, a baseline of time spent by clinicians on direct care was established in 1994 and is to be remeasured following the opening of the care centre. It is anticipated that, with the implementation of team midwifery and team nursing, the time spent on direct patient care will increase.
- **Reduced unit costs.** Although one of the more difficult elements to measure, reduced unit costs have been demonstrated in maternity and neonatology. It was difficult to measure in ophthalmology due to a 16% increase in day surgery and a 19% increase in outpatient visits (Towers, 1998).

CONCLUSIONS

IPC is a philosophy of care which puts the patient at the centre of the health service. Such an ethos is not new; it is a central tenet underpinning the professional working within the health service. As patients' expectations continue to rise (partly owing to the influence of pressure groups seeking greater involvement with the way services such as HIV/AIDS care and midwifery are delivered; and partly owing to government initiatives such as the *Patients' Charter*), the need to review services continuously to take account of patients' views is inevitable.

IPC (as used in our Trust) provides a vehicle for delivering changes, both those identified internally and those that may be dictated from outside the Trust. It provides a structured framework for analysing current services; identifying recommendations for change; implementing these; and evaluating the impact. This is done in collaboration with clinical staff, and facilitated by a central team who have developed expertise in the process.

This is not to suggest that many clinicians and managers working in the health service do not continuously improve services using their own initiative. However, the difficulty in a large and complex organization is to ensure that changes in practice are incorporated into the strategic planning of the Trust and are not developed incrementally without wider reference to the impact both on other services or specialties and on use of resources.

Considerable funding and efforts are being expended on BHC's new capital redevelopment. For a truly efficient and effective service to be delivered within the new infrastructure, effort needs to be made to ensure that care processes in the new building are designed and implemented around the best interests of the patient. IPC allows the fundamental principles underpinning patient care to be examined and reconfigured; hence it is a means to an end – not an end in itself. It provides the framework for delivering our corporate aim, 'Putting patients' interests first'.

The process of implementing IPC has created opportunities. Our evaluation of IPC shows that the broad aims of the project were realized. Some of the more ambitious claims for PFC, cited both in the literature and by management consultants, were, however, overstated, since the healthcare system in the USA is fundamentally different from the NHS in the UK. Indeed, as, will been seen from the case study and the findings from the nine UK pilot sites, the differences between the UK and US systems has meant that many of the claims for PFC have not been realized in the UK, for the following reasons. First, UK hospitals are heavily unionized, whereas their US counterparts do not recognize either trades union or professional organizations. Second, UK hospitals have only limited scope to develop remuneration strategies, and plans to expand this under the previous Conservative government were revoked by the new Labour government. Third, UK hospitals have significantly lower staffing levels than similarly configured hospitals in North America. As so much of the projected cost savings claimed by PFC are dependent on reducing labour costs through skill mix and staffing levels, it is perhaps not surprising that savings on the scale predicted in the US sites have not been replicated in the UK (Buchan, 1995). Nevertheless, there are benefits – additional to the advantages cited in the case study – and these are outlined in our final summary below. In terms of the 'evidence base' for supporting PFC as a management tool, further empirical work is needed. Funding for the case study site was insufficient to allow the wholesale application of all the principles set out in the PFC literature. One needs to be mindful of the latter points when drawing general conclusions about PFC benefits in the case study.

FINAL SUMMARY

Chapters 1 and 2 explored how clinicians can ensure that their care and treatment of patients is based on the best evidence. This is achieved through reviewing the literature to identifying and document best practice. Chapters 3 and 4 then outlined how to audit current practice. Chapter 5 identified strategic planning as a tool that can be used to improve practice, and described some of the change management theories that can assist clinicians in closing the audit loop to improve clinical practice. Throughout the book, it has been noted, in the words of a number of commentators, that the quality of patient care, although heavily influenced by the competence of the individual clinician, will also be influenced by numerous other factors that are often outside the scope of the healthcare professional; for example, availability of beds, timely access to diagnostic tests and treatment, and the quality of support services, to name but a few. Chapter 1 cited a number of criticisms by professionals that the strong emphasis on robust evidence in clinical decision making was not always replicated when it came to setting health policy at a national level, or strategic planning at an organizational level. Chapter 5 therefore examined strategic planning and change management theories to determine how these can be utilized to support and inform practice development. Chapters 6 and 7 looked at organizational approaches that create an organizational framework to support and encourage the application of best practice for both clinicians and management. Hence, in the PFC model, the diagnostic phase will review literature on known best practice for the principles outlined above (e.g. what work is published on the numbers of staff and the skill mix ratio for a given area; how this service is delivered in other similar units elsewhere), and collect information on current practice and use this to inform potential areas for change and improvement. Hence the PFC phases closely mirror the audit cycle, albeit on a much larger scale. Guidelines, protocols and pathways, outlined in Chapter 2, are also building blocks for PFC. However, organizations adopting the PFC approach implement these in a systematic way, as part of a wider strategy.

In many ways, we have found that PFC, as an organizational development tool, is a logical extension of addressing the numerous issues that start to become evident as clinicians develop their skills in applying evidence in practice. As multidisciplinary teams start to develop guidelines, protocols and pathways, we have found it inevitable that questions are raised about the underpinning processes that support the clinical pathway. For example, why does it take x days for a diagnostic test result to return? Are there ways this can be reduced? Does the patient need several outpatient visits, or could their care be streamlined into one episode? Does it have to be a doctor, nurse or physiotherapist (for example) who undertakes this aspect of the care? Would it be more efficient if someone else did it? Could others do these tasks with additional training? Are patients giving informed consent for treatment, or is there potential to develop further a genuine partnership, with both parties understanding their respective responsibilities?

Without an organization-wide approach to addressing these questions as they arise, it is our experience that professionals become disenchanted with what they perceive to be bureaucratic intransigence that undermines their attempts to put evidence into practice. Patient focused care, when implemented well, does, we believe, offer a systematic way of supporting clinicians in delivering high-quality patient care based on best evidence, while subjecting non-clinical functions to the same level of rigorous review.

In practice, any of the key principles of IPC outlined above can be developed at an organizational, departmental or individual level as stand-alone options, and have some impact if done well. However, we believe that addressing all of them simultaneously has distinct advantages, since they are all interrelated. The literature clearly identifies the importance of top managers' commitment and front-line workers' involvement to make the most impact . The phases outlined in the case study (i.e. diagnostic, planning, implementing and evaluation) ensured that these latter factors were present. Importantly, it also provided a structured approach and framework for undertaking an extremely complex change initiative.

If we have one criticism of PFC, it concerns the paradox of an approach aimed at making the patient the focus of care, which then focuses on an organization-ally deterministic model of delivering that care. Hence, by and large, our care pathways, redesigned processes and care centre teams have been constrained within the organizational boundaries of our acute hospital. Shifting from this organizational mindset to one working across acute primary and social care offers potentially even more creative and innovative opportunities, such as cross-boundary pathways with evidence-based practice used by clinicians and social services in both primary and secondary care. The evidence for this proposition as an approach to improving the quality of healthcare is certainly worth exploring. But that is, possibly, the topic for another book.

REFERENCES

Audit Commission (1997) *First class delivery: improving maternity services in England and Wales*, Audit Commission, London.

Bevan, H., Cullen, R. and Windess, P. (1997) *Evaluating outcomes of the Leicester Royal Infirmary Re-engineering Programme*, Leicester Royal Infirmary NHS Trust, Leicester.

Booz-Allen and Hamilton (1990) *Operational Restructuring: The Patient Focused Hospital*, Booz-Allen & Hamilton, London.

Braithwaite, J. (1995) Organisational change, patient-focused care: an Australian perspective. *Health Services Management Research*, August, 172–84.

Buchan, J. (1995) Patient-focus Pocus? *Nursing Management*, 2(7), 6–7.

Department of Health (1993a) *Changing Childbirth, Part I: Report of the Expert Maternity Group*, Department of Health, London.

Department of Health (1993b) *Changing Childbirth, Part II: Survey of Good Communication Practice in Maternity Services*, Department of Health, London.

Hart, A. (1997) *Team Midwifery: An Evaluation of a Pilot Scheme – The Impact on Women, Practitioners and Practice*. Brighton Health Care, in collaboration with the Centre for Nursing and Midwifery Research, University of Brighton, Brighton.

Hurst, K. (1995) *Progress with Patient Focused Care in the United Kingdom*, NHS Executive/Nuffield Institute for Health, Leeds.

Langan, J. (1993) *Kingston Hospital Presentation on Patient-Focused Care*, Kingston Hospital NHS Trust, Kingston-upon-Thames.

Layton, A. and Morgan, G. (1994) *Managing NHS Trust Release*, Longman, Harlow, ch. 20, section 3.

Mang, A. (1995) Implementation strategies of patient-focused care. *Hospital and Health Services Administration*, Fall, 426–35.

Moffit, G.K. and Galloway, M. (1992) Patient focused care and total quality management. PFCA Review, Summer, 2–6.

Nuffield Institute of Health and NHS Centre for Reviews and Dissemination (1996) *Effective Health Care Bulletin*, Vol. 2, No. 3: *Management of Cataract Care*, Churchill Livingstone.

Royal College of Ophthalmologists (1995) *Cataract Care Practice*, Occasional Paper, Royal College of Ophthalmologists, London.

Towers, J. (1998) *Ophthalmology Integrated Patient Care: Project Closure Report*, Brighton Health Care NHS Trust Board, Brighton.

Appendix*

Objectives of the BHC Strategy for Nursing and Midwifery

– Strategy IV –

Back to the Future

Dear colleagues,

It is my very great pleasure to write the preface of this document, *Strategy IV: Back to the Future*. It seems appropriate, as we are celebrating 50 years of the NHS, that we also take the opportunity to celebrate the significant contribution nurses and midwives have made both nationally and within Brighton Health Care NHS Trust to a health service that is the envy of many countries. It is a chance for us to look back on our achievements and anticipate the successes of the future.

Many of you will recall earlier versions of this Strategy document, the first having been produced in 1993 and followed in 1995 by *Strategy II*. We liked the idea of having a subtitle for sequels, like a cinema blockbuster, as we believed our Strategy was going to run and run! And so it did, with the launch of *Strategy III: The Next Generation*. This title was apt, as – following research which high-lighted what was working well about the Strategy (fortunately most of it!) and what needed to change – nurses and midwives throughout the Trust had worked together in eight focus groups to update their objectives. We listened to what people had to say and made changes based on the research.

In seeking a sub-title for Strategy IV, I felt *Back to the Future* seemed apt at a time when we are looking back on the collective successes of the NHS and looking forward to how the service might evolve into the future. Reflections on the past are important since, in the words of Sigmund Freud, *'Those who do not understand their past are forced to relive it'*. Furthermore, as Churchill stated, *'The more one looks back, the further one can see forward'*. In the *Back to the Future* films, this is what makes Doctor Emmett Brown and his attempts at time travel so intriguing for us. He had the advantage of a DeLorean to travel back into the past, with the benefit of today's knowledge, and made changes which would significantly influence both the future and the present.

The importance of learning from our past experiences cannot be underestimated. In Brighton Health Care NHS Trust we are committed to continually reviewing and updating our Strategy to take account of the rapid changes which constantly challenge the Health Service. This includes changes at a political level, advances in medical science, advances in technology, and developments within our own

---

* Reproduced with the permission of Brighton Health Care NHS Trust.

profession as we grasp opportunities afforded us through our scope of professional practice.

I'm sorry to say that I don't own a DeLorean! However, I believe our Brighton Health Care NHS Trust Strategy for Nursing & Midwifery offers an equally impressive and reliable vehicle to take us forward to meet the challenges for the future. As any race-driver knows, the skills of the person in the driving seat are only one of a number of important factors that will determine whether or not the race is won. It is the combined efforts of a dedicated, knowledgeable and enthusiastic team – from managers to those in the pit stops – which will ultimately determine the outcome. So it is with our Strategy. I can say with sincerity (and I often do) that I am genuinely proud to be Director of Nursing in Brighton Health Care NHS Trust. The commitment and enthusiasm of nursing and midwifery staff does us all great credit. This is evident from the numerous innovative projects that have evolved through the Strategy (not just in the senior nurse groups, but throughout all the nursing focus groups) and the projects I see being developed at ward level when I come and work a shift with staff.

I did start to do a list of acknowledgements for Strategy IV, but stopped when I got to the end of the second page, as the number of contributors to this work are too numerous to mention. To all of you I say a big thank you on behalf of myself, the Trust Board and, perhaps more importantly, the numerous patients who write to me praising the excellent nursing care they have received in Brighton Health Care NHS Trust.

Let's keep up the good work into the future – and remember: the more people we can actually get involved in developing nursing practice across the Trust, the greater impact we can have on continually improving the services we offer to patients.

Karen Parsley
Director of Nursing.

INTRODUCTION

This document outlines the key objectives for nursing and midwifery practice development for the period 1998/99. It builds on the successes of Strategies I, II and III and has been designed following a review of the national and local issues requiring a practice development response by the two professions. As in previous years, a review of progress in relation to the objectives identified in Strategy III was undertaken to inform the development of this new document.

We recognise that it is important to learn from both the successes and the difficulties encountered, if the practice development agenda is to be set in a way that is realistic, achievable, timely, measurable and specific to the needs of the nursing and midwifery professions, the Trust strategic plan, and – importantly – the health care needs of patients accessing Brighton Health Care NHS Trust.

The background paper accompanying this document gives the details of the review of Strategy III which took place on 9th February 1998. The Director of Nursing, Assistant Director of Nursing, Patient Services Development Group, heads of nursing, ward managers, focus group members and link worker representatives all participated in this process. It is their deliberations that have informed the Strategy IV objectives.

Subsequent sections show the actions that the focus groups are taking to support the sister, charge nurses and link workers in achieving their group's broad objectives. It is expected that each clinical area will develop their own action plan on how they will work towards achieving their objectives. Workshops for sisters/charge nurses are being run over the summer where focus group members will assist them in developing their local plans.

There are eight nursing focus groups in total. Research carried out into the Strategy in 1996 indicated that one of the factors influencing link workers' commitment to achieving the objectives was how relevant they found them to their everyday work. It was clear that although the objectives of some groups were vitally important for the nursing and midwifery professions, these were best addressed at a corporate level (for example identifying how many student nurses we need to commission over the next five years to meet our projected workforce demand in the Trust). Such issues were best tackled by a few nurses on behalf of the Trust.

For this reason, it was agreed that the Workforce Planning and the (then) Marketing groups would become 'corporate groups' and disseminate their work via our nursing newsletter, *The Lamp*, as well as through the senior nurse network. Following suggestions from the link workers this year, it has also been decided to make the Equal Opportunities Focus Group a 'corporate group'. Therefore link workers are required only for the remaining five groups which have direct impact at a clinical level.

GUIDE TO USING THE STRATEGY PORTFOLIO

Why a portfolio format?

The portfolio format has been designed so that ward managers and link workers can tailor the document to suit their ward/departmental needs and practice development priorities. We hope that ward managers will encourage link workers and other staff members to use this portfolio to accumulate evidence of progress on strategy objectives. This can be accessed readily by the whole team and promotes interaction between project-specific focus group work. Just as we are encouraged by the UKCC to demonstrate our individual portfolios of evidence on continuing education, the ward manager is responsible for ensuring that the Strategy IV portfolio is the source of evidence of the continuing practice development agenda being achieved in their designated area.

Quick reference

The summary focus group objectives are produced in table format to facilitate a quick review. The focus group members and contact numbers are also produced in this way, and have been included to encourage staff to use members for advice and support in developing local action plans.

Adding to the portfolio

Ward managers should encourage link workers to include copies of all work they do in relation to their roles – for example copies of focus group notes, copies of workshop programmes, copies of link worker meeting notes, action plans and so on. This makes it possible for such information to be fed back to directorate service planning reviews, so that the strategy work and emerging resource requirements can be built into the business planning process in a systematic way.

Using Strategy IV as evidence for PREP

For many nurses and midwives, determining the best way to meet their PREP requirements remains a little mysterious. The UKCC has decided not to specify the sort of activity that must be undertaken to satisfy re-registration requirements for the evidence of continuing professional education.

Whilst this absence of strict guidelines has been confusing to many, it offers the opportunity for creativity and a great deal of freedom for the individual nurse in choosing what activities best meet PREP needs.

The UKCC has specified that each nurse should complete a minimum of five days (or equivalent hours) of study every three years to demonstrate a commitment to continuing education.

Strategy activities can all be used by link workers, focus group members, and any other nurses involved, as evidence towards the mandatory five days of study. Anyone wishing to use Strategy IV activities towards their PREP can seek advice from focus group members, particularly the Staff Development Focus Group. They can offer help in:

- identifying the relevance of link worker activity to the individual's own area of practice and development, and how this should be documented;
- identifying the anticipated learning outcomes of strategy activities;
- providing a certificate of attendance for all educational activities;
- identifying approaches to recording time spent on strategy activities and any time spent in follow-up activities appropriate to meeting the UKCC requirement for five days (or equivalent hours).

While it is necessary to keep a profile to provide evidence of continuing education activities undertaken between each registration period, link workers will be encouraged to use their experience of these roles for a wider variety of additional purposes – such as building their link worker activities into an up-to-date curriculum vitae, or when making APEL bids.

Action planning

An action plan proforma is available for use by ward managers and link workers. It provides a summary of key planned activities against time available to carry out identified actions.

Resource guide

In addition to the structure of link workers and focus group members, the Director of Nursing and Assistant Director of Nursing are available for advice and support in taking the strategy objectives forward in your area – please use them!

There are also some funds available to support link workers and focus group members who attend study days such as external conferences, seminars, site visits, and workshops, in addition to the in-house provision co-ordinated by the focus groups. Approach the Director of Nursing in the first instance for further details of these.

Conclusion

We hope you will find the revised format of the strategy document helpful. Please let us know by completing the attached evaluation form. We will be grateful for all comments and suggestions, and endeavour to incorporate these in future strategy documents.

QUICK REFERENCE

The objectives for the 98/99 Strategy for Nursing are:

Clinical leadership

- To develop guidelines relating to ethical issues arising from 'Duty of Care' and 'making concerns known'.
  Time scale: March 99
- To design creative approaches to recruitment and retention of nursing staff and associated support worker roles.
  Time scale: Ongoing
- To explore and clarify the local framework for professional nursing contribution to clinical governance.
  Time scale: March 99
- To develop nursing practice through a framework of clinical supervision.
  Time scale: Ongoing

Advancing nursing practice

- To promote effective nursing documentation practices throughout Brighton Health Care NHS Trust for the purpose of supporting continuity and consistency of patient focused care.
  Time scale: Ongoing
- To further develop the Trust agreed infrastructure for the development of nursing roles, taking into consideration any recommendations from statutory bodies.
  Time scale: Ongoing
- To design and implement education which supports staff in achieving clarity about the nature of accountable practice across key professional activities; i.e. Records and Record Keeping, Administration of Medicines, Guidelines for Professional Practice, giving professional advice, and Trust clinical policies and procedures.
  Time scale: March 99

Putting research into practice

- To support the application of relevant research to practice ensuring evidence-based nursing practice.
  Time scale: Ongoing
- To develop educational approaches to promote skills necessary to critically appraise and implement relevant research
  Time scale: Ongoing
- To work in collaboration with other research and development forums within the trust to establish the nursing contribution to Culyer recommendations.
  Time scale: March 99

Staff development

- To continue to support staff in meeting UKCC Prep requirements for evidence of continuing professional development.
  Time scale: Ongoing
- To enhance effectiveness of preceptorship preparation for clinical placements of students at both pre and post registration levels, and for staff new in post.
  Time scale: Sept 98

- To explore the training needs for Bank nurses and raise awareness amongst this group of staff regarding the in-house and external provision of nurse education. *Time scale: Sept 98*
- To further develop competency-based training and assessment expanded role activities. *Time scale: Ongoing*

Quality into nursing practice

- To communicate the systematic approach to the setting and auditing of nursing and midwifery standards across Brighton Health Care NHS Trust. *Time scale: Ongoing*
- To develop outcome measures for nursing and midwifery activities. *Time scale: Ongoing*
- To facilitate standards and outcomes work in the following areas: Cancer pain; Acute pain; Chronic pain; Discharge; Wound Care; and Nutrition. *Time scale: Ongoing*
- To be a resource for the link workers and ward staff for any other quality improvement work they may wish to undertake. *Time scale: Ongoing*

Equal opportunities

- To continue to raise awareness of best practice in Equal Opportunities at ward/departmental level through continuing education of link workers. *Time scale: Ongoing*
- To review the work and recommendations from Care of the Dying and Bereavement and Loss Group and develop action plan to address these across the Trust. *Time scale: Sept 98*
- To update, with direction from Personnel, existing ward-held information on equal opportunities in light of recommendations from recent national and local reports. *Time scale: Sept 98*
- To explore and clarify the nursing contribution to effective risk management and make recommendations regarding any training needs emerging. *Time scale: Sept 98*

Communication

- To publicise Strategy for Nursing and Midwifery (IV) objectives to Brighton Health Care nursing and midwifery staff. *Time scale: Sept 1998*
- To communicate information on Strategy (IV) progress throughout Brighton Health Care. *Time scale: Ongoing*
- To disseminate information, internally and externally, on positive developments in nursing and midwifery within the Trust *Time scale: Ongoing*
- To raise awareness of marketing concepts within the nursing and midwifery profession. *Time scale: Ongoing*

Workforce planning

• To identify, collect and analyse available quantitative and qualitative data/information for the purpose of providing an ongoing baseline on the current workforce.	*Time scale: Ongoing*
• To develop a robust methodology for calculating multidisciplinary skill mix and service delivery	*Time scale: June 99*
• To provide local nursing professional advice to the educational consortia	*Time scale: Ongoing*
• To co-ordinate the educational commissioning process.	*Time scale: Ongoing*

CLINICAL LEADERSHIP

Purpose

To develop clinical and professional leadership and promote clinical supervision for nursing and midwifery staff within Brighton Health Care.

Objectives

1. **To develop guidelines relating to ethical issues arising from 'Duty of Care' and 'making concerns known'**
   Actions will include:
   • Review of existing local approaches to triggering requests for professional advice.
   • Identification of training needs for nursing staff within this area and development, in conjunction with the Advancing Nursing Practice Focus Group, of appropriate education to meet needs arising.
   • Design for approval of Patient Services Development Group broad trust guidelines for staff to refer to in the event of such situations arising.
2. **To design creative approaches to recruitment and retention of nursing staff and associated support worker roles**
   Actions will include:
   • Ongoing development of 18 month staff nurse rotation programme in conjunction with Personnel Department. Establish a flow chart of events to guide recruitment officer in maintaining this programme.
   • Establish a clear diary of events for the recruitment to the Return to Practice Programme in conjunction with programme co-ordinators at INAM.
   • Establish a subcommittee to design, implement and evaluate Brighton Health Care Return to NHS Practice course in conjunction with NVQ department.
   • To continue the Career Development Programme for Nurses and Midwives in Brighton Health Care.
   • Liaise with the Workforce Planning Focus Group in relation to the development of a clear strategy for recruitment and retention of nurses.
3. **To explore and clarify the local framework for professional nursing contribution to clinical governance**

Actions will include:
- Establish a project plan of how this work is to be taken forward.

4. **To develop nursing practice through a framework of clinical supervision**
Actions will include:
- Review progress of action research project with Heads of Nursing and identify forward plan for implementing clinical supervision.

ADVANCING NURSING PRACTICE

Purpose

To lead and support nurses and midwives in developing professional practice within Brighton Health Care.

Objectives

1. **To promote effective nursing documentation practices throughout Brighton Health Care for the purpose of supporting continuity and consistency of patient focused care**
Actions will include:
- Promoting the Trust wide standard for nursing documentation and ensuring its inclusion in the ward audit calendars.
- Designing, delivering and evaluating a programme of workshops to raise awareness of the Trust wide standard and the implications for practice of the UKCC standards for records and record keeping.
- Promoting integrated patient care concepts in any recommendations for developing nursing documentation.
- Examining the relationship between documentation practices and systems of organising care.

2. **To further develop the Trust agreed infrastructure for the development of nursing roles, taking into consideration any recommendations from statutory bodies**
Actions will include:
- Receiving reports from the Assistant Director of Nursing and Clinical Nurse Specialist member regarding the progress of nurse practitioner and clinical nurse specialist forum, with particular reference to mapping the education and training needs of post holders and their need for support and supervision.
- Contributing to the membership of PAPER Group.
- Receiving reports from the non-medical led drug administration group.
- Develop a position statement in relation to the use of complimentary therapies by nursing staff in the Trust.
  - Establish a subgroup to develop a project plan for this work.
  - Prepare a paper for consideration by PSDG and CMT.

3. **To design and implement education which supports staff in achieving clarity about the nature of accountable practice across key professional activities; i.e.**

Records and Record Keeping, Administration of medicines, Guidelines for Professional Practice, giving professional advice, and Trust clinical policies and procedures
Actions will include:
- Contribute to monthly Safe & Secure Handling of Medicines workshop in conjunction with Clinical Nurse Specialist IV Therapy.
- Contribute to New Nurse Induction programme session on Accountability and Trust Clinical Policies & Procedures.

PUTTING RESEARCH INTO PRACTICE

Purpose

To facilitate the dissemination, implementation, communication and evaluation of nursing research. This involves a cycle of activity aimed at creating a culture where the questioning approach and ongoing evaluation will perpetuate the cycle, ensuring evidence-based nursing practice is delivered to patients, and where appropriate, the initiation of new research is supported.

Objectives

1. To support the application of relevant research to practice ensuring evidence-based nursing practice
   Actions will include:
   - Work collaboratively with other focus groups in identifying the underpinning research evidence where requested.
   - Further develop the research journal club, encouraging presenters to prepare material for wider distribution outside the journal club assisting other clinical areas in assessing relevance of research findings for changes in practice.
   - Support link workers in building area specific evidence-based practice resources within the strategy portfolio and evaluate usefulness of such resources to staff working in the designated area.

2. **To develop educational approaches to promote skills necessary to critically appraise and implement relevant research**
   Actions will include:
   - Review and update content of the link worker resource pack.
   - Explore research awareness of link workers, with specific reference to research training needs. Inform the contract monitoring process with Institute of Nursing and Midwifery, via Trust account management meeting accordingly where gaps identified. Liaise with INAM re-provision of 2 day research awareness workshop.

3. **To work in collaboration with other research and development forums within the Trust to establish the nursing contribution to Culyer recommendations**
   Actions will include:
   - Identify focus group link person responsible for maintaining strong links with Centre for Research at INAM.

- Explore the implications of the Culyer report for nursing and examine what other organisations are doing in relation to this important area.
- Prepare an advisory paper for Patient Services Development Group on the basis of actions taken in 3.3.

STAFF DEVELOPMENT

Purpose

To encourage staff development within Brighton Health Care to meet the needs of patients (now and in the future) and promote a learning culture within the nursing and midwifery professions.

Objectives

1. **To continue to support staff in meeting UKCC Prep requirements for evidence of continuing professional development**
   Actions will include:
   - Review the content of the existing workshop pack in light of evaluations from previous participants and presenters. Update the materials as indicated.
   - Identify forward plan of workshops for 98/99, disseminate revised publicity materials to all clinical areas.
   - Explore the necessity of a workshop designed specifically to meet the needs of sisters/charge nurses, senior nurses and those with a nursing background no longer in nursing posts.
   - Prepare new focus group members to deliver the workshops.
   - Continue with the sales of the Trust PREP Profile File and floppy disc version. Explore market for further external workshops by way of income generation.
   - Work with link workers and sisters/charge nurses to develop their understanding of individual profile-building principles can be applied to developing the practice development evidence in Strategy IV ward profiles.
2. **To enhance effectiveness of preceptor preparation for clinical placements for students at both pre and post registration levels, and for staff new in post**
   Actions will include:
   - Work collaboratively with Institute of Nursing and Midwifery (INAM) to review current half day workshop 'Making Preceptorship Work' and prepare focus group members to co-facilitate the workshop.
   - Identify forward plan of workshops for 98/99, disseminate relevant publicity materials to all clinical areas and establish appropriate person training days accounting mechanism for this with INAM.
   - Evaluate effectiveness of workshop in changing perceptions of preceptorship preparation for preceptors, students and link teachers.
   - Link with work being undertaken by Clinical Educators Forum in developing preceptors guidelines for ENB 998 as required.

3. **To explore training needs of bank nurses and raise awareness amongst this group regarding the in-house and external provision of nurse education**
   Actions will include:
   - Identify ways of communicating with bank nurses.
   - Explore their perceptions of access to educational provision.
   - Develop appropriate forward plan on basis of results to 3.2. Plan to go as recommendation paper to Patient Services Development Group.
4. **To further develop competency-based training and assessment strategies**
   Actions will include:
   - Involving Personnel, plan a systematic way forward that is in line with Trust objectives.

QUALITY IN NURSING PRACTICE

Purpose

To encourage and support the delivery of high quality nursing and midwifery care, and evaluate the care patients receive through audit and the development of measurable outcomes.

Objectives

1. **To communicate the systematic approach to setting and auditing of nursing and midwifery standards across Brighton Health Care**
   Actions will include:
   - Evaluate the recent content update of existing Trust Standard Setting Workshop, which now includes outcome measurement.
   - Agree programme of workshops, facilitators, venues and dates for the next 12 months. Mailshot wards and departments with details of the workshop's applications. Generate interest via poster campaign. Monitor attendances and develop mechanism for targeting future participants.
   - Review the nursing and midwifery standards database held in Department of Clinical Audit and make recommendations on the actions necessary.
   - Continue to develop the role of Head of Nursing as audit lead and evaluate effectiveness of Audit Lead Resource and utilisation of Nursing Audit Information Resource. This will necessitate close working with the Department of Clinical Audit.
2. **To develop outcome measures for nursing and midwifery activities**
   Actions will include:
   - Continue to promote awareness and understanding of nursing outcomes measurement, and the mechanisms for carrying out this work.
   - Lead the development of nursing outcomes measurement in specific areas of: pain; discharge; nutrition and wound care.
   - Provide advice and support (where possible) for nursing outcomes measurement in other nursing and midwifery topic areas.
3. **To facilitate standards and outcomes work in the following areas: Cancer pain; Acute Pain; Chronic Pain; Discharge; Wound Care and Nutrition**

Actions will include:
- Continue work of pain subgroups based on the pain audit recommendations and international pain guidelines work.
- Continue work of discharge planning subgroup in collaboration with Discharge Planning Manager.
- Establish Nutrition subgroup in collaboration with dieticians and identify action plan for future work.
- Establish the Wound Care subgroup in collaboration with Wound Care Nurse Specialist, review terms of reference and identify action plan of way forward.
- Liaise with Heads of Nursing, link workers and ward sisters to ensure departmental audit calendars identify forward plan of audit activity.

4. **To be a resource for link workers and ward staff for any other quality improvement work they may wish to undertake**
Actions will include:
- Identify each focus group member's geographical area of responsibility in the Trust. Each focus group member will contact the link workers in their area at least quarterly, to act as a 'buddy' and ensure ward based quality issues are raised with the focus group.
- Ensure link worker details are kept up to date.
- Devise flyer for departments identifying what the focus group is about and how it can help address quality issues.
- To assist link workers and ward staff to fulfil their role in updating the Nursing Audit Information Resource.

EQUAL OPPORTUNITIES

Purpose

To ensure that nurses and midwives working within Brighton Health Care are aware of the principles of equal opportunities in relation to the care of patients, and in working relationships and conditions of colleagues.

Objectives

1. **To continue to raise awareness of best practice in equal opportunities at ward/departmental level through continuing education of Sisters/Charge Nurses**
Actions will include:
- Distribute Equal Opportunities learning pack to Sisters/Charge Nurses in every ward/department throughout the Trust.
- Under direction from Personnel representative, continue with awareness training for Sisters/Charge Nurses.

2. **To review the work and recommendations from the Care of the Dying and Bereavement and Loss Group and develop an action plan to address these across the Trust**

Actions will include:
- Develop a project plan for improving care of the dying in Brighton Health Care.
- Implement and evaluate the project plan.

3. **To update, with direction from Personnel, existing ward held information on equal opportunities in light of recommendations from recent local and national reports**
Actions will include:
- Review and standardise existing ward-held information in all areas.
- Work with the new Director of Personnel to agree on the re-issue and re-formatting of existing information resources.

4. **To explore and clarify the nursing contribution to effective risk management and make recommendations regarding any training needs emerging**
Actions will include:
- Work with the Senior Nurse Manager responsible for risk management within each directorate to action current concerns arising from their review of risk management issues.
- Work with Risk Management (Clinical and Non-Clinical) to agree ways of addressing proposals from the Senior Nurse Managers and prioritising training issues.
- Develop action plans with ward Sisters/Charge Nurses.

COMMUNICATION

Purpose

To raise awareness of the contribution of nursing and midwifery practice to the delivery of high quality patient care, both within Brighton Health Care and to external agencies.

Objectives

1. **To publicise Strategy IV objectives to Brighton Health Care nursing and midwifery staff**
Actions will include:
- Producing leaflets and posters about the Strategy for Nursing and Midwifery.
- Publicising conference and forthcoming Nursing and Midwifery practice development events.
- Identifying resources required to publish *The LAMP* nursing and midwifery newsletter.
- Producing *The LAMP* and distributing to staff throughout Brighton Health Care.
- Designing templates for articles in *The LAMP* and posters to update focus group activities.

- Review production process and distribution of *The LAMP* and carrying out cost analysis, with a view to improving production efficiency and extending distribution.

2. **To communicate information on Strategy IV progress throughout Brighton Health Care**

   Actions will include:
   - Installing permanent boards in clinical areas to display information on strategy work carried out.
   - Providing guidelines to ensure regular update of strategy displays in clinical areas.
   - Identifying and maintaining central areas on each site for general poster displays on strategy work.
   - Planning programme for bi-monthly poster feature for each focus group in rotation.
   - Identifying key link members from all other focus groups who will co-ordinate their group's update on activities and co-ordinating this work.
   - Designing questionnaire for gathering focus group updates in standard format.
   - Promoting the use of the ward portfolios and monitoring their use.
   - Organising conferences to share the work carried out in relation to Strategy IV.

3. **To disseminate information, internally and externally, on positive developments in nursing & midwifery within the Trust**

   Actions will include:
   - practice achieved through the realisation of strategy objectives.
   - *[via Press & PR]* Offering advice and proof-checking resource to Brighton Health Care nurses wishing to submit articles for publication in professional journals.
   - *[via Press & PR]* Disseminating internally and externally any articles on nursing developments in Brighton Health Care published in professional journals.
   - Providing bi-monthly update for *GP News* on good nursing practice and innovations in Brighton Health Care relating to GPs.

4. **To raise awareness of marketing concepts within the nursing and midwifery profession**

   Actions will include:
   - Acting as Nursing advisory resource for marketing initiatives such as conferences.
   - *[via Press & PR]* Acting as collection point for any articles on nursing issues which have been written by Brighton Health Care staff and published externally.

Note: The group may co-opt the skills and experience of non-members for specific projects.

WORKFORCE PLANNING

Purpose

To review, evaluate and strategically plan the nursing workforce agenda and education requirements in Brighton Health Care within the context of the national workforce agenda to deliver safe, effective patient care.

Objectives

1. **To identify, collect and analyse available quantitative and qualitative data for the purpose of providing an ongoing baseline on the current workforce**
    Actions will include:
    *   A review of the Nursing Information Systems (NIS) data where this is fully operational. This will be carried out by Patient Services Development Group member in conjunction with the NIS co-ordinator and ward managers. The review will include:
        - Monthly review of all NIS information and ward templates within each directorate.
        - Identification of actions to be taken following the review.
        - Quarterly Trust-wide report of NIS information with trends and recommendations for presentation to PSDG, and directorate service planning reviews.
        - Convene benchmarking subgroup.
    *   A further review of the current workforce data for each directorate indicating:
        - Numbers and grades of nurses, midwives and care assistant roles and where they are working.
        - Bank, agency and overtime usage.
        - Sickness and absence data.
        - Study leave taken, how much and what sort.
        - Maternity leave, annual leave, carers leave, compassionate leave, unpaid leave, other leave.
    *   Develop the Quality Pointers Tool programme.
2. **To develop a robust methodology for calculating multidisciplinary skill mix and service delivery requirements**
    Actions will include:
    *   Establish a subcommittee to oversee the project plan for the consortia funded project.
    *   Establish a project plan for benchmarking our nursing information against other comparable trusts.
3. **To provide local professional nursing advice to the educational consortia groups, namely the Professional Nursing and Midwifery Advisory Group and the Strategy Group**
    Actions will include:
    *   Reviewing the relevant papers and preparing responses on behalf of Brighton Health Care.

- Members deputising for the Director of Nursing at meetings.

4. **To co-ordinate the education commissioning process**
   Actions will include:
   - Developing and monitoring the new Person Training Days data base.
   - Developing the annual commissioning plans for nurse education.
   - Promoting the educational contract and service level agreement on behalf of Brighton Health Care.
   - To review Brighton Health Care commissioning plan.

5. **To develop a strategy for nurse recruitment and retention**
   Actions will include:
   - Establish subcommittee to develop strategic plan in conjunction with representation from Directorate of Personnel.

Index

03968862

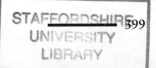
STAFFORDSHIRE
UNIVERSITY
LIBRARY